Piety and Patienthood in Medieval Islam

How did pious medieval Muslims experience health and illness? Rooted in the prophet's experiences with medicine and healing, Muslim pietistic literature developed cosmologies in which physical suffering and medical interventions interacted with religious obligations and spiritual health. This book traces the development of prophetic medical literature and religious writings around health and disease to give a new perspective on how patienthood was conditioned by the intersection of medicine and Islam.

The author investigates the early and foundational writings on prophetic medicine and related pietistic writings on health and illness produced during the Islamic Classical Age. Looking at attitudes from and toward clerics, physicians, and patients, sickness and health are gradually revealed as a social, gendered, religious, and cultural experience. Patients are shown to experience certain sensoria that are conditioned not only by medical knowledge, but also by religious and pietistic attitudes.

This is a fascinating insight into the development of Muslim pieties and the traditions of medical practice. It will be of great interest to scholars interested in Islamic Studies, history of religion, history of medicine, science and religion, and the history of embodied religious practice, particularly in matters of health and medicine.

Ahmed Ragab is the Richard T. Watson Associate Professor of Science and Religion, Affiliate Associate Professor at the Department of the History of Science, and Director of the Science, Religion and Culture program at Harvard University, USA. He is a physician, a historian of science and medicine, and a scholar of science and religion.

Routledge Studies in Religion

Religion, Culture and Spirituality in Africa and the African Diaspora
Edited by William Ackah, Jualynne E. Dodson and R. Drew Smith

Theology and Civil Society
Edited by Charles Pemberton

Neoliberalism and the Biblical Voice
Owning and Consuming
Paul Babie and Michael Trainor

European Muslims Transforming the Public Sphere
Religious Participation in the Arts, Media and Civil Society
Asmaa Soliman

Radical Orthodoxy in a Pluralistic World
Desire, Beauty, and the Divine
Angus M. Slater

Spiritual and Social Transformation in African American Spiritual Churches
More than Conjurers
Margarita Simon Guillory

Liberal Religion
Progressive Versions of Judaism, Christianity and Islam
Emanuel de Kadt

Piety and Patienthood in Medieval Islam
Ahmed Ragab

For more information about this series, please visit: www.routledge.com/religion/series/SE0669

Piety and Patienthood in Medieval Islam

Ahmed Ragab

Routledge
Taylor & Francis Group
LONDON AND NEW YORK

First published 2018 by Routledge

2 Park Square, Milton Park, Abingdon, Oxfordshire OX14 4RN
52 Vanderbilt Avenue, New York, NY 10017

Routledge is an imprint of the Taylor & Francis Group, an informa business

First issued in paperback 2020

British Library Cataloguing-in-Publication Data
A catalogue record for this book is available from the British Library

Library of Congress Cataloging-in-Publication Data
Names: Ragab, Ahmed, author.
Title: Piety and patienthood in medieval Islam / Ahmed Ragab.
Description: New York, NY : Routledge, [2018] | Series: Routledge studies in religion | Includes bibliographical references and index.
Identifiers: LCCN 2018002572 | ISBN 9780815361282 (hardback : alk. paper) | ISBN 9781351103534 (ebook)
Subjects: LCSH: Suffering—Religious aspects—Islam. | Diseases—Religious aspects—Islam. | Medicine, Arab.
Classification: LCC BP190.5.S93 R34 2018 | DDC 297.2/66—dc23
LC record available at https://lccn.loc.gov/2018002572

ISBN: 978-0-8153-6128-2 (hbk)
ISBN: 978-0-367-59103-8 (pbk)

Typeset in Times New Roman
by Apex CoVantage, LLC

To Soha, Carmen
and my grandmother Nabawiyya

Contents

Coda 213

Piety 213
Patienthood 217
Medieval Islam 220

Acknowledgments

It takes a village to write a book. It must be a nice village, though. It must have supportive family, friends, colleagues, and mentors and grants from generous institutions. It must have loved ones who are willing to take the emotional ups and downs, the anxiety, the self-doubt, and the evolving ideas and the evolving self that produces and is being produced by these ideas. It must have sources of inspiration from these same loved ones and from students and friends as well, all of whom have to be willing to read and listen and talk ideas through. And, of course, this village has to have a publisher and a talented, supportive editor. I was able to write this book because I had this village.

I am grateful to my editor, Joshua Wells, and the remarkable team at Routledge Press for all of their hard work in bringing this book to life. I am also grateful to the anonymous reviewers for their remarks and suggestions. The generous support from Harvard University's Provost Office's research-enabling grant supported my research travels and the collection of needed materials and texts. The Weatherhead Center for International Affairs at Harvard University also supported this research at a crucial time, providing a generous grant that allowed me to review important texts and sources and to spend important time charting the course of the book. The generous and encouraging community of the Max Planck Institute for the History of Science – Department II, which supported and hosted me in the spring of 2016, provided me with time and a remarkable scholarly community that significantly helped the development of this book. I am also grateful for David Hempton, Janet Gyatso, Willaim Graham, and Janet Browne for their support and care.

I am indebted to my friend and co-author (in another book), Katharine Park, for her advice and help and for the inspiration that her work always provides. I am beholden to my students Shireen Hamza, Eli Nelson, Juanita Becerra, Angel Rodriguez, Gili Vidan, Joseph Vignone, and Brittany Landorf for the stimulating and inspiring environment that their work continues to provide and for the fresh and insightful ideas generated by talking to them. Shireen copyedited parts of this manuscript, helping me refine its arguments and bring out its voice. Brittany also copyedited and proofread the rest of the book and its revisions. Her remarkable work is an integral part of the making of this book.

I am very grateful to John Harvard Brewery and Cambridge Common restaurant – in particular, the talented performer and inspired bartender at

Cambridge Common, Julee Antonellis – who provided a refuge for thinking, reflecting, and writing through some particularly difficult and challenging parts. I am also grateful for *Rogue One* (directed by Gareth Edwards) which was released at a crucial moment in my thinking and research. *Rogue One* provided a different image of the Force. In *Rogue One*, the Force was not only "an energy field created by all living things. It surrounds us, penetrates us, and binds the galaxy together" as Obi Wan Kenobi calls it in *New Hope*; it was also a locus for religious meaning-making and devotion among those who are not bluebloods, Jedis, or Skywalkers. Chirrut Imwe's (played by Donnie Yen) mantra, "I am one with the Force and the Force is with me," animated a layer of Force-piety that has never been explicitly explored in the Star Wars universe before. Although this book, unfortunately, does not explore this Force-piety, this new valence of the Force and how different beings related to it helped the conceptualization of my arguments about piety and illness. I am also deeply indebted to my dear friend, Sophia Roosth, for listening, discussing, and helping me bring these ideas to meaningful fruition. Our discussions about time, queer theory, embodiment, and Star Wars honed my thinking about piety, illness, and care of the self. Sophia's work continues to inspire my work in this book and beyond.

The slow metamorphosis of a book is fraught with anxiety, fears, worries, and uncertainties, all of which take a tremendous toll on one's life and on the lives of their loved ones. My love, partner, and interlocutor, Soha Bayoumi, was there every step of the way, with comments, critiques, and ideas that helped clarify my thinking and sharpen my arguments. She was the force that guided me and provided the love and care that powered us through the book's evolution. My daughter Carmen's wit, humor, and interest in the subject of this book were breaths of fresh air, inspiring much of this book and giving me the momentum to continue. Carmen and I exchanged notes about this book and a book she was writing, which was coincidentally also about patients, albeit animal ones.

As I thought about prophetics (or *nabawiyyāt*), my late dear grandmother, *Nabawiyya*, was a constant presence in my mind. This book is dedicated to her memory.

Introduction

How does a person become sick? How does one make sense of the physical, emotional, and psychological experience of sickness? On one hand, sickness is rooted in embodiment. Physical, spiritual, emotional, and other forms of ailments are conceived within embodied experiences at the heart of the making of the body as a social, gendered, sexualized, and racialized entity. Moreover, the embodied experience of sickness is produced through the confines of medical knowledge and experience with their dynamic history. On the other hand, sickness is also a site of production of social and cultural knowledge. Being sick entails a set of relations, rituals, and interactions that condition how one can inhabit and perform sickness as a locus of social experience and communication. Over the past few decades, historians and anthropologists of medicine explored how historical, social, and cultural contexts influenced the making of illness – both as a category of medical knowledge and practice, and as a site for the cultural and social production of meaning.[1] This book is about how medieval pious Muslims became sick.

The question of illness and the experiences of how one encountered diseases, why diseases happened, and how to deal with them were central to an expanding corpus of works in the early medieval Islamic period. *Ḥadīth* (Prophetic Traditions) collections produced in the ninth and tenth centuries contained chapters that were dedicated to illness, health, and medicine.[2] There, ḥadīth scholars and compilers collected traditions and anecdotes that addressed illness and explained how the prophet and his companions experienced diseases or sought cures. Moreover, the genres of pietistic writings such as *zuhd* (renunciation of earthly goods or asceticism) and *raqāʾiq* (exhortations) emerging and expanding during the ninth century reserved a place for questions of health and disease.[3] In these works, health was presented as a gift from God that required care and maintenance and conditioned specific forms of pietistic practice rooted in using one's strength and health to obey God. This pietistic understanding of health and the duties that it incurred relied on understanding human bodies as always prone to ills. As such, illness was an important category to be analyzed on its own. It provoked key questions about causality and about the pietistic behaviors pious Muslims needed to adopt during episodes of hardship.

Throughout the medieval and early modern periods, a number of scholars of ḥadīth, Islamic law, and other religious sciences produced volumes on medicine that constituted a corpus known as "prophetic medicine" (*Ṭibb al-Nabiyy* or *al-Ṭibb al-Nabawī*).[4] Historians have traced the origins of this literature to the ninth-century major collections of ḥadīth where compilers dedicated chapters to discussing the prophet's experiences with illness and his recommendations in relation to health and medicine. Irmeli Perho explained that these early manifestations of the prophet's medicine lacked serious and sustained engagement with learned Galenic medical knowledge, which was the dominant medical paradigm in the Islamic world beginning in the ninth and tenth centuries and extending into the nineteenth century. She argued that the sustained engagement with medical theory and practice commenced with the works of two physicians: ʿAbd al-Laṭif al-Baghdādī (d. 1231) and Ibn Ṭarkhān (d. 1320), who wrote volumes on prophetic medicine that included deeper and more substantive discussions of medical theory and practice.[5] Perho, followed by other scholars, focused primarily on the writings of al-Dhahabī (d. 1348), Ibn Mufliḥ (d. 1362), Ibn Qayyim al-Jawziyah (d. 1350), and others in the late medieval period as central examples of prophetic medicine at its zenith. In most of the studies addressing this literature, historians looked to the potential contradictions between medical theory and religious views expressed in these traditions, the potential medical theoretical interventions presented by religious scholars, and the legal implications of some of these texts, including how they influenced non-Muslim medical practitioners, among other related issues.[6] Little attention was devoted to the early formative periods that extend from the ninth century to the twelfth century. Even less attention was devoted to how writings on prophetic medicine, particularly in the early period, could be understood within the context of ḥadīth sciences or how they participated in the emerging pietistic and religious discourse of the time. This book looks at the production of pietistic narratives that addressed and conditioned the experience of patienthood in the early Islamic medieval period. At the intersection of medicine and Islam, this book investigates how pious Muslims experienced illness, how they perceived their pietistic duties, and how they understood their physical ills from a pietistic perspective.

The study of Islamic piety has focused primarily on four areas. First, piety and asceticism, among other religious practices, continue to be explored within Islamic mysticism or Sufism.[7] There, many scholars have investigated the production of selfhood and the meaning of religious observance and of piety in Sufi discourses and practices across different historical periods. Second, works similar to Daniela Talmon-Heller's *Islamic Piety in Medieval Syria: Mosques, Cemeteries and Sermons Under the Zangids and Ayyūbids* focused on the institutions that constituted the pietistic infrastructure in the medieval period.[8] Talmon-Heller, along with a number of other scholars, investigated how these institutions and structures provided spaces and modes of pietistic performance that were connected to political, social, and individual practices. Third, Annemarie Schimmel's *And Muhammad Is His Messenger* presented a different view on the study of piety.[9] Schimmel crafted a narrative that included a variety of texts and a series of conversations that animated the meaning and the role of Muḥammad as an object of veneration. Schimmel's work attempted to investigate the production of pietistic meanings within learned discourse with the understanding that such learned discourse manifested in preaching as well as in political and social institutions. In a similar vein, Christopher Melchert's work on piety has looked at the meaning of piety as an ethic, a mode of comportment, and a social performance for different groups, including scholars of ḥadīth, among others.[10] Finally, and with a focus on the modern and contemporary, the works of Saba Mahmood, Talal Asad, and Charles Hirschkind have contributed to the understanding of piety as social and political agency deployed through the consumption and production of particular narratives, texts, and behaviors.[11]

This book is situated at the intersection of the last two trends of studying piety. On one hand, I look at piety as represented in the textual tradition with attention to the roles that these texts play in the construction of social practice. Although institutions remain key to the development of different social and individual pietistic performances, I argue that the construction of meanings around specific practices through the production of authoritative texts was part of the infrastructure in which these institutions developed and influenced pietistic practice. Schimmel's work provides overarching narratives that are built on the commonalities of practices from the medieval to the modern period, but this book investigates the classical period as a moment where the archive of pietistic meaning was developed and from which the authority that legitimized later iterations of this archive emerged. Similar to the work of Saba Mahmood in the contemporary, I am equally interested in investigating the layers of agency embedded in pietistic narratives. Here, however, I do not look at how performances of piety created modes of agential practice. Instead, I investigate how these narratives relied on and cultivated certain modes of agency deemed central to the production of the pious agent.

As such, the book investigates the early and foundational pietistic writings on illness, health, and medicine to explore the pietistic and religious dimensions of the experience of health and disease. Although medical knowledge provided important narrative, intellectual, and practical resources that constructed the experience of illness, pietistic and religious writings created a thick web of meanings and references that influenced how people understood their afflictions, how they experienced their own sick bodies, and what behaviors they deemed pious or socially acceptable in the event of sickness. Here, patienthood is understood as a social, gendered, religious, and cultural experience where patients experienced certain sensoria that were conditioned not only by medical knowledge (or the medical knowledge that they had access to) but also by religious and pietistic attitudes. This dynamic space of patienthood was populated by stories of prophets and saints and filled with prayers and incantations as well as with honey, black seed, and other material objects that were featured within prophetic narratives about medicine. In this context, the prophetic narratives that engaged with health and illness should not be solely viewed in relation to contemporaneous medical knowledge, but also in connection to the emerging practices of piety and observance and with the developing ritual practices and spaces that conditioned what it meant to be a pious Muslim at that time.

In short, this book explores how a pious Muslim got sick. It investigates how religious writings created pietistic spaces that the sick pious inhabited and cosmologies that conditioned their views, perceptions, and reactions to the experience of illness and to the encounter with learned medicine. In this context, the importance of the classical period is paramount. In addition to being central to the formation of Muslim pieties and to the construction and development of sectarian identities, legal schools, and institutional frameworks, the writings of this period created an archive of prophetic materials that came to supply pietistic and religious writings on health and diseases for centuries to come.[12] This archive was composed of prophetic narratives, anecdotes, legal questions, and pietistic habits and rituals. It contributed to ascribing specific meanings to health and disease that Muslims needed to grapple with as these texts came to acquire increasing intellectual authority.[13]

In exploring early collections of ḥadīth and other pietistic writings, I argue that these texts provided for systems of self-care whereby pious Muslims understood their bodies and their behaviors and aimed to care for themselves in a pietistic manner. Building on the Foucauldian and post-Foucauldian discussions of self-care, I argue that these narratives constructed habits and ritualized perceptions, sensoria, acts, and rhetorics that influenced how pious Muslims understood themselves and contributed to the construction of common identities rooted in the specificities of the individual body and soul. These pietistic spaces were rooted in ambivalent positions that understood God's role in causing illnesses and granting healing and held in tension the necessity to rely on God for wellbeing and the need to seek earthly care. At another level, this ambivalence conditioned practices of reflexivity and self-awareness that individualized pietistic practices of patienthood at the same time that it provided for the social life of this patienthood. This reflexivity, necessary for maintaining the tension of ambivalent practices of piety, relied on the cultivation of virtues of sovereignty over one's body that emanated from God's ultimate sovereignty over the bodies that He created.

Book structure

The book traces a historical arc explored through thematic discussions. The first chapter commences in the ninth century and focuses on the production of Muḥammad's image in early ḥadīth compilations. The ninth century witnessed important debates around the legal and pietistic roles of the sunna (literally defined as 'way,' it often refers to legacy and tradition) of the prophet and his companions and the ḥadīths (prophetic traditions) and anecdotes that made up this sunna. These debates contributed to the flourishing of the sciences of prophetic traditions and the emergence of recognizable groups of scholars specializing in the study of ḥadīth and its criticism. In this burgeoning environment, scholars contended with the legal and pietistic dimensions of a few central questions, including: What was the prophet's sunna? How should it be reported and discussed? And what obligations did this sunna constitute? The sunna and the prophet's sayings and deeds that constituted most of its amorphous corpus formed part of a pietistic discourse that identified what pious Muslims were supposed to do and how they were required or asked to behave. In this regard, knowledge about the prophet and the early community became an important tool in creating a pietistic environ that Muslims were asked to inhabit. This environ was structured around the prophet as a moral and pietistic example and, as the Quran put it, "a beau ideal for whosoever fears God" [Q33:21]. The prophet's example did not only inform legal debates or discussions of religious rituals and obligations, but was also important for various daily activities from eating to drinking, to having sex, or to getting sick and receiving treatment.

The first chapter focuses on the construction of the prophet's persona as a *beau ideal* in relation to questions of health, disease, and medicine. First, it addresses the making of the sunna and its evolving relation to ḥadīth in the ninth century. It then discusses the relation between ḥadīth and adab, understood as a literary and epistemic discipline and a locus of self-fashioning. In its second half, the chapter looks at the medical sections in the major ḥadīth collections of the ninth century. Here, it investigates the beginning of interest in *medical prophetics* from the works of Muʿammir ibn Rāshid (d. 770) and his student ʿAbd al-Razzāq al-Ṣanʿānī (d. 826) and in the works of Abū ʿAbd Allāh ibn Saʿd (d. 845). It then analyzes the medical chapters of some of the major ḥadīth compilations, including those of Ibn Abī Shaybah (d. 849), al-Bukhārī (d. 870), Muslim ibn al-Ḥajjāj (d. 875), and al-Tirmidhī (d. 892), among others.

A distinguishing feature of these writings on medical prophetics, or the medical chapters in ḥadīth compilations, is that they were not about medicine. Rather, they were rooted in the prophetics genre and interested first and foremost in producing knowledge about the prophet. This literature paid little attention to the composition of the body, the physical reasons behind diseases, or the manners of treating different diseases. Instead, it focused on the illnesses suffered by Muḥammad himself or by his companions and diligently followed the events of their lives. Although this literature intersected with medicine, the intersection was circumstantial and occasional. The second chapter traces a second episode in the development of this archive of prophetic materials on health and disease. In these works, the logic of organization that governed these texts was not coming from the prophet's life but rather from medical literature. Texts were attentive to medical theories and descriptions of the composition of bodies. The discussion of diseases, treatments, and manners of health preservation followed what was deemed medically more significant or was perhaps more urgent from the viewpoint of readers interested in health and disease over what was deemed important in the prophet's and companions' lives. To be sure, many of the anecdotes and narratives that figured in the medical chapters of ḥadīth compendia continued to figure in these volumes of prophetic medicine. The difference, however, resided in the organizational schema and epistemic priorities – both now came to be more aligned with medical knowledge. The second chapter investigates some of the earliest writings of this genre, namely the works of the Andalusian scholar ʿAbd al-Malik ibn Ḥabīb al-Qurṭubī (d. 853), that of the two Shiite Twelver brothers Abū Ṭālib and Muḥammad ibn Bisṭām, and those of the renowned Sunni scholars Ibn al-Sunnī (d. 1003) and Abū Nuʿaym al-Iṣfahānī (d. 1038), as well as a treatise attributed to the Shiite Twelver Imām ʿAlī al-Riḍā (d. 813) but that was likely produced in the eleventh century. The chapter argues that these texts were central to the production of an archive of prophetic traditions, narratives, and anecdotes that will continue to populate narratives on medicine and piety. Because of the influence and importance of these authors, these texts provided important resources for other scholars addressing questions related to illness, health, and medicine in prophetic and Imami narratives. The chapter also looks at the production of a Galenic pious body, which entailed specific understanding of health that was conditioned by Galenic medical knowledge as well as by prophetic narratives.

The third and fourth chapters focus on specific themes that constituted the experiences of piety and patienthood. The third chapter looks at the pietistic space of illness and how pietistic texts aimed to produce a cosmology that provided meaning to the experiences of illness and that influenced the sensoria that characterized these experiences. The chapter focuses on some of the earliest and most central texts on piety and zuhd (renunciation of earthly pleasures), which outlined how pious Muslims needed to deal with a variety of religious and pietistic questions. These texts included the writings of Ibn al-Mubārak (d. 798), Wakīʿ ibn al-Jarrāḥ (d. 813), Ibn Wahb (d. 813), Aḥmad ibn Ḥanbal (d. 855), and Hannād ibn al-Sarī (d. 858), all of whom composed texts under the title of *zuhd*. Along with these texts, the chapter pays special attention to the chapter on illness in al-Bukhārī's (d. 870) ḥadīth compilation *al-Ṣaḥīḥ*, analyzing it in light of some of its earliest commentaries such as that of Ibn Baṭṭāl (d. 1058) and Ibn Abī al-Dunyā's book on *Al-Marad wa al-Kaffarat* (diseases and penance), which was deeply influenced by the previously mentioned texts on zuhd and was also one of the earlier and more widely cited texts dedicated particularly to illness. The chapter locates the authorial voice in these compilations and discusses how the authors' selections of prophetic narrations produced coherent pietistic narratives. It then investigates the question of diseases and their connection to sins and reward. It concludes with a discussion of the behavior that was recommended of pious Muslims when sick.

Engaging with a different dimension of patienthood, the fourth chapter looks at spiritual medicine as a genre of medicalized ethical writings which addressed the pietistic dimensions of spiritual ills. One of the earliest treatises entitled *Spiritual Medicine* was produced by the famous physician Abū Bakr al-Rāzī (d. 925). Al-Rāzī's work was part of a longer tradition of Hellenistic-Galenic ethics that can be traced back to Galen's commentary on the Timaeus, which was translated to Arabic in the ninth century. In the Islamicate context, al-Rāzī's work was preceded and influenced by al-Kindī's (d. 873) treatise on dispelling sorrow. Al-Kindī's student, Abū Zayd al-Balkhī (d. 934), who was also a physician and may have been one of al-Rāzī's teachers, included a section on spiritual medicine, virtues, and ethics in his medical encyclopedia *Manāfiʿ al-Abdān wa al-Anfus* (*Benefits for Bodies and Souls*). Similar discussions could also be found in the writings of Miskawayh's (d. 1030), such as *Tahdhīb al-Akhlāq* (*Refinement of Manners*). Alongside this Hellenistic narrative, religious scholars produced similar texts that addressed questions of spiritual medicine. For instance, the Ismāʿīlī scholar Ḥamīd al-Dīn al-Kirmānī (fl. 996–1021) composed a text on spiritual medicine that was a direct critique and refutation of Abū Bakr al-Rāzī's *Spiritual*

Medicine. Ibn al-Jawzī (d. 1201) followed al-Rāzī's example and composed his own *Spiritual Medicine* in which he relied heavily on al-Rāzī, organizing his book in the same manner. For both al-Kirmānī and Ibn al-Jawzī, not to mention al-Balkhī and al-Rāzī, this ethical discussion was imbued with significant medical meanings and was rooted in a belief that in guaranteeing the health of the body, these recommendations also guaranteed the health of the soul, as both composed the full person. This chapter looks specifically at four works that presented themselves as writings on spiritual medicine: al-Balkhī's *Manāfi'*, al-Rāzī's *Al-Ṭibb al-Rūḥānī*, al-Kirmānī's *Al-Aqwāl*, and Ibn al-Jawzī's *Al-Ṭibb al-Rūḥānī*, locating this discussion of spiritual health in the Galenic ethical tradition and in the context of other pietistic writings, such as those of Ibn Abī al-Dunyā, al-Ḥakīm al-Tirmdhī, and others.

The final chapter (Chapter 5) looks at the making of the pious physician. Here, the chapter engages with medical biographies as a mode of ethical writings that intended to provide models of how one could be a good pious medical practitioner. The chapter then moves to discuss the works of two physicians who wrote on prophetic medicine and engaged with the prophetic and pietistic literature directly. The works of the two physicians 'Abd al-Laṭif al-Baghdādī (d. 1231) and Ibn Ṭarkhān (d. 1320) were seen as significant moments in the history of prophetic medicine. Known for their religious knowledge and their experience in ḥadīth and other religious sciences, the two physicians were able to compose treatises on prophetic medicine. Al-Baghdādī dictated a commentary on the medical chapter of Ibn Mājah's ḥadīth compilation, and Ibn Ṭarkhān compiled his own collection of medical traditions, which became rather popular in the following decades and helped inform later writings in the thirteenth and fourteenth centuries. This chapter explores how these physicians understood their own professions from a pietistic viewpoint, with a focus specifically on al-Baghdādī and Ibn Ṭarkhān as examples of pious physicians who composed texts that intended to provide a narrative of pietistic medical practice. The chapter demonstrates how their work provided a template for how Muslim physicians should understand their own practice, how they should practice pietistically, and how they should attend to the pietistic needs of their patients.

In discussing piety and patienthood, the book proposes two connected historiographic and methodological points. Although the production of Islamic pietistic narratives, practices, and institutions is located at the intersection of various concerns and different debates, I argue that the image and character of Muḥammad as a figure to be emulated and to be revered and loved as a matter of faith continued to play a central role in the construction of these modes of piety. In this view, and as I will demonstrate, the collection of materials that described and illustrated the prophet's life was in itself a form of pietistic practice that rendered the archival making of Muḥammad a ritualistic and iterative act of salvage. Here, I use the term salvage to refer to the belief that governed much of the early endeavors of ḥadīth collection that the legacy of the prophet was in danger and required significant energy, dedication, and responsibility to be collected. At another level, salvage as an analytical term portrays how these scholars and compilers of ḥadīth purported that their roles had no influence on the integrity of the salvaged prophetic materials. In a process of salvage, the best collector is always the one that had the least impact on the salvaged materials. Because of the nature of these materials, as will be explained in the book, Muḥammad's image was not drawn as a grand narrative but rather as a collection of little narratives (*petits recits*), each of which was a localized, event-connected, and specific narrative that, when woven together, formed the tapestry that was the prophet's character. In the following chapters, I will investigate how this peculiar nature of the prophetic pietistic archive engendered specific modes of thinking and behavior and particular types of pietistic performance.

Perceiving the prophetic legacy and the pietistic structures, narratives, and performances that were based on it as an archive places a premium on investigating moments of beginning, collecting, and construction, as well as on the manners through which the archive was organized. As such, I argue that the study of the earlier and classical period from the ninth century and into the eleventh century allows us to better understand the making of this pietistic archive that continues to influence pietistic performances and hermeneutics today. Moreover, this investigation requires a deeper understanding of the authorial voice of curators and editors and how they chose to compile their texts and their little narratives. Here, the materials analyzed in the book are almost all claimed to have descended from the prophet and his companions. In this book, I will not investigate the accuracy of these claims or build historical narratives about the prophet's life based on these narratives. In fact, the authors of these texts and the collectors of ḥadīth in the period from the ninth century and into the thirteenth century and beyond would not make certain claims of authenticity either. As will be demonstrated later, these authors and collectors perceived the value of pietistic ḥadīths to be precisely in their pietistic content and in the charismatic power imbedded in the prophet's name. As such, they were willing to allow many traditions that they believed were inaccurate or even fabricated in order to benefit from them in the making of a larger pietistic narrative. Instead of investigating truth claims, this book will follow the lead of the authors that it investigates and will analyze the pietistic import and messages that these traditions aimed to deliver. The authority of these traditions is located in their attribution to the prophet, but is applicable only to their time of emergence whether it was in the ninth century or in the fourteenth century. Regardless of whether Muḥammad indeed experienced these events, pious Muslims continued to hope they would.

Notes

1 See, among many others, Kleinman, *Patients and Healers in the Context of Culture*; Kleinman, *The Illness Narratives*.
2 See, for instance, the ḥadīth collections produced by Ibn Abī Shaybah, al-Bukhārī, Muslim, and others.
3 On these writings, see Kinberg, "Zuhd;" Marín, "Zuhd in al-Andalus;" Yaldiz, "Afterlife."
4 Some of the more prominent examples of this subgenre are the works of Ibn Mufliḥ, Ibn Qayyim al-Jawziyah, and al-Dhahabī. See Ibn Qayyim al-Jawzīyah, *Al-Ṭibb*

al-Nabawī; Al-Maqdisī, *Khamsūn Faṣlan fī al-Tadāwī wa-l-ʿIlāj wa-l-Ṭibb al-Nabawī*; Al-Dhahabi, *Al-Ṭibb al-Nabawiyy*; Ibn Ṭūlūn, *Al-Manhal al-Rawī fi al-Ṭib al-Nabawī*; Al-Suyūṭī, *Al-Raḥmah fī al-Ṭib wa-l-Ḥikmah.*

5 Perho, *The Prophet's Medicine*, 53–62 especially 57–8.

6 Although Perho produced the single comprehensive monographic study on prophetic medicine, other scholars contributed significantly to this debate. Examples include Elgood, "Tibb-ul-Nabbi"; Rahman, *Health and Medicine*; Dols, "Islam and Medicine"; and Perho, "Koran and the Sunna in the Medicine of the Prophet." More recently, see, among others, Fancy, "Virtuous Son of the Rational"; Stearns, *Infectious Ideas*; Lewicka, *Medicine for Muslims?*; Fancy, *Science and Religion in Mamluk Egypt*; and Zinger, "Tradition and Medicine." In relation to Shiite writings, see Newman, "Islamic Medical Wisdom"; "Baqir al-Majlisi and Islamicate Medicine"; and "Recovery of the Past." Prophetic medicine also figured in writings about medicine, science, and Islam in general. Central examples include Morrison, *Islam and Science*; and Hogendijk, Sabra, and Morrison, "Enterprise of Science in Islam."

7 See, for instance, Baldick, *Mystical Islam*; Bin ʿĀmir, *Dirāsāt fī al-Zuhd wa-al-Taṣawwuf*; Bin Ramli, "Rise of Early Sufism"; El-Leithy, "Sufis, Copts and the Politics of Piety"; and Hoffman-Ladd, "Mysticism and Sexuality."

8 Talmon-Heller, *Islamic Piety in Medieval Syria.* See also, Talmon-Heller, "Society and Religion in Syria" and Frenkel and Lev, eds., *Charity and Giving in Monotheistic Religions.* Similarly, and in relation to institutions, see Ragab, *The Medieval Islamic Hospital*; Bonner, Ener, and Singer, eds., *Poverty and Charity in Middle Eastern Contexts*; Tabbaa, *Constructions of Power and Piety in Medieval Aleppo*; and Fernandes, "Evolution of the Khānqāh Institution."

9 Schimmel, *And Muhammad Is His Messenger.* See also Schimmel, *My Soul Is a Woman*; Schimmel, *Mystical Dimensions of Islam.*

10 Melchert, "Piety of the Hadith Folk;" "Aḥmad ibn Ḥanbal's Book of Renunciation;" and "Exaggerated Fear."

11 Mahmood, "Ethics and Piety" and *Politics of Piety*; Omer, "Modernists Despite Themselves"; Asad, *Formations of the Secular*; and Hirschkind, "Is There a Secular Body?"

12 See Schimmel, *And Muḥammad Is His Messenger*; Duderija, "Evolution in the Canonical Sunni Ḥadīth"; Lucas, *Constructive Critics, Ḥadīth Literature, and the Articulation of Sunnī Islam*; Melchert, *The Formation of the Sunni Schools of Law*. Brown, *The Canonization of al-Bukhārī and Muslim*; Newman, *The Formative Period of Twelver Shī'ism*; and Melchert, "Piety of the Ḥadīth Folk."

13 On the implications of these writings in the contemporary, see Ragab, "Prophetic Traditions and Modern Medicine." In another vein, but also connected to the impact of classical and postclassical icons and archives on contemporary thought, see Pormann, "Arab 'Cultural Awakening (Nahda)'"; Najjar, "Ibn Rushd"; and Elshakry, "Gospel of Science."

1 "A beau ideal for whosoever hopes for God"

The making of medical prophetics in the ninth and tenth centuries

The middle of the ninth century witnessed a number of watershed moments for the development of ḥadīth sciences. The work of al-Shāfiʿī, as many contemporary and later scholars explained, helped consolidate the importance of ḥadīth in legal jurisprudence. Ibn Ḥanbal's work helped solidify some of the emerging methods and tools of ḥadīth criticism in a variety of ways, including training a group of scholars and reporters who would dominate the scene of ḥadīth reporting and criticism for the rest of the ninth century and whose work would come to constitute important milestones in the sciences of ḥadīth. Ibn Ḥanbal's position during the *miḥna* (the trial or testing) and his vicious attacks against Shiites and Muʿtazilites helped solidify a new theological and sectarian position for the emerging group that came to be known as the people of ḥadīth (*ahl al-ḥadīth*).[1] Other scholars like Isḥāq ibn Rāhawayh (d. 853), Abū Zarʿah al-Rāzī (d. 878), Abū Ḥātim Muḥammad ibn Idrīs al-Rāzī (d. 890), and Muḥammad ibn Naṣr al-Marwazī (d. 907) played important roles in consolidating some of the traditions of ḥadīth sciences, which would continue to influence scholars for centuries to come and, in many cases, continue to resonate today. In this same period, the collections of al-Bukhārī (d. 870), Muslim ibn al-Ḥajjāj (d. 875), Abū Dawwūd (d. 889), al-Dārimī (d. 868), al-Tirmidhī (d. 892), and al-Nasāʾī (d. 915) were produced. Although almost a century would pass before most of these compilations acquired the respect and reverence that they enjoyed later on as some of the central collections of Sunnī ḥadīths,[2] the rise of these rather selective collections marked an important moment in the history of ḥadīth sciences and indicated a level of maturity in the epistemic and professional practices of these scholars. The rise of these collections was also a sign of a slow but steady transition toward privileging the *marfūʿ* (elevated) over *mawqūf* (arrested) ḥadīths – the former being ones that go back (elevated up) to the prophet himself and the latter as ones whose chains of transmission stop at one of the companions and do not reach the prophet. To be sure, the *mawqūf* traditions continued to play a significant role in the production of legal and pietistic discourses and continued to be subject to scrutiny, criticism, and analysis in ways similar to the *marfūʿ* traditions. However, the shift in the number of *mawqūf* traditions from the early collections of Mālik ibn Anas to the collections of Ibn Abī Shaybah and then of al-Dārimī, al-Bukhārī or Muslim ibn al-Ḥajjāj mark this growing interest in preserving the legacy of the prophet himself in a manner that would be distinguishable from those of even his closest companions.[3]

At the heart of this burgeoning environment, scholars contended with the legal and pietistic dimensions of a few central questions: What was the prophet's sunna? How could it be reported and discussed? And what obligations were constituted by this sunna? The sunna, and the prophet's sayings and deeds that constituted its amorphous corpus, functioned as part of a pietistic discourse that identified what pious Muslims were supposed to do and how they were required or asked to behave. In this regard, knowledge about the prophet and the early community became an important tool in creating a pietistic environ that Muslims were asked to inhabit. This environ was structured around the prophet as a moral and pietistic example and, as the Quran put it, "a beau ideal for whosoever hopes for God" [Q33:21]. Such a legacy did not only involve legal questions or issues related to religious rituals and obligations, but was also important in relation to various daily activities, from eating to drinking to having sex or getting sick and receiving treatment. Although many of the reported narratives about the prophet's daily life did not constitute *furūḍ* (religious obligations), they contributed to the making of a pietistic narrative, which included *sunan* and *nawāfil* (supererogatory acts), among other nonmandatory rituals, that influenced how pious Muslims understood their relationship to the religious past.

This chapter focuses on the construction of the prophet's persona as a beau ideal in relation to medicine. In its first half, it starts by addressing the making of the sunna and its evolving relation to ḥadīth in the work of al-Shāfiʿī and other ninth-century scholars. Here, I look at the connections between ḥadīth and adab and the attending practices of collecting and categorization. It then moves to discussing the relation between ḥadīth and adab, understood as both a literary and epistemic discipline, as well as a locus of self-fashioning. In the second half, the chapter looks at the medical sections in the major ḥadīth collections of the ninth century. Here, I investigate the beginning of the interest in these medical questions in the works of Muʿammir ibn Rāshid (d. 770) and his student, ʿAbd al-Razzāq al-Ṣanʿānī (d. 826), as well as in the works of Abū ʿAbd Allāh ibn Saʿd (d. 845) and their contemporaries. I then analyze the medical chapters of some of the major ḥadīth compilations, including those of Ibn Abī Shaybah (d. 849), al-Bukhārī (d. 870), Muslim ibn al-Ḥajjāj (d. 875), and al-Tirmidhī (d. 892), among others. Here, I first analyze the main themes and common tropes in these various compilations before concluding with an examination of the "materia prophetica," or the materials used and mentioned in these texts as treatments. In mapping the "materia prophetica" in these compilations, I attempt to reproduce the material space of this prophetic narrative.

The emergence of Muḥammad

The development of ḥadīth sciences in the seventh and eighth centuries was connected to the development of the *sīra* and *maghāzī* literature chronicling the life of the prophet and his companions. For instance, some of the earliest examples of a systematic effort to collect ḥadīths and to record them was undertaken by the famous author of sīra, Ibn Shahāb al-Zuhrī (d. 742). Al-Zuhrī worked under the patronage of the Umayyad court as an educator to the Umayyad Caliph Hishām ibn ʿAbd al-Malik's (r. 724–743) sons. Al-Zuhrī used this opportunity to collect and record ḥadīths aided by a number of students.[4] Sīra and maghāzī books included collections of ḥadīths attributed to Muḥammad along with anecdotes that were reported by eyewitnesses or attributed to other important companions who were close to events in the life of Muḥammad.[5] With the rise in importance of ḥadīth and the sunna as sources for interpreting the Quran and for the law, the importance of sīra and maghāzī rose as well.

The development of the maghāzī and sīra literature from the mid-seventh to the ninth and tenth centuries further demonstrates the increasing interest in the details of Muḥammad's life in connection to the emerging importance of the sunna at the legal and pietistic levels.[6] The beginning of this literature on Muḥammad's history was in the maghāzī accounts, which focused on the battles and wars that Muḥammad waged and other central events in his life.[7] The maghāzī literature had its roots in Arabian tribal accounts of battles and conquests known as *ayyām al-ʿArab* or *Battles of the Arabs*. The new Islamic rendition, however, extolled a significant pietistic dimension. In maghāzī works, divine interventions, the causes of various events or actions taken by the prophet, and the consequences of these events presented an important pietistic background that supplanted the tribal heroisms of *ayyām al-ʿArab*.[8] For instance, al-Zuhrī was reported to have said that "'the science of maghāzī is the science of both this world and the Hereafter'; ʿAlī b. al-Ḥusayn is recorded as saying, 'We used to learn maghāzī of the prophet as we learnt a sūrah of the Qur'ān.'"[9]

Moreover, Muḥammad's life and the early days of the Muslim polity carried significant political implications under first, the Umayyads, and then, the Abbasids. The stories of different companions, their connections to Muḥammad, and the different roles that they played or that were assigned to them significantly influenced how they and the legitimacy of their political positions and acts were perceived in the following centuries. Thus, these stories, the perceptions of them, and the legitimacy they proffered came to form the claims of the various reigns and polities that followed Muḥammad's death. Ultimately, the strongest claim to legitimacy was one related to tribal origin (namely, belonging to Quraysh, with preference awarded according to the clan and family) and to precedence in accepting Islam and migrating from Mecca to Medina, known as *al-sabq fī-l-Islām wa-l-hijra*.[10] Those who believed in Muḥammad first, who accompanied him, and who emigrated with him were awarded more legitimacy and more authority retrospectively.[11]

This ranking of the companions based on precedence in Islam and migration carried particularly significant political weight for the Umayyads, whose forefathers were mostly late-comers to Islam and had fought against Muḥammad for a decade or more before joining his victorious polity. Facing Alid opposition, which was bolstered by ʿAlī's kinship, companionship to the prophet, and his precedence in Islam, the Umayyads relied on the legitimacy of the first three caliphs, particularly ʿUthmān ibn ʿAffān, who was their closest of kin, and in whose assassination they implicated ʿAlī.[12] In his *Maghāzī*, Ibn Shahāb al-Zuhrī paid special attention to the place of ʿAlī and ʿUthmān and their various claims to precedence. For instance, in discussing who the first Muslim was, al-Zuhrī dismissed the claim that ʿAlī was the first to convert, attributing this honor to Muḥammad's adopted son Zayd ibn Ḥāritha.[13] The choice of Zayd is significant for a number of reasons. On one hand, his close association with Muḥammad made this anecdote plausible. On the other, Zayd passed away during Muḥammad's life and was not party to the conflicts between ʿAlī and Muʿāwiyah (r. 661–680). His son, Usāma ibn Zayd (d. 673), who was an important companion in his own right and was appointed by Muḥammad to lead the last campaign dispatched shortly before his death, refused to fight alongside ʿAlī, casting significant doubts on his support for the Alid cause.

The same sensitivity can be seen in the discussion of the battle of Uḥud (ca. 625), which constituted Muḥammad's first defeat and a moment of great distress to the emerging community. Al-Zuhrī paid attention to how Abū Sufyān (the father of Muʿāwiyah, the Umayyad first caliph), who was among the leaders of the Meccan armies fighting against Muḥammad, acted gallantly, and was even remorseful for the calamities that befell the Muslims:

> Abū Sufyān said, "You will find that some of your dead were mutilated. [Know] that this was not decided by us or by our leaders." He then said, "May Hubal (a Meccan deity) be glorified." ʿUmar ibn al-Khaṭṭāb said, "Allah is mightier and holier." Abū Sufyān said, "Your dead are for our dead in the battle of Badr." ʿUmar replied, "The two are not equal. Our dead will be in heaven and yours will be in hell." So Abū Sufyān said, "We have failed then!" and he went back to Mecca.[14]

In the same vein, the roles played by different companions, their closeness to the prophet, and the details of their lives influenced how later scholars of law and ḥadīth judged their piety and integrity and accepted them as sources for ḥadīth or for the law. G.H.A. Juynboll has argued that ḥadīth transmitters and compilers of the eighth century engaged in discussions around the role and trustworthiness of the prophet's companions and showed significant interest in defending the collective integrity of the companions, especially those involved in the first *fitna* or civil war (656–661 AD) as well as in other conflicts in the first century of Islam.[15] In his *Sunnah*, Ibn Ḥanbal employed many traditions to explain the hierarchy of the prophet's companions, insisting that Abū Bakr, ʿUmar, ʿUthmān, and ʿAlī – the first four caliphs – were the most important authorities in matters of religion and the best people in the nation after the prophet.[16] Although Sunni scholars ultimately agreed on expanding pietistic authority (*taʿdīl al-ṣaḥāba* or proving the integrity of the companions) to include all the prophet's companions, earlier works up to the tenth century paid special attention to certain events in the prophet's life that distinguished certain companions over others and proved their particular worth.

One of the clearest examples of how sīra influenced views on the companions is related to some of the major battles that Muḥammad witnessed. For instance, in his *Tabaqāt*, Ibn Saʿd considered attending Badr as well as the truce of al-Ḥadaybiya to be central conditions in defining who counted as an actual companion of the prophet.[17] Although the definition of companionship expanded in later writings to include all those who came in contact with the prophet, Nancy Khalek explained that the battle of Badr and similar significant events were still central in constructing a narrative of excellence that differentiated the companions.[18] As a result, different sīra authors took pains to enumerate the participants in the battle of Badr. Equally important was the analysis of the reasons why some people failed to join the battle. For instance, Ibn Qutaybah (d. 889) dedicated a chapter in his book, *al-Maʿārif*, to those who failed to join Badr, explaining their reasons and the prophet's response to their absences. Implied in this discussion was the belief that failing to join the first battle of this nascent community while able-bodied represented a significant blemish on a person's piety and integrity. Ibn Qutaybah started his chapter with ʿUthmān ibn ʿAffān (d. 656), the third caliph and an important figure in Sunni–Shiite polemics, who had failed to attend the battle of Badr. Ibn Qutaybah explained that ʿUthmān, who was married to Muḥammad's daughter Ruqayyah, was asked by the prophet to stay in Medina to care for his ill wife. The prophet guaranteed ʿUthmān both his share of the spoils and his divine reward as if he were a participant.[19] Similarly, Ibn Qutaybah explained that Ṭalḥah ibn ʿUbayd Allāh and Saʿīd ibn Zayd were excused by the prophet and guaranteed their share in spoils and in divine reward.[20] The fact that these men were excused by the prophet and guaranteed their divine reward meant that they remained on the same level as other companions who participated in this battle in terms of their integrity, their trustworthiness as ḥadīth reporters, and the worthiness of their legal opinions. Proving or explaining a connection to Badr was even more complicated with regard to the prophet's uncle and namesake of the Abbasid dynasty, al-ʿAbbās, who did not publicly convert to Islam before Badr. Some authors, like Ibn Saʿd, explained this by claiming that al-ʿAbbas had secretly converted to Islam and was serving as a spy in Mecca, therefore indicating that he still played an important role in the battle of Badr.[21] At another level, the details of the prophet's life provided further insights into the occasions in which certain traditions were uttered and on how these traditions can be interpreted. Ibn Qutaybah, one of the earlier authors who discussed contradictory and odd traditions in his *Taʾwīl Mukhtalif al-Ḥadīth* or "Interpretation of contradictory traditions," emphasized the importance of knowing when a tradition was spoken and the circumstances surrounding it to better understand its meaning and legal or pietistic significance.[22]

Although al-Zuhrī's main focus was on Muḥammad's battles and major events in his career, he did not begin with Muḥammad's birth or his prophethood but rather with his grandfather's renovation of the Meccan sanctuary and the birth of Muḥammad's father. This point, which continued to be the beginning of the story for many authors and compilers after al-Zuhrī, was important in linking Muḥammad to the Meccan sanctuary and foregrounding the honor and privileged status of his family. Al-Zuhrī's narrative glossed over many details, explaining only the most important battles, wars, and major events in Muḥammad's life. The political nature of al-Zuhrī's text is unmistakable. On one hand, the text attempted to produce the foundational narrative of the Islamic empire by rooting it in the early battles of Muḥammad's polity and the history of his successors. On the other, the author appeared keenly aware of the political implications of his text regarding claims to authority made by the Umayyads and their detractors in the first half of the eighth century. Although the character of Muḥammad was central to the narrative, his character was viewed primarily through these politically and militarily charged moments. Al-Zuhrī barely referenced his physical description and offered a sparse discussion of his personal habits or even method of governance. The narrative was primarily a political history that happened to occur around the life of the prophet.

The next well-known sīra compendium followed al-Zuhrī's narrative structure, albeit with a few departures. Ibn Isḥāq's (d. 768) *sīra*, which was reported on and edited by Ibn Hishām (d. 834), also focused on the major events that punctuated the life of the prophet.[23] Ibn Isḥāq was respected by al-Zuhrī and others. He lived most of his life in Medina, and his grandfather was a companion of the prophet who would have witnessed much of what the grandson wrote about.[24] Among scholars of law and ḥadīth, like Mālik ibn Anas and Ibn Ḥanbal, Ibn Isḥāq did not enjoy a similar repute. Mālik was known to have despised him and to have attacked him in public, and Ibn Ḥanbal criticized him for reporting ḥadīths without clear chains of transmission – a method deemed more acceptable in transmission of sīra and maghāzī.[25]

Ibn Isḥāq's *sīra*, in the recension of Ibn Hishām, combined varying tastes and catered to changing interests. On one hand, it followed a very similar arc to that of al-Zuhrī's text, focusing on battles and major events, many of which had been previously selected by al-Zuhrī. However, in his edition, Ibn Hishām managed to remove many anecdotes that were not directly related to the prophet, making the text more focused on the prophet. For instance, Ibn Isḥāq, in Ibn Hishām's reporting, started his *sīra* with Muḥammad's mother and her death, as opposed to the story of his grandfather in al-Zuhrī. More importantly, and also in keeping with the rising interest in the occasions of revelation, Ibn Hishām's *sīra* paid special attention to the occasions where some of the more important verses of the Quran were revealed – something that cannot be found in what survived of al-Zuhrī's *maghāzī*. For instance, Ibn Isḥāq/Ibn Hishām explained the occasion on which the Quranic chapter *al-Kawthar* or "Abundance" was revealed [Q: 108]. The importance of this sura might be related to its being a divine promise of heaven to the prophet. Furthermore, the occasion for revealing *Sura al-Kahf* or "the Cave" was also emphasized because it was seen as involving specific challenges by the Meccans to Muḥammad that the *sura* responded to. In these examples and others, the interest in linking sīra literature to the Quran seemed to have emerged from the rising importance of ḥadīth in understanding the Quran and the emerging interest in *asbāb al-nuzūl* (occasions of revelation), which relied more heavily on sīra in understanding the Quran.[26] Similar to al-Zuhrī, Ibn Isḥāq's *sīra* did not include any descriptions of Muḥammad as a person, his daily activities, or any of his actions beyond battles and major religious questions (such as the occasions for revealing the previously mentioned verses).

Ibn Hishām's contemporary, Ibn Saʿd (d. 845), who also authored an important volume that dealt with the life of the prophet, took a markedly different approach from al-Zuhrī, Ibn Isḥāq, al-Wāqidi, and Ibn Hishām. Ibn Saʿd's text was neither a maghāzī nor a sīra text. Instead, it was one of the earliest texts of *ṭabaqāt* (generations) literature.[27] From the outset, the focus of Ibn Saʿd's collection was directed toward scholars of ḥadīth and their emerging concerns about lines of transmission.[28] Ibn Saʿd's *Tabaqāt* included close to 2,000 biographies of companions and followers arranged in different generations (ṭabaqāt) – a useful arrangement for the emerging disciplines of ḥadīth criticism. As previously mentioned, Ibn Saʿd's work was not without political significance as the precedence and importance of particular companions carried significance in legitimacy debates under the Abbasids. A prominent example is Ibn Saʿd's detailed analysis of the life, precedence, and religious authority of Ibn ʿAbbās (d. 687), who was Muḥammad's cousin, the grandfather of the Abbasid Caliphs, and the source of their claims to legitimacy as members of the prophetic family. In his biography, Ibn Saʿd was concerned about the question of Ibn ʿAbbas's age. Because Ibn ʿAbbās was ten years old when the prophet died, his knowledge of the sunna, his ability to report traditions, and his legal erudition and authority could come under scrutiny. To dispel any doubts, Ibn Saʿd proceeded to explain how Ibn ʿAbbas was particularly precocious, that the prophet prayed that his young cousin be learned in religion, and that he was consulted by many of the major companions, including ʿUmar ibn al-Khaṭṭāb, who held him in the same regard as he held the companions who witnessed Badr.[29] Ibn Saʿd illustrated Ibn ʿAbbas's unique piety and his selection by God by recounting how he was the only one to see the archangel when he was meeting with Muḥammad. This anecdote signified how the young companion was endowed with wisdom and chosen by God for a great destiny to come.[30]

The first treatise of Ibn Saʿd's book, entitled "The sīra of the prophet," focused on the prophet's life and was composed of two main sections. In the first, Ibn Saʿd traced the main events in the prophet's life in a manner similar to al-Zuhrī and Ibn Isḥāq. In the second part, Ibn Saʿd focused on details of the prophet's habits and his behavior. For instance, one finds a chapter on "the prophet's manners" (*akhlāq al-rasūl*), including traditions about the way he spoke, how he walked, how he prayed, how his hair grayed, what he wore, how he slept, etc. Throughout the thirty-five chapters, Ibn Saʿd used traditions reported by the prophet's companions and wives to explain many details about his life and habits. Following these chapters, he included twenty-three other chapters that described the different objects that he used, such as his swords, spears, horses, camels, combs, shields, etc. In the first chapter of the second section, Ibn Saʿd came close to explaining the purpose behind these various chapters detailing the prophet's life. He commenced the chapter with a number of ḥadīths in which ʿĀʾisha was asked about the prophet's manners. She replied, "His manners were [like] the Quran."[31] This tradition became ubiquitous in the literature discussing the prophet from the ninth century until today and showed how the prophet's behavior explained and embodied the Quran. Thus, Ibn Sa'd invokes this tradition to assert that by following and discussing the manners and behaviors of the prophet, no matter how minute in detail, one approaches the true meaning of the Quran.

In the writings of Ibn Saʿd, Muḥammad's character emerged in an unprecedented manner. The sīra became the vessel for understanding Muḥammad as a person. The details of his life – from his manners to how he walked, had sex, and dyed his hair – were described vividly, illustrating his life as a walking embodiment of the Quran. Ibn Saʿd's concern was not solely legal but also largely pietistic. Although some of his accounts and anecdotes had some legal implications (in the sense of individual or communal obligations and normative legal rules), many did not. For instance, none of the twenty-three chapters discussing tools and animals used by Muḥammad had any immediate legal implications. Yet all of these chapters and anecdotes carried important pietistic implications, as they drew the image of the prophet as one who should be emulated and loved as a matter of belief.[32] In part, emulating the prophet was following the Quran incarnate; however, it was also a pietistic endeavor that went beyond what is required and mandated into what is worthy of a believer.[33] Moreover, the epistemic exercise of knowing about the prophet and of faithfully and indiscriminately transmitting his traditions was in itself a pietistic exercise. A believer should be motivated by the desire to know about the prophet and to understand all the details of his life.[34]

Ibn Saʿd's magnum opus was part of a corpus of literature that served the emerging ḥadīth sciences. The majority of its content was dedicated to the different generations of reporters of ḥadīth and to analyzing and discussing their trustworthiness. In this framework, his pronounced interest in the details of Muḥammad's life and behavior, which was unique in its scope and detail, reflected the interests of both the emerging community of ḥadīth scholars and preachers and legal scholars, among others.[35] This interest in the details of Muḥammad's life was also emphasized by Ibn Saʿd's near contemporary, Ibn Qutaybah (d. 889). In his own book on *Mukhtalif al-Ḥadīth* or "The Contradictory Traditions," Ibn Qutaybah started by defending the people of ḥadīth against attacks from many others, while also criticizing those he considered to be unworthy of belonging to the ranks of the *Muḥaddithīn* or the people of the ḥadīth. He writes that those people:

> were satisfied by the appearance of knowledge and the title that comes with studying ḥadīth, and were content if they were mentioned as knowledgeable about the methods and the narrations of ḥadīth, but were disinterested in their being known as having followed what was written or applying what was known [of the sunna].[36]

Thus, the knowledge of ḥadīth and the transmission of sunna was not simply an act of accumulating anecdotes and knowing the tools and methods needed to verify and rectify ḥadīth. It was also a pietistic endeavor that required the knower to follow the example of the prophet and to embody the sunna in their own lives.

In the same vein and following in Ibn Saʿd's footsteps, many scholars and ḥadīth compilers produced volumes that highlighted specific aspects of the prophet's life. For instance, Ibn Sawrah al-Tirmidhī (d. 892) composed a book entitled *Al-Shamāʾil* or "The [Prophetic] Characteristics" which explored the prophet's manners and behaviors through different ḥadīths and anecdotes.[37] Al-Tirmidhī started by discussing Muḥammad's shape and appearance, moved to his hair, his garments, his footwear, his greying hair and dyes, swords, shields, different animals, etc. He then proceeded to discuss various aspects of his behavior such as how he ate and what food he preferred, how he washed and prayed, how he joked and talked, and how he slept, among many other things. In addition to these chapters, al-Tirmidhī collected traditions and anecdotes to address some directly pietistic questions such as the prophet's humility, his fear of God, and his manners and ended with the division of his inheritance. Here, as well, the legal significance of these traditions seemed to be less important than the pietistic implications.[38] *Al-Shamāʾil* was intended to present the prophet to the readers as a divine person: a personification of the Quran. It proceeded to satisfy intellectual and pietistic needs for knowing about the prophet and to push an ever-evolving argument about his perfection, both at the physical and spiritual levels. At the same time, this book and others like it further solidified the position of the Muḥaddithīn as the heirs and guardians of Muḥammad's legacy and the keepers of prophetic knowledge. Similar to al-Tirmidhī, Abū Nuʿaym al-Isfahānī's (d. 1038) "The Manners of the Prophet (*Akhlāq al-Nabiyy*)" and Imam al-Bayhaqī's (d. 1066) "Proofs of Prophecy (*Dalāʾil al-Nubuwwa*)" narrated ḥadīths and accounts that discussed the details of Muḥammad's life, physical appearance, and the objects that he used. In these later volumes, the *shamāʾil* were combined with detailed discussions of proofs (*dalāʾil*), miracles, and admissions of Muḥammad's prophecy. In essence, the prophet's *shamāʾil* (characters) were also part of the *dalāʾil* (proofs).[39]

This evolving trend continued in the writings about Muḥammad in the tenth century and beyond. Ibn Jarīr al-Ṭabarī's (d. 923) *Tārīkh al-Rusul wa al-Mulūk* or "The History of Prophets and Kings" represents an important example of how this growing interest in the details of Muḥammad's life and behaviors made its way to the heart of the historiographic tradition of sīra. Al-Ṭabarī followed the same overall chronological arc laid out by al-Zuhrī and Ibn Isḥāq in Ibn Hishām's recension. Starting with Muḥammad's life before prophecy, he recounted how a monk recognized the signs of prophecy in Muḥammad when the prophet accompanied his uncle on a trade journey to the Levant. Yet unlike al-Zuhrī or Ibn Hishām, al-Ṭabarī was more interested in the details of this recognition and how the signs of prophecy were imprinted on Muḥammad's body and visible in his manners:

> When Buḥayrā [the monk] saw the prophet, he stared at him, and kept observing him very closely. He looked at things in the [prophet's] body that he had read in his books. After [. . .], he asked the prophet about specific things in his manners, his wake and his sleep. Each time the prophet told him [about something], he found it similar to what he had [in his books]. [Buḥayrā] then looked at [the prophet's] back and saw the sign of prophecy between his

> shoulders. Then Buḥayra said to the [prophet's] uncle, Abī Ṭālib, "What is this boy to you?" Abū Ṭālib said, "He is my son." Buḥayrā said, "He is not your son. This boy should not have a living father." Abū Ṭālib said, "He is my nephew." Buḥayrā [asked], "What happened to his father?" [Abū Ṭālib answered,] "He died while his mother carried him." [Buḥayrā] said, "[This is right!]. Take him back to your land and be careful of Jews. If they see him and know what I knew, they would hurt him. By God, he will have a great destiny."[40]

Although the narrative of recognition remained the same, al-Ṭabarī highlighted the interest in Muḥammad's appearance and physical qualities and how they informed the monk's recognition.

Notably, he also attends to how the monk asked about details of Muḥammad's life and his different habits. In al-Ṭabarī's view, the signs of prophecy were to be found on Muḥammad's body and in his manners, even before he became a prophet,[41] signifying that, from birth, he was ordained and protected by God. Al-Ṭabarī reported a tradition where Muḥammad explained how, as a boy, he was tempted to join his peers in drinking and in seeking women, but miraculously fell asleep on his way so that he failed to commit these acts.[42] The prophet's body and his manners were therefore purified, protected, and perfected by God even before his prophecy: this emphasized the perfect example that he was. These same accounts were reported with similar details in Ibn Ḥibbān's (d. 965) *Sīra* as well.[43]

With the increased interest in ḥadīth and ḥadīth compilations, Muḥammad emerged as an infallible *beau ideal*, to use the Quranic expression, who should be known and emulated. His behavior embodied the Quran and exemplified proper, if not always attainable, model behavior. This pietistic orientation was built on what scholars, such as Armand Abel and Annemarie Schimmel, described as *imitatio muhammadi* – an orientation to imitate the prophet in all his acts as a sign of ultimate piety.[44] At another level, following the prophet's example was seen to come from a particular disposition that characterized the true believer. In his compendium, al-Bukhārī (d. 870) dedicated a chapter to the foundations of true faith, discussing in a subchapter "that loving the prophet is part of the faith." The subchapter included two similar traditions (with different *isnāds* [chains of narration]), in which the prophet said, "By God! None of you truly believes until he loves me more than his parents and offspring."[45] Loving the prophet, and by relation his companions,[46] was emerging as Muslim pietistic disposition. This literature, I termed prophetics, was a product of, and contributed to, this interest and emphasis on such pietistic dispositions. Prophetics included anecdotes, stories, ḥadīths, and various accounts that circulated within ḥadīth, sīra, and other genres and that attempted to provide detailed knowledge of Muḥammad's life, his preferences, and his manners without seemingly immediate theological or legal implications. Instead, they served a learned and pietistic purpose that took on an increasing importance in the ninth and tenth centuries.

Thus, at the pietistic level, prophetics helped create the image of the prophet as a person who could be emulated in all his actions and behaviors. Moreover, the interest in these details and seeking this knowledge were in themselves signs of the love for the prophet and the desire to emulate him. At a learned level, prophetics were undoubtedly part of the emerging adab (etiquette; *belles lettres*) culture, parallel and similar to the wealth of anecdotes and trivia that the literati sought and memorized about kings, princes, saints, and other historical figures. The difference between these anecdotes and narratives that formed adab culture and prophetics was that the mention of the prophet and the interest in his life was a sign of faith and was to be rewarded by God.[47]

The normativity of the prophet's behaviors and his recommendations reported through ḥadīths and transmitted through inherited communal behavior also formed part of the debates around the meaning and legal role of the sunna. Al-Shāfiʿī (d. 820) provided some of the more important arguments for the importance of sunna and of ḥadīths in legal reasoning. In both his *Al-Risālah* (Epistle), of which he wrote two different versions in first Iraq and then in Egypt, and *Jāmiʿ al-Umm* (The Comprehensive Exemplar), al-Shāfiʿī argued for a divine origin for the sunna and for the obligation of Muslims to follow the sunna. In *Al-Risālah*, relying on a number of verses from the Quran, al-Shāfiʿī argued that the sunna was one part of a bipartite revelation that explained how Muslims should conduct their lives in accordance with God's will. First, he expounded the notion that the sunna was what the Quran referred to as *ḥikma* (wisdom) and which was consistently coupled with the Quran in a number of verses. As such, al-Shāfiʿī awarded the words and deeds of the prophet with the sanctity of revelation expanding the scope of the revelatory message to include both the Quran and the Sunna.[48] Al-Shāfiʿī argued that this dual nature of revelation indicated that obeying the sunna is tantamount to obeying the Quran and that this obligation was not bestowed on anyone but Muḥammad, "[God] has paired the [knowledge of the sunna] with His book, and did not grant this to any of his creatures but to his prophet."[49]

Therefore, not only was following the sunna a divine obligation that was paired with obeying the Quran, but the sunna was also necessary for understanding the Quran. The sunna created an operative text out of the scripture.[50] Al-Shāfiʿī argued that the sunna was necessary to understand how particular rulings in the Quran should be applied and to understand the details of rulings that were mentioned only in general terms.[51] Moreover, the sunna was necessary to understand which of the rulings in the Quran was operative and which was abrogated (*mansūkh*). Although al-Shāfiʿī strongly believed that a Quranic verse could only be abrogated by another Quranic verse, he saw the sunna as the only means by which one could know which verse came before the other, and therefore, which abrogated which.[52] He used the example of different types of prayers that were mandated before the five daily prayers to explain that people could argue about which verses abrogated which and whether the later verses added requirements, rather than abrogating them:

> Therefore, it was necessary to find evidence in the sunna for one of these views. We therefore found that the prophet's sunna indicated that there are only five mandatory prayers. So we settled that the mandate is for the five prayers and that all other [mentioned] prayers were abrogated.[53]

With this and a few other examples, al-Shāfiʿī made the argument that the sunna was indeed necessary for understanding the Quran properly. Foremost, the ḥadīth and the sunna represented the key evidence for exegesis because the prophet was the one with the clearest understanding of the Quran. Moreover, the sunna demonstrated the intentions behind different verses and showed with the prophet's example the manner by which one should live in accordance with God's will. Here, al-Shāfiʿī was confronted with the fact that some *sunan* (pl. of sunna) mandated what was never mentioned in the Quran. He returned to the earlier pairing of the Book and the Wisdom:

> Part of what was revealed to [the prophet] was his sunna, which is the Wisdom that God mentioned [along with] the Book, which is the book of God, which was also revealed to [the prophet]. All that has come to him is part of God's blessings and in accordance with what God willed. These blessings that came to him are similar in their being all blessings [from God] and are different in relation to some issues.[54]

This view of ḥadīth that al-Shāfiʿī and others espoused was directly connected to a specific historical consciousness that highlighted the difference between the prophet's generation and the ones following him. This view elevated the legitimacy and normative power of prophetic traditions reported by single companions or through singular transmitters (*aḥādīth al-āḥād*) as well as partially undermined the legitimacy of shared communal practices. For al-Shāfiʿī, and in agreement with the emerging scholars of ḥadīth, these reports carried the same normative power at the legal level that communally transmitted (*mutawātir*) sunna had.[55]

Ḥadīth as adab

The discussion of Muḥammad's qualities, the details of his life, and his behaviors constituted an important topic in adab writings.[56] In sīra as early as the surviving fragments of Wahb Ibn Munabih's writings, stories about the prophet and about the early community shared in the narrativistic and literary framing of adab, and authors paid significant attention to entertainment as part of the goals of these writings alongside pietistic and political roles that these narratives were intended to play. In the same way, poetry was also a form in which the prophet's life and the history of the early community was told.[57] At another level, the evolution and flourishing of adab in the eighth and ninth centuries and beyond contributed to the formation of discourses of elite morality alongside the epistemic and professional formation that these writings offered. This is evident in some of the earliest writings in adab, such as those by Ibn Qutaybah or al-Jāḥiẓ, who highlighted how their books intended to educate scribes, scholars, and the learned elites in manners, histories, and other virtues that constituted the refined urban traditions of ninth- and tenth-century Baghdad. In this context, the term *adab* itself, as well as the verb *taʾaddab*, referred simultaneously to the practice of *belles lettres* as well as to the practice of acquiring good manners.[58] Not only did authors and books of adab reference their role in providing moral education, ḥadīth compilations also used the term *adab* to refer to certain sections in the compilations that focused on acquiring good manners and behaving appropriately in society.[59]

Tarif Khalidi and Stefan Sperl explained that ḥadīth materials also constituted part of the sources used in adab. In addition to providing sources for moral and pietistic narratives explored in adab, ḥadīth represented texts that survived from the oft-revered early periods of Arabic writings, allowing for utilizing these materials to explore different linguistic themes common in adab writings. The prophet himself was revered and praised for his eloquence by various adab authors, such as al-Jāḥiẓ.[60] Khalidi argued that, unlike adab authors, scholars of ḥadīth were rather concerned with questions of authenticity in the materials that they reported.[61] However, the interest in authenticity was limited to certain types of compilations which came to characterize what Jonathan Brown has called the *ṣaḥīḥ movement*.[62] Although this "movement" influenced compilers of ḥadīth and produced more heightened awareness around questions of authenticity, this did not in any way expunge the ḥadīth corpus from seemingly doubtful materials. In fact, such materials continued to circulate in various compilations. Moreover, more latitude could be observed in writings about manners and about miracles or other pietistic writings, as Brown notes, "Sunni ḥadīth critics and jurists of the third/ninth and fourth/tenth centuries advocated relaxing authenticity requirements for topics such as manners (adab, raqāʾiq) or exhortatory (targhīb) and dissuasive (tarhīb) homiletics."[63] In other words, although some ḥadīth compilations may have departed from the collecting impulse of adab authors, other compilations, particularly those concerned with manners, stories, and/or miracles (or in other words, materials closer in topic to the traditional topics of adab), continued to circulate a larger corpus of prophetic materials that paid less attention to questions of authenticity.

Of course, adab, as writings but also as a professional activity, figured rather prominently in the works of many ḥadīth scholars, not least of which is Ibn Qutaybah. Scholars like Ibn Khallād al-Rāmahurmuzī (d. 970), who was credited by later ḥadīth scholars such as al-Dhahabī with writing the first treatise dedicated to ḥadīth sciences,[64] had a rather illustrious career in adab. Although his reputation in later biographical dictionaries resided primarily on his renowned *al-Muḥaddith al-Fāṣil* (The Discerning Scholar), earlier biographers, such as his contemporary Ibn al-Nadīm (d. 990), presented him as a poet and a litterateur who was connected to the famous literary circles around the Buyid viziers, Ibn al-ʿAmīd (d. 970) and Yazīd ibn Muḥammad al-Muhallabī (d. 963).[65] Ibn Khallād wrote on table manners, on youth and old age, and on travels. Following in the footsteps of al-Jāḥiẓ, to whom he was likened in his style and erudition, he wrote compendia of anecdotes on lovers, of poetry and anecdotes about nostalgia to homeland, of funerary poetry, and of strange and funny anecdotes. He also wrote on the manners necessary to dealing with viziers – an insightful volume likely based on his own experience – and on the proper training of speakers. Along with these different books, Ibn Khallād wrote a treatise on Quranic sciences and another that was entitled "the two flowers (*al-rayḥānatayn*; lit. sweet basil); al-Ḥasan and al-Ḥusayn," which was likely a biography of Muḥammad's grandchildren.[66]

At the same time, combining careers in adab and ḥadīth did not come without tensions, which seemed to grow along with the gradual professionalization of ḥadīth. Ibn Khallād himself might have seen some tension between a career in adab and the pursuit of ḥadīth. In a chapter of his ḥadīth science compendium that discussed intentions (*al-niyyah*), he reported an anecdote involving the famous ḥadīth scholar, later known as *shaykh al-Islām*, Sufyān ibn ʿUyaynah (d. 814):

> Ḥafṣ ibn Māhān said, "We were once in the gathering (*majlis*) of Sufyān ibn ʿUyaynah when a man came up to him and asked, 'O Abā Muḥammad, [. . .] did you seek this knowledge [i.e. ḥadīth], when you did, for God's sake?' Sufyān looked away from him so the man asked him a second time. [Sufyān] looked away again so the man repeated his question [a third time]. So Sufyān said, 'By God no! We [first] sought [ḥadīth] for [the purpose of] literary refinement and entertainment (*taʾadduban wa taẓarrufan*). But God [turned the pursuit] to be only for His sake.'"[67]

Sufyān ibn ʿUyaynah did not seem to be the only one who entertained earthly motives connected to adab in his original pursuit of ḥadīth. A similar account is reported about Simāk ibn Ḥarb (d. 741), another reputable reporter of ḥadīth of a generation even earlier than Ibn ʿUyaynah.[68] Simāk was approached by some people who wanted to learn ḥadīth. When his students raised doubts about the seekers' dedication, Simāk said, "Speak well [of these people]. We [first] sought [ḥadīth] not for the sake of God. When I had learned it, it showed me what truly benefits me and protected me from what harms me."[69] Ibn Khallād cited yet another anecdote in the same vein – this time from Mujāhid ibn Jabr (d. 721), who said, "We have sought [ḥadīth] when we had little by way of good intentions. God purified [our] intentions after that."[70]

These three anecdotes involved people whose knowledge and dedication to ḥadīth were beyond doubt. All three were not only important authorities and remarkable reporters, but also acquired undeniable reputation for their piety and dedication. In this context, discussing their intentions becomes particularly important, as these men stood to be role models for young students and scholars of ḥadīth. The accounts followed a similar pattern and delivered similar messages. First, all three scholars had earthly motives for learning ḥadīth, mostly related to adab, as explained by Ibn ʿUyaynah. Not only were these scholars aware and honest about these earthly motives for learning ḥadīth, they also seemed to accept that earthly concerns may inspire some of their students as seen in Simāk's anecdote. In recounting these anecdotes while discussing intentions, Ibn Khallād may have shown that he, too, was accepting of these motives among his own students and readers.

Second, all three scholars reported a pietistic journey where God intervened, using ḥadīth itself, to purify their intentions and reinforce their dedication.[71] These pietistic journeys underscored a few significant points. On one hand, and despite their acceptance of people seeking ḥadīth for earthly reasons, the anecdotes insisted that the truly worthy endeavor was one dedicated to God alone and thus devoid of any earthly intentions. Among the many people who may seek ḥadīth for earthly reasons, only a select few would be endowed with the pure intentions that would allow them to achieve true knowledge and the well-earned repute that comes with it. In the same chapter, Sufyān ibn ʿUyaynah was also reported as saying, "I do not know of a more worthy endeavor than seeking knowledge and ḥadīth – for those whose intentions are pure."[72] On the other hand, this gift of pure intentions was portrayed to be a blessing from God to particular people. Simāk explained that this purification of intentions, which was a blessing, was rooted in the knowledge of ḥadīth itself. In this view, which Ibn ʿUyaynah expressed as well, the pietistic nature of learning ḥadīth was highlighted not only in terms of good intentions and dedication, but, more importantly, in terms of ḥadīth being itself a conduit to better faith and better intentions. Learning ḥadīth was, therefore, a form of spiritual exercise that made a person more faithful and more pious. However, this effect of ḥadīth was not available to all – it was only available to those who had pure intentions and piety underneath the façade of earthly desires.[73]

At another level, the source materials for both adab and ḥadīth compilations existed in a similar form: small, self-contained narratives capable of being repurposed in a variety of ways.[74] These small narratives provided authors and compilers with enormous power in structuring narratives based not on their own writings but on selecting, cataloguing, and curating other works.[75] Ḥadīth compilers continued to produce compilations with shortened chains of transmission or devoid of chains of transmissions altogether, further shortening the narrative unit and making it discursively more manageable. In the same vein, the genre of *aṭrāf al-ḥadīth* (ḥadīth signifiers), where scholars arranged ḥadīths using only the most significant part of their *matn* (text of the ḥadīth), utilized this heightened awareness of the existence of a core narrative in every ḥadīth to allow scholars to trace the isnāds of traditions based only on a tradition's core narrative. Moreover, the earlier *muṣannafāt* (compilations) of ḥadīth, which arranged traditions based on topics, closely mirrored the arrangement of adab encyclopedias. Khalidi noted that the division of Ibn Qutayba's *uyūn al-akhbār* (The Best of Anecdotes) paralleled the division of the *ṣaḥīḥ*s of al-Bukhārī and Muslim ibn al-Ḥajjaj, which in turn paralleled earlier muṣanafāt such as those of ʿAbd al-Razzāq al-Ṣanʿānī and Ibn Abī Shaybah, not to mention Mālik's *Muwaṭṭa*ʾ.

While developing as a specialized epistemic practice, *ḥadīth*, as a field of knowledge, continued to be part of the intellectual lives of Arabic-speaking and Muslim elites from the middle of the eighth century onward. Primarily, ḥadīth and anecdotes about Muḥammad and his companions represented part of a cultural heritage of Arabic linguistic arts that was being organized during this period.[76] It was also a major source for the history of early Islam, including Muḥammad's battles (maghāzī).[77] At these two levels, *ḥadīth* emerged as part and parcel of the adab tradition – preoccupied with similar concerns, studied, produced, and consumed by the same people. With al-Shāfiʿī's work, ḥadīth acquired even more importance in relation to law and as a source of legal precedence. Although this new function contributed significantly to the gradual professionalization of Muḥaddithīn and to ḥadīth occupying an increasingly important place in jurisprudence, it did not affect the life of ḥadīth outside of the law and in the learned culture of the period. Across its different iterations and its different functions, ḥadīth remained a pietistic literature by virtue of its connection to Muḥammad and his early companions. Interest in ḥadīth was always seen as a fine endeavor and a worthy study which helped one get closer to God and gain His favor. Ḥadīth acquired this devotional significance from its connection to Muḥammad and his companions. At the same time, it was the source through which the image of Muḥammad, his nature, and the role of his and his companions' legacy were discussed, understood, and formulated. Although Muḥammad was presented as the "beau ideal" for Muslims in the Quran, it was ḥadīth that gave substance to the pietistic endeavor of following and embodying Muḥammad's example.[78] The interest in ḥadīth was connected to the interest in Muḥammad and his early companions, and the manner by which ḥadīth was consumed corresponded to the manner by which Muḥammad's character, as a *beau ideal*, was understood and his legacy utilized by the believers.

Medical prophetics

The interest in Muḥammad's life and character (including his physical characteristics) appeared in "little narratives" that spread across different genres from ḥadīth compilations, to sīra, *shamāʾil* (prophet's characters), and *dalāʾil* (proofs of prophecy) and other *raqāʾiq* (exhortations) and adab volumes. These narratives, which can be referred to as prophetics, helped to paint detailed images of the prophet and inscribed practices of reverence and imitation. These narratives were just as rooted in the practice of adab as they were rooted in the pietistic love for the prophet.[79] In all the previously mentioned examples, such as the compendia of ʿAbd al-Razzāq al-Ṣanʿānī (d. 826), Ibn Shaybah (d. 845), Ibn Saʿd (d. 845), al-Bukhārī (d. 870), Muslim ibn al-Ḥajjāj (d. 875), and al-Tirmidhī (d. 892), in which prophetics became a subject of interest and occupied an increasing number of pages, health, disease, and medicine were also featured as part of the habits of the prophet. Embedded in some texts, inside discussions about his food and drink, or separated in independent chapters, these accounts intended to discuss how the prophet fell sick, what diseases affected him, and how he sought treatment or attempted to get better. Like other sections on the details of Muḥammad's life, these chapters and narratives were not primarily or solely interested in legal questions, but rather, they carried important pietistic and epistemic implications that conditioned the narratives of prophetics. At the same time, this literature on health and disease intersected with existing fields of knowledge, namely learned medicine, which was becoming increasingly part of the learned culture in Abbasid centers over the ninth century.[80]

To be sure, these narratives about the prophet's illnesses and his seeking medical care, or what we can describe as medical prophetics, were not professional medical writings. Whereas later writings on *prophetic medicine* (*al-ṭibb al-nabawī*), or the prophet's medicine (*ṭibb al-nabiyy*), were explicitly connected to medical literature, as will be explained later, medical prophetics were not.[81] Instead, medical prophetics were part of a body of literature that addressed the habits, customs, recommendations, and preferences of the prophet in all aspects of life, of which medicine was only a part. As such, these materials existed in the same field as traditions and anecdotes about the prophet's habits in eating and drinking and in the same vein as accounts on his animals, swords, or spears. Similar to writings in adab compendia and encyclopedia, these narratives also intersected with more specialized fields of knowledge, from knowledge about animals to weapons, among other things. However, they remained rooted in the prophetic corpus and in its epistemological and pietistic orientations. As will be seen later, the arrangement of traditions in medical prophetics collections and the editorial voice embedded in the selection and curation of these "little narratives" reflected the organizational priorities of ḥadīth scholars.

One of the earliest appearances of some traditions and accounts about medicine (or narratives of medical prophetics) can be seen in Abd al-Razzāq al-Ṣanʿānī's (d. 826) compendium, in a dedicated chapter entitled "Treatments that were prescribed [by the prophet and his companions]," which contained six traditions.[82] He also had a chapter on plague (ten traditions), on cupping *ḥijāmah* (six traditions), and a longer chapter on ruqya (incantations) and the evil eye (twenty traditions) – topics that were often included in medical prophetics. ʿAbd al-Razzāq also had a brief chapter on "treatment" in another treatise of his entitled, *Athār al-Ṣaḥābah* or "The Anecdotes of the Companions," which recounted anecdotes, often with legal or pietistic significance, from the history of major companions. However, the chapter included only one anecdote where dieting (*al-ḥimyah*) was recommended to ʿUmar I.[83] Although it is hard to determine with certainty whether ʿAbd al-Razzāq was indeed the first to be interested in questions of medicine, alongside other issues related to the prophet's habits and comportments, it is instructive to note that none of the earlier, better-known ḥadīth compilers included chapters on medicine in their work. This applies to the compilations (known as *athār*) of Abū Yūsuf Yaʿqūb ibn Ibrāhīm al-Anṣārī (d. 798),[84] Muḥammad ibn al-Ḥasan al-Shaybānī (d. 805),[85] and ʿAbd Allāh ibn Wahb al-Miṣrī (d. 813).[86] The notable exception is the collection *Al-Jāmiʿ* (The Comprehensive) of Muʿammir ibn Rāshid (d. 770), which included chapters on leprosy and contagion[87] and another on cautery,[88] both of which were areas discussed in subsequent compilations, as will be discussed later. Muʿammir's collection, however, was reported and compiled by his student, ʿAbd al-Razzāq al-Ṣanʿānī himself. It is difficult to ascertain whether the interest in medicine, even at this very limited level, went back to Ibn Rāshid or started with his student, ʿAbd al-Razzāq.

Moreover, the chapters on medicine contained a much higher number of *marfūʿ* traditions (traditions that go up to the prophet) than the overall collections or other chapters addressing legal matters. Although Harold Motzki found that there were very few traditions that went back to the prophet in the overall muṣannaf of ʿAbd al-Razzāq,[89] my analysis of the medical chapters revealed that 69% of these traditions went back to the prophet or reported directly about him (marfūʿ ḥadīths). This significant disparity in the ratio of marfūʿ traditions further emphasizes the distinct role that traditions played in these different chapters. Whereas chapters addressing legal questions looked to provide precedence, whether coming from the prophet himself or from companions and important followers, chapters addressing other issues related to the details of the prophet's life focused more on traditions that went back to the prophet himself. Even within the medical chapters, this phenomenon could be attested. For instance, the chapter on plague, which dealt primarily with legal questions, contained only 30% marfūʿ traditions. This ratio rises to 66% in the chapter addressing the medications that the prophet used and up to 80% in the chapter about cupping, which focused primarily on the prophet's preference for this procedure. The chapter on incantations and evil eye contained 85% marfūʿ traditions, most of which listed the specific prayers that the prophet himself used. The remaining *mawqūf* traditions (traditions that stop at one of the companions) were all connected to the legality or illegality of using these methods.

The interest in medicine in ʿAbd al-Razzāq's works was only the beginning as medical questions increasingly came to occupy the writings of ḥadīth and sīra scholars, who gradually included traditions without clear legal or historical significance. In his *Ṭabaqāt*, Ibn Saʿd (d. 845) dedicated a few chapters to discussing how the prophet was bled and how he considered bloodletting to be a very useful treatment.[90] Ibn Abī Shaybah (d. 845), whose muṣannaf was much lengthier than ʿAbd al-Razzāq's, dedicated far more space to these questions than his predecessors, in both his ḥadīth compendium and his book on adab. In the ḥadīth compendium, he dedicated an entire treatise to medicine entitled *Kitāb al-Ṭibb* or the treatise of medicine, which included close to forty chapters addressing various questions in great length.[91] In this treatise, Ibn Abī Shaybah gathered the disparate materials and topics found in various chapters in Ibn Rāshid's and al-Ṣanʿānī's compendia. In his adab volume, he focused instead on questions of contagion, plague, and leprosy, which seemed to fit better in his narrative surrounding public issues and questions.[92] Similar to ʿAbd al-Razzāq's compendium, Ibn Abī Shaybah's included a much higher ratio of marfūʿ traditions in the medicine treatise compared to the rest of his compendium. Scott Lucas has examined the legal chapters in Ibn Abī Shaybah's muṣannaf and found that only one in eleven traditions (9%) went back to the prophet.[93] In examining the chapters included in the book on medicine, the number of marfūʿ (elevated) traditions ranged from 40% to 60% depending on the topic of the chapter. In chapters discussing legal questions, such as two chapters addressing the legality of using amulets, most of the traditions tend to be mawqūf. In other chapters addressing more pietistic questions or focusing on details about the prophet's life, such as ones that addressed his illnesses, the number of marfūʿ traditions rose to 60% or more. This pattern mirrors the one observed in al-Ṣanʿānī's muṣannaf.

Medical prophetics occupied a consistent space in the following compendia of the ninth century. For instance, al-Bukhārī (d. 870) dedicated two treatises in his compendium to medicine and diseases. The first, *Kitāb al-Maraḍ* or the treatise of illness, discussed different illnesses and the prophet's behavior around sick people.[94] The second was dedicated to medicine and treatment and addressed most of the questions that Ibn Abī Shaybah had discussed before.[95] As al-Bukhārī was more selective, his compendium contained fewer traditions compared to Ibn Abī Shaybah's.[96] Moreover, in legal issues discussed later, al-Bukhārī often chose a particular legal stance and reported the traditions that supported it. This was contrary to Ibn Abī Shaybah, who reported traditions on both or all sides of any given legal question without ostensibly supporting any. Muslim ibn al-Ḥajjāj's (d. 875) compendium followed al-Bukhārī's example in discussing medicine more briefly than Ibn Abī Shaybah and in choosing specific positions in matters of legal importance. However, Muslim's discussion of medicine extended over twenty chapters within a treatise on safety (*Al-Salām*), which may have meant safety in person, possession, and body.[97] Ibn Sawra al-Tirmidhī (d. 892) also followed the same pattern with an entire treatise dedicated to medicine in his *Al-Jāmiʿ al-Kabīr* (The Comprehensive).[98] In his book *Al-Shamāʾil al-Muḥammadiyyah* (Muḥammadan Manners), he included a chapter on bloodletting, which acquired special importance as will be shown later.[99]

Although these authors and others following them showed interest in questions of medicine, this interest was not conditioned by the organization of medical knowledge. Instead, one finds different patterns of organization and classification that reflect the compiler's view on traditions and the overall vision of their volume. Al-Bukhārī and Muslim ibn al-Ḥajjāj paid more attention to legal questions and preferred to remove contradictory traditions. Ibn Abī Shaybah and al-Tirmidhī were more inclusive and included more diverse sets of traditions. For Ibn Saʿd, Ibn Abī Shaybah, and al-Tirmidhī, books that addressed Muḥammad's life, sīra, or behaviors and were more located in the tradition of adab or history had less space for medical questions than ḥadīth compilations. The latter seemed to operate under an encyclopedic impulse where authors collected as many traditions that fit their criteria as they could. Other books seemed to have a less inclusive purview and to focus on very specific questions – namely bloodletting.

For ḥadīth compilers, medicine included a number of practices that extended beyond learned medical knowledge and included magic, amulets, and other charms. This was not only because amulets and magic were part of existing treatment modalities.[100] It was also related to how these amulets were used to treat diseases. Moreover, the word *ṭibb* and the verb *ṭabb* in pre- and early Islamic Arabic referred both to medicine and magic. For instance, most authors reported a tradition about Muḥammad being a victim of magic. In this report, compilers used the verb *ṭabb*, to mean *to charm* or make someone the object of a magical spell. The linguistic connection and the larger meaning of *ṭibb* also explains why chapters on prognostication, astrology, and fortunetelling were placed among chapters on treatments and diseases, even when fortunetelling had nothing to do with health and disease. This wider definition further highlights how the authors of ḥadīth compilations were rooted in their own local categories, recalled from linguistic knowledge and from the early Islamic heritage. In all cases, authors relied on a similar set of traditions and anecdotes and operated under the same premise of what constituted relevant issues to their discussion of medicine and of health and disease. These traditions formed the infrastructure for medical prophetics. In the following pages, we will investigate some of these major themes that characterized writings on medical prophetics.

The central anecdotes

Different compendia tapped into a similar set of traditions and anecdotes which revolved around a few anecdotes that stood as central to the overall narratives of medical prophetics. These central anecdotes were consensual, in the sense that all compilers referred to and reported traditions about them and connected them to clear and definable moments in Muḥammad's life. Thus, they were found not only in ḥadīth compilations but also, importantly, in sīra and maghāzī literature. These central anecdotes were deeply important in defining the very meaning of health and disease in a manner that regulated and disciplined the entire literature of medical prophetics, particularly from a pietistic perspective. Four main anecdotes could be classified within this group of central narratives: Muḥammad's exposure to poison, Muḥammad's exposure to magic, his final illness, and, to a lesser extent, the injuries that he endured during the battle of Uḥud.

In all these anecdotes, the object of health and disease was the prophet's own body. The causes of the illness, the prophet's behavior as a sick man, the way he sought or did not seek cure or medical care, and the people who cared for him became parts of the prophetics tradition. Although other anecdotes in which the prophet described or recommended treatments and cures were also important and repeated in many places, these four anecdotes carried more weight, possibly because of the wealth of details they included and because of their more direct connection to the body and life of the prophet. The fact that the anecdotes were repeated in almost identical detail among these different Sunni compilations further added to their importance in the making of the medical prophetics archive. It is not unreasonable to suppose that the prophet's suffering in all of these incidents added to the pietistic emotions that believers were supposed to experience. These ranged from anger against his enemies to mourning for losing him in his last illness. In these cases, such emotions would also be governed and regulated by the same prophetic accounts that mandated and explained the proper emotions to feel and the correct manner to experience and express them.[101]

The first two anecdotes, the poisoning and the charming, were connected to Medinan Jews and the hypocrites *(al-Munāfiqīn)*, who were accused of attempting to poison and charm Muḥammad. Both groups were cast as the main enemies to Muḥammad's emerging polity in Medina.[102] Both anecdotes were important in the maghāzī lore as they were connected to Muḥammad's war against the Jews of Medina and Arabia. In the first anecdote, Muḥammad was presented with a luxurious meal cooked by a Jewish woman. Before eating, he was warned by God, through the Archangel Gabriel, that the food was poisoned. He summoned the woman, or her family, and demanded to know why they attempted to poison him. Far from denying responsibility, the woman explained that she thought, if he was indeed a prophet, God would save him and he would not be harmed. If he was a liar and a false prophet, he would die and they would be rid of him.[103] Although the anecdote fed into the anti-Jewish lore that emerged in maghāzī literature around the eighth century,[104] it also served to illustrate a miracle and a proof of the truthfulness of Muḥammad's claims. Protected as he was by God, his prophecy was further illustrated and proven by this divine intervention. Although the anecdote itself played little role in illustrating medical treatments or questions related to cures, it invariably served as an entryway to discussing poisons, including using poisons in preparing treatments. The importance of this anecdote is precisely in its being a moment in which the prophet encountered poison, even though the manner by which he survived would not be helpful for the Muslims reading these traditions.

The second anecdote is more significant because Muḥammad was indeed affected by a magical charm. In this case, Muḥammad suffered mightily from various mental (and in some accounts, physical) ailments that could not be cured:

> A man called Labīd ibn al-Aʿṣam, from the tribe of Banī Zurayq, worked magic on the prophet till the prophet started imagining that he had done things that he had not really done. One day or one night he was with me [ʿĀʾishā, Muḥammad's wife], he invoked God for a long period, and then said, "O ʿĀʾishā! Do you know that God has instructed me concerning the matter I have asked him about? Two men came to me; one of them sat near my head and the other near my feet. One of them said to the other, "What is this man's [Muḥammad] ailment?" The other replied, "He is under a spell (*maṭbūb*).' The first one asked, 'Who cast the spell on him?' The other replied, 'Labīd ibn al-Aʿṣam.' The first one asked, 'What did he use [to cast the spell]?' The other replied, 'A comb and the hairs stuck to it and the skin of pollen of a male date palm.' The first one asked, 'Where is [the cast]?' The other replied, 'in the well of Dharwān'" So the prophet went there with some of his companions. When he came back, he said, "O ʿĀʾisha, the color of [the well's] water is like the infusion of Henna leaves. The tops of the date-palm trees near it are like the heads of the devils." I asked. "O prophet of God, why did you not show it (to the people)?" He said, "Since God cured me, I disliked to let evil spread among the people." Then he ordered that the well be filled up with earth.[105]

Although here again the prophet was cured by divine intervention that revealed the place and nature of the cast, the anecdote served to lead the discussion on magic. It showed that magic was indeed real, and having affected the prophet, it could affect other people.[106]

Along with these anecdotes, the prophet's final sickness, which ended in his death, was an equally important account for these compilers. The prophet's final sickness served as a conduit for a number of important issues that the compilers aimed to address and, therefore, was repeated several times. The overarching theme that governed the different iterations about Muḥammad's final sickness was how severe and difficult it was and how he withstood such terrible pain. In some accounts, traditions showed that Muḥammad suffered more than any other person in his sickness, in part because suffering in sickness is a conduit to God's reward.[107] In other accounts, Muḥammad's wives and his companions used his own prayers and invocations to attempt and help him in his suffering.[108] In some of these accounts, especially the ones closer to the end of his life, he refused to receive treatment or relief even in the form of prayer as he prepared to depart this world.[109] The account was also a narrative site to include discussion of recipes, preferences for treatment, and ethical discussions related to visiting patients and praying for them. Although it is difficult to determine whether some of these accounts that narrated Muḥammad's sickness were indeed about his final sickness or about other bouts of ailment, the final sickness, its difficulty, and its implications for the community continued to loom large over these discussions of medical prophetics and to condition many of the topics addressed by the compilers.

Finally, Muḥammad's injury in the battle of Uḥud also figured in the majority of these compilations. The battle of Uḥud, which represented the first defeat that Muḥammad and his young polity endured and where he suffered from the most serious injuries in all of his military expeditions, persisted at the heart of many narratives in maghāzī and in ḥadīth. Similar to the battle of Badr, the names and roles of those who participated in this battle were important for establishing the precedence and authority of different companions.[110] In part because of this importance, and in part because of the severity of the injuries that Muḥammad endured during the battle, the account of the battle and his injuries were repeated in chapters related to medicine. In most cases, the anecdotes were means to discuss treatment of injuries, use of cautery for treating cuts and wounds, and whether women can medically treat men (because Muḥammad and others were nursed by women during the battle).[111] Ultimately, the prominent place that the battle of Uḥud occupied in the well-known maghāzī tradition helped lend it more importance in this neighboring literature of medical prophetics.

Along with these four main anecdotes, compilers discussed other questions through the use of multiple ḥadīths, many of which were repeated from one theme to the next, and most of which were conserved in the works of most, if not all, ḥadīth compilers. In general, the arrangement of these traditions helped to serve a number of central themes: illness and the pietistic attitude toward ailment and suffering, the habits and preferences of the prophet in relation to treatment, and a number of questions with legal significance.

Materia prophetica: the prophet's cures

Compilers were also interested in discussing specific cures and preparations that the prophet seemed to prefer or use frequently. Despite the wealth of prophetic traditions, relatively few cures and preparations were mentioned in the different compilations. The most famous and important among these cures was cupping (*ḥijāmah*), which was repeatedly and consistently discussed. For instance, Ibn Saʿd dedicated a chapter to discussing the prophet's cupping, showing that he paid the cupper and how the practice was legally permitted.[112] Similarly, Ibn Abī Shaybah reported traditions about the prophet's preference for cupping and how he thought it was the best cure to many diseases.[113]

In these various accounts, and in addition to narrating the prophetic practice, most compilers were interested in a number of specific questions. First, they focused on how the prophet favored the practice and thought highly of it. In one tradition, the prophet explained that, during his night journey to heaven early in his career, angels recommended cupping to him and told him to advise his people to use it to cure their ailments.[114] Second, and following the interest in the details of the prophet's actions and behaviors, they were interested in reporting how many times the prophet was cupped, how often, if he did so on specific days of the week, in which part of his body, and how much blood was cupped.[115] Third, other traditions were related to a number of questions with particular legal significance, namely whether one can be bloodlet while remaining ritually pure. This was discussed particularly in relation to the ritual purity during pilgrimage, where stricter rules of dress and purity applied (*iḥrām*). Compilers were interested in reporting that the prophet was bloodlet while in *iḥrām*.[116] Similarly, Ibn Saʿd and others explained that the prophet was cupped while fasting and while in the mosque, indicating the legality and permissibility of these behaviors.[117] Ibn Saʿd also explained that the prophet ordered the blood to be buried "so that it may not be found by a dog."[118] Most of these questions were motivated by the fact that blood was ritually impure, therefore raising a series of questions about how to best perform bloodletting.

Unlike the overwhelming preference for cupping, cautery seemed to elicit mixed responses. Compilers reported different traditions, some of which supported and others which rejected cautery.[119] A similar response could be found in relation to dieting. Al-Tirmidhī started his chapter on medicine with a tradition on dieting where the prophet orders his cousin ʿAlī to eat specific things and not eat others as part of his convalescence from a particular disease.[120] This tradition was not referenced by other compilers in this same context. Al-Tirmidhī also reported traditions that recommended soups and light feeding for patients[121] and others that warned against forcing patients to eat specific foods or drink particular drinks because God instructed the body to seek the foods that they need and that best suit them.[122]

Alongside these practices, specific materials played significant roles in the narratives reported by these compilers and seemed to occupy a particularly important space in the prophetics tradition. The most important materials were black seed, honey, palm dates, al-Qasṭ al-Hindī (costus), and snuffs. Muḥammad was reported to have favored both honey and black seed and to have thought very highly of them as cures for all diseases. The case for honey was further strengthened by the fact that it was mentioned in the Quran as being "a cure for all people" – a verse that was recalled by al-Bukhārī in the beginning of his short chapter on honey.[123] One of the main traditions reported about honey also addressed the question of efficacy:

> A man came to the prophet and told him, "My brother has diarrhea." The prophet said, "Give him honey." The man did and then came back and said, "O prophet of God, I gave him honey but it only increased his diarrhea." The

> prophet said, "Give him honey." The man did and then came back and said, "O prophet of God, I gave him honey but it only increased his diarrhea." The prophet said, "God has spoken the truth and your brother's belly has lied. Give him honey." The man did so and [his brother] was cured.[124]

This anecdote served to link the prophetic recommendation of honey to the divine promise of cure – something that could not be said except, perhaps, about cupping when taking the angels' recommendations in mind. The actual efficacy of honey, and whether or not it led to curing the ailing belly, was recast in terms of God's will and the faith in God's words. In the prophet's words, the immediate evidence of the honey's inefficacy was a 'lie' in that it contradicted the true order of the world that was revealed and promised by God. Ultimately, the belly responded and honey provided the cure that was promised.

In highlighting the significance of these particular practices and materials for the prophet, compilers were constructing a pietistic material space that was populated by Muḥammad's material preferences and his different habits. Cupping, both as a choice of treatment and as a preventive measure, would occupy a central place in this pietistic space. Although this did not mean that Muslims were obligated to use cupping or were even necessarily rewarded for doing so, the procedure acquired an aura by being linked to Muḥammad and his practice, placing it within the narratives of *imitatio muhammadi*.[125] This aura was perhaps more pronounced when it came to honey, dates, and black seed, all of which were regular food stuffs and components of recipes. Emulating the prophet in consuming these food stuffs was easier and more accessible to daily practice. Moreover, this growing pietistic material space also regulated the emotions and feelings that faithful Muslims could and should harbor towards particular practices and food items. Rejecting cupping, honey, black seed, or other similar items, or doubting the overall efficacy of these treatments (though not necessarily their specific efficacy in treating particular conditions) would constitute a rebuke to the practice of the prophet.[126] Whether or not one was able to follow the prophet's practice, admiring this practice and believing in its divine nature were signs of proper faith.

In addition to these specific procedures and materials, compilers explained in detail some of the prophet's other behaviors in relation to health and sickness. These included his various prayers, the Quranic verses he often recited, the type of ruqya (incantation) that he used or recommended, and his use of the *maʿudhatayn*, which are two chapters in the Quran that were believed to expel the evil eye.[127] Even more so than the material objects and medical procedures, these prayers and specific sayings served to better delineate the prophetic behavior in relation to health and disease. Although these prayers and readings represented the prophet's response to illness, there is no indication that they were the sole response or that the compilers of these traditions intended them to be viewed as such. Instead, they existed alongside traditions about cupping, cautery, snuffs, and other medical techniques. Specifically, these prayers and chosen verses created a pietistic textual environment that conditioned the manner by which a person could get sick, as will be shown later. This space surrounded and contained all other medical practices and procedures and contributed to the making of the pietistic manners of health and illness.

Legal questions

Although the interest in legal questions was not equal in all compendia, all compilers paid attention to a number of questions that may have animated important legal debates around health and disease. Almost all compilers commenced their chapters or treatises on medicine with a discussion of the legality and the legitimacy of seeking cure and of practicing medicine. This was particularly important as it laid the ground for the entire chapter and legitimized the discussion and the practice of medicine. Accepting God's will and the place of illness in discussions about fate were also important, in part, because of their connection to medical knowledge and to the role of medicine in society, and also, because of contemporary debates on fate and on God's role in inflicting harm. Compilers largely agreed that seeking medicine was permissible, that this did not constitute a violation or a rejection of God's will, and that treatment as well as learning about medications and about medicine was part of God's will and His design. In other traditions, the prophet was shown to advise people to benefit one another and help one another in curing illnesses.[128]

There were a few practices which seemed to have been a subject of debate that these compilers intended to intervene in. The first of these is *al-ruqya*, which refers to specific readings and incantations that could be recited to prevent illness or to treat it. Here, scholars were interested in first, discussing whether it was legal or not; second, how it should be performed; and third, how the legal ruqya could be differentiated from other illegal behaviors. Both Ibn Abī Shaybah and al-Tirmidhī included traditions that showed the legality of *al-ruqya*, whereas others rejected its legality or at least considered it to be largely undesirable.[129] On the other hand, Al-Bukhārī and Muslim ibn al-Ḥajjāj seemed convinced of the legality of *al-ruqya* and its role in prophetic practice as they included only traditions that proved its legality.[130] Regardless of their differing positions, all compilers seemed to agree on a few traditions that indicated the proper way for *al-ruqya* and that focused mainly on using Quranic verses in *al-ruqya* and not any other incantations. For all of them, differentiating this practice from other non-Muslim incantations and charms was a crucial condition of its legality, regardless of how convinced they seemed of the practice's overall legality.

They also focused on the use of *al-ruqya* for specific conditions and the actual texts that were used to address these specific conditions. Central among these conditions was scorpion and snakebites, which had particular ruqyas that the prophet consistently used.[131] Similarly, *al-ruqya* was linked to the evil eye, and specific ruqya traditions were reported to avert the evil eye.[132] In discussing the evil eye, compilers included a few traditions that indicated that the evil eye indeed existed and that the prophet had accepted the effects of the evil eye. The tradition most frequently cited compared the evil eye to fate, "The prophet said, 'If there were a thing that preceded (interrupted) fate, it would be the evil eye.'"[133] This concern with the reality of the evil eye and with its relation to fate reflected anxieties around views, beliefs, and practices that were inherited from the pre-Islamic period. Compilers used a number of traditions where new Muslims explained to the prophet their pre-Islamic habits and practices and asked for his opinion. Compilers were also keen on showing that accepting fees for performing *al-ruqya* was legal and was sanctioned by the prophet.[134] They also discussed the practice of breathing in the hands or spitting in them after performing *al-ruqya* in a manner that would put the words in the hands that would rub the affected body. Here, compilers reported various traditions supporting and prohibiting the practice. Finally, and as explained before, the chapters on *al-ruqya* ended with discussions about the habits and the manners that the prophet followed in performing *al-ruqya*. Such details included the actual texts and verses that he used and the fact that he used his hand to rub the place of pain. When the prophet himself was sick, his wife read his ruqya but used his own hand to rub his body, as his was more blessed than hers.[135]

Magic and prognostication were areas which all compilers agreed were outlawed and were contrary to the tenets of monotheism. Many traditions were reported to indicate that consulting with fortunetellers, trusting them, or paying them would amount to abandoning faith.[136] Similarly, compilers were adamant in rejecting amulets, with most of them rejecting even those that had verses from the Quran written in them.[137] Using the Quran as a cure was discussed, albeit not in a dedicated fashion. Rather, it was discussed and accepted as part of *al-ruqya* and rejected in relation to amulets by most compilers. Ibn Abī Shaybah discussed a practice in which written verses would be put in water and then the water consumed by the sick person, bringing traditions that supported and rejected this practice into his text.[138] Compilers were largely in agreement that using wine to treat diseases was unlawful and largely not useful.[139] Although most compilers did not allow for treatment with poisons, their rationale seemed to be related to the risk of killing oneself, because they all reported traditions prohibiting suicide in discussing treatment using poisonous materials.[140] It appears that they believed that using poison for treatment was similar to suicide in that the individual consumed poison knowingly and willingly. The desire for death clearly mattered as discussed before; however, treading too close to such lethal materials was seen to be unlawful or at least unbecoming of a true believer. Along with these questions, compilers discussed a number of other legal questions that ranged from cupping while fasting to using camel urine, milk, and asses' milk for treatment. The legal issues related to these materials (blood, urine, and asses' milk) likely stemmed from these materials being otherwise a source of ritual impurity.[141]

Compilers were generally interested in collecting every mention of illness in the prophetic corpus that met their compilation criteria. Although many of these mentions were secondary to a given tradition and were largely cursory, they were important in serving the encyclopedic purpose of these compilations. Ultimately, their aim was not only to collect what seemed important for a specific purpose, but also to collect the traditions that they saw as fitting within the theme that they addressed – namely, health and disease.

Conclusion

The interest in sīra and sunna was not only legal or even just pietistic. Instead, it emerged as part of the adab culture that flourished in the late Umayyad period and under the Abbasids.[142] As authors of adab continued to collect anecdotes and exhibit their linguistic abilities in focusing on early and pre-Islamic textual heritage, anecdotes around the prophet's life and the lives of his companions were part of this emerging corpus of adab epistemology.[143] Such epistemology was conditioned by the appreciation of the linguistic heritage of early and pre-Islamic Arabia (or al-Jāhiliyyah period).[144] This adab epistemology was encyclopedic in nature, in the sense that it aimed to provide access to extensive frameworks of knowledge without necessarily developing depth in any one of them.[145] The work of these authors of adab allowed for the making of what can be called an 'adab archive,' where a certain number of historical figures (such as famous pre-Islamic poets and 'funny men'), particular anecdotes, and specific themes and topics were repeated consistently in various writings, regulating the adab landscape.

Ḥadīth and sīra anecdotes were perfect specimens for this archive. They were inherently worthy because of their authors and subjects (the prophet and his companions); they descended from a period of linguistic excellence and could serve, alongside pre-Islamic poetry and the Quran, as evidence for linguistic authenticity; and, they were "little narratives," which could be moved and curated in a variety of ways. The self-contained aspect of each anecdote or ḥadīth and their connection to various aspects of the reader's daily life made them useful for recalling and deploying in accordance with the performative and oral nature of adab. The fact that they were dispersed among reporters spread in the empire's different regions emphasized the ability of the collectors and their commitment to the ideals of searching for knowledge.[146] Of course, the fact that these anecdotes and ḥadīths contained instructions for proper manners spoke to one of the immediate purposes of the adab culture – the refinement of morals and behaviors. As seen before, many famous scholars of ḥadīth seemed to have started their careers and their engagement with prophetic traditions from this adab vantage point. Many continued to write on adab even as they emerged as bona fide Muḥaddithīn.[147]

Take the example of Ibn Abī Shaybah. He was one of the earliest authors of ḥadīth compendia. He composed a *musnad* as well as one of the earlier muṣannafāt. Ibn Abī Shaybah wrote a treatise on adab which included ḥadīths and prophetic accounts but was also arranged to suit the needs of adab authors and readers. For Ibn Abī Shaybah and other scholars and authors of ḥadīth, both ḥadīth and adab existed on a continuum and were deeply connected. Although the pietistic nature of ḥadīth could not be overemphasized and helped to set it apart from other adab materials, the epistemic and intellectual impulses that motivated adab authors were very similar to those that motivated and preoccupied ḥadīth scholars. More importantly, the scholars composing texts in these two genres were often the same people.

The arrangement of ḥadīth along adab epistemic priorities and the rise in importance of ḥadīth and the sunna in the making of law and in formulating the Muslim pietistic discourses contributed to the making of Muḥammad's new persona as a living example, or a *beau ideal*. There was growing interest not only in the major events of his life or in ḥadīths that explained important legal points, but also in the details of his daily behavior – what he ate, how he ate and drank, how he had sex, how he spoke or slept, etc. One of the earliest examples of this interest can be seen in Ibn Saʿd's *Ṭabaqāt* where he dedicated chapters to explain such details in the life of the prophet. This continued in ḥadīth compilations as well as in sīra volumes for the coming two centuries and beyond. I propose the term prophetics (nabawiyyāt) to describe this subgenre of literature that was increasingly more preoccupied with anything and everything related to Muḥammad.

The materials for this subgenre were and continued to be found in chapters of different ḥadīth compilations, sīra, and maghāzī. They also emerged in specific volumes dedicated simply to these details of the prophet's life, such as Muḥammad ibn Ḥabīb al-Hāshimī's (d. 859) *Ummahāt al-Nabiyy* (The prophet's mothers), Ḥammād ibn Isḥāq Al-Azdī's (d. 880) *Tarikat al-Nabiyy* (The prophet's heritage), al-Tirmidhī's (d. 892) *Al-Shamāʾil al-Muḥammadiyyah* (The Muḥammadan manners), Ibn Abī ʿĀṣim's (d. 900) *Al-Ṣalāt ʿalā al-Nabiyy* (Praying for the prophet), Muḥammad ibn Hārūn ibn Shuʿayb al-Anṣārī's (d. 946) *Ṣifat al-Nabiyy* (Describing the prophet), and al-Isfahānī's (d. 979) *Akhlāq al-Nabiyy* (The prophet's manners), among others. Ultimately, these books satisfied this emerging thirst for knowledge about Muḥammad as they constructed the character of the prophet.

Within these volumes and in the major ḥadīth compilation, one can see the proliferation of medical prophetics. These were chapters that addressed Muḥammad's health and the diseases he endured and his various recommendations and personal preferences in relation to health and disease. Similar to other prophetics writings, these medical prophetics had some anecdotes with legal significance, but most anecdotes carried only the pietistic import of the prophetics narratives. They were obviously connected to medical knowledge and professional medical practice, but only marginally, as their main priorities were dictated by the priorities of knowledge about the prophet and not by the priorities of medical knowledge. For instance, there was no discussion of medical theory, of the composition of the body, or of origins of diseases. There was also no reference to any sophisticated or complex recipes and little desire to engage in discussions about health preservation. Instead, authors constructed their narratives around specific anecdotes that were central in thinking about the prophet's health and disease and highlighted only a few materials and procedures that Muḥammad preferred. They were interested in a number of legal questions, but this interest stemmed from the legal and prophetic tradition and not necessarily from the concerns or demands of the medical profession.

Medical prophetics conditioned a pietistic landscape where pious Muslims were to exercise and perform their sickness and respond to the sickness of their fellow Muslims. Specific procedures carried a prophetic aura that made them particularly favorable, although not mandated. Certain food stuffs and preparations acquired value and continued to survive in the center of this pietistic space of health and illness. Muslims were asked to embody a particular attitude toward sickness that involved patience, endurance, a belief in the blessing that is embedded in the most difficult episodes of sickness, and a resignation to the will of God – all while knowing that treatment and seeking cure is also part of the will of God. I do not wish to argue that all Muslims, regardless of their views and the times and conditions they lived in, followed these recommendations or even inhabited this performative space – even as dissidents. There is no evidence to support such an assumption, and there is hardly any reason to believe that these writings had any oversized influence on the lives of Muslims. Instead, I argue that the emergence of this particular genre and this new archive (or subarchive) of medical prophetics created a pietistic space that was inhabited by some, especially committed and pious Muslims, and that it became part of the overall performance of piety, along with other public acts such as prayer and charities. In all these cases, prophetics played a role in drawing this type of behavior and in conditioning the meaning of public piety. Equally pertinent to the book's overall story, medical prophetics provided the matter of origin for the emergence of prophetic medicine *tout court*. Although this chapter analyzed only a few ḥadīth compilations, these compilations and the medical chapters within contributed to the construction of an archive of medical prophetics that underwrote later writings on the topic and helped delineate the priorities of related discussions of medicine, health, and disease, which will be explored in the coming chapters.

Notes

1 See, for instance, Michael Cooperson, "Ibn Ḥanbal and Bishr al-Ḥāfī," 79.
2 On the process of the canonization of these ḥadīth compilations, see Brown, *The Canonization of al-Bukhārī and Muslim* and Brown, "Canonization of Ibn Mājah." It is worth noting that the earliest commentaries on al-Bukhārī's *Ṣaḥīḥ* were authored by Abū Sulaymān al-Khaṭṭābī (d. 988), who also wrote a commentary on Abū Dāwūd's compendium, followed by Ibn Baṭṭāl (d. 1058). On al-Khaṭṭābī's commentary, see Tokatly, "A'lām al-Ḥadīth of al-Khattābī."
3 Brown, "Critical Rigor vs. Juridical Pragmatism," 9.
4 Abbott, "Hadith Literature – II," 294–5.
5 See Görke, Motzki, and Schoeler, "First Century Sources for the Life of Muḥammad?" See also Hinds, "'Maghazi' and 'Sira.'"
6 The meaning and limits of the sunna developed and changed throughout the eighth and ninth centuries as it came slowly to be restricted to the prophet's sayings and deeds (Duderija, "Evolution in the Canonical Sunni Ḥadīth," 393–4). On the various types of sunna and its connection to the deeds and sayings of the prophet, see Duderija, "Understanding the Concept of Sunnah." On the pietistic role of the sunna and in the making of Muslim identity, see Shoemaker, *The Death of a Prophet*. At the legal level, see, for instance, Picken, "Sunna in the Early Shāfi'ī Madhhab." See also Schacht, *The Origins of Muhammadan Jurisprudence*.
7 Jones, "Chronology of the Maghāzī;" Hinds, "'Maghazi' and 'sira.'"
8 Sizgorich, "Community in Islamic Late Antiquity," 21–2.
9 Cited in Jones, "Maghazi Literature," 344.
10 On the role of history in making claims to authority, see Graham, "Traditionalism in Islam." See also Mottahedeh, *Loyalty and Leadership in an Early Islamic Society*.
11 Afsaruddin, *Excellence and Precedence*.

12 On Alid-Umayyad polemics, see Alajmi and Keshk, "Umayyad Ideology." Along with the first three caliphs, and particularly ʿUthmān, number of less known figures from Muḥammad's life were mobilized in these political debates, see Urban, "Identity Crisis of Abū Bakra."

13 Al-Zuhrī, *Al-Maghāzī al-Nabawīyah*, 46. See Powers, *Zayd*.

14 Al-Zuhrī, *Al-Maghāzī al-Nabawīyah*, 78. This is quite different from how the same account was presented by al-Wāqidī (d. 822), writing under the Abbasids, who emphasized Abū Sufyān's glorification of the Meccan deities and continued the anecdote to include sacrifices that Abū Sufyān made in Mecca in gratitude for defeating Muḥammad. Al-Zuhrī was respected by many contemporary ḥadīth scholars (see Abbott, 295–6). However, his closeness to and association with the Umayyad court motivated some suspicion and criticisms from contemporary and later ḥadīth scholars, Kister, "The Sirah Literature," 365.

15 Juynboll, *Muslim Tradition*. Juynboll highlighted the efforts made by early compilers to rehabilitate the image of Abū Hurayra, who was the subject of much criticism. In the same vein, Lucas argued that the evolving notion of *adālat al-ṣaḥāba* (or the integrity of the companions) emerged in the ninth century to deal with the problems emerging from reports of conflicts between them, Lucas, *Constructive Critics, Ḥadīth Literature, and the Articulation of Sunnī Islam*, 221–5. Dickinson argued that the doctrine of ʿadālat al-ṣaḥābah was consolidated in the work of Abū Ḥātim al-Rāzī and that it was one of the ways that ḥadīth scholars resorted to solve problems with the inconsistency of some chains of transmission, Dickinson, *The Development of Early Sunnite Ḥadīth Criticism*. See also Osman's analysis of the construction of the concept of ʿadālat al-ṣaḥāba, particularly in the works of al-Baghdādī and al-Juwaynī, Osman, "ʿAdālat al-ṣaḥāba." Also, Khalek investigated the development of this concept (ʿadālat al-ṣaḥābah) and traced its gradual dominance through the fourteenth and fifteenth centuries, Khalek, "Medieval Biographical Literature," 280–81. On the question of the ṣaḥāba among Shiites, see Kohlberg, *The Attitude of the Imami-Shiʿis to the Companions of the Prophet*; "Some Zaydi Views;" Amir-Moezzi, "Seul l'homme."

16 Ibn Ḥanbal, *Kitāb al-Aunnah*, 208–10.

17 Ibn Saʿd, *Al-Ṭabaqāt al-Kubrā*.

18 Khalek relied on Ibn ʿAbd al-Barr and Ibn Ḥajar in her discussion of the ṣaḥāba, Khalek, 287–8.

19 Ibn Qutaybah, *Kitāb al-Maʿārif*, 153. See discussion of ʿUthmān's absence in ʿUthmān's biography, 193.

20 Ibid., 153–4.

21 Kister, "The Sirah Literature," 362–3.

22 Ibn Qutaybah, *Taʾwīl Mukhtalaf al-Ḥadīth*. Ibn Qutaybah's method, which was similar to other scholars of ḥadīth, was mocked by al-Jāḥiz among others who argued for testing these traditions against the Quran. See Brown, "Matn Criticism," 166.

23 Al-Wāqidī's (d. 822) *maghāzī* probably appeared in writing at the same time as that of Ibn Isḥāq edited by Ibn Hishām. Based on simple chronology, al-Wāqidī has been accused of copying Ibn Isḥāq without referring to him. Jones investigated these accusations and argued that both authors likely relied on similar heritage of story-telling *qaṣaṣ* materials. See Jones, "Ibn Isḥāq and al-Wāqidī."

24 Al-Dhahabī, *Siyar Aʿlām al-Nubalāʾ*, 7:34–45. Al-Dhahabī reported a few anecdotes to indicate that Ibn Shahāb al-Zuhrī respected Ibn Isḥāq, allowed him in his company without permission (7:37), and considered him the remaining repository of knowledge about the battles of the prophet in Medina (7:37). Al-Shāfiʿī was also reported to consider Ibn Isḥāq the most knowledgeable person about maghāzī (7:37).

25 Jones, 347. Al-Dhahabī summarized the overall opinions about Ibn Isḥāq, "[He was] an elevated figure to a certain degree especially in sira. However, in ḥadīths of

legal significance (*aḥādīth al-aḥkām*), his ḥadīths drop from the degree of 'correct (*al-ṣiḥah*)' to the degree of 'good (*al-ḥusn*)'." He attributed this in part to Ibn Isḥāq's alleged alid sympathies. However, al-Dhahabī admitted that Mālik's opinions of Ibn Isḥāq influenced how he was viewed by later scholars, al-Dhahabī, 7:40–2.

26 While the genre under the name "asbāb al-nuzūl" did not appear as such until the writings of al-Wāḥidī (d. 1075), Andrew Rippin has convincingly argued that the materials as well as the desire to include the occasions and times of the revelation within the exegetical literature could be traced as far back 'Ikrimah's (d. 723) and al-Ḥasan al-Baṣrī's (d. 728) books under the same title *Nuzūl al-Qurān (the Revelation of the Quran)* and 'Alī ibn al-Madīnī's (d. 848) *Kitāb al-Tanzīl (Book of Revelation)*. See Rippin, " 'Asbāb al-nuzūl,' " 2–3. In this framework, the works of al-Zuhrī, Ibn Isḥāq, and Ibn Hishām coincided with and contributed to the growing interest in these materials to varying degrees.

27 See Makdisi, " 'Ṭabaqāt'-biography." Ibn Sa'd was not a stranger to the maghāzī literature. In fact, he was a known student and companion of al-Wāqidī to the extent that he was nicknamed *kātib al-Wāqidī (al-Wāqidī's Scribe)*. The differences between his and his master's and contemporaries' work, which are discussed later, are therefore a function of the evolution of this literature and not one of rupture or separation.

28 Khalek, 272–3.

29 Ibn Sa'd, 2: 278; 2: 282.

30 These anecdotes were mentioned in a more detailed biography of Ibn 'Abbās, which was part of an annex to the *Ṭabaqāt* dedicated to the companions who were young when the prophet passed. *Al-Mutamim li-Tabaqāt ibn Sa'd*, 127.

31 Ibn Sa'd, 1: 273.

32 See Annemarie Schimmel, *And Muhammad Is His Messenger*.

33 See Melchert, "Piety of the Hadith Folk." Melchert argued that *ḥadīth folk* presented a model of ascetic pietism that contrasted with the mystical piety of Sufis or popular preachers. Regardless, both models of piety drew from the image of the prophet and relied on his precedence to create their own pietistic paradigms.

34 Many scholars from Mālik ibn Anas to Aḥmad ibn Ḥanbal expressed the pietistic dimensions to knowing about the prophet and to transmitting this knowledge to others. See Duderija, "Evolution in the Canonical Sunni Ḥadīth," 412; Abbott, 290.

35 Sperl, "Man's "Hollow Core," 461.

36 Ibn Qutaybah, *Ta'wīl Mukhtalaf al-Ḥadīth*, 58.

37 Apart from Ibn Sa'd's sections, to my knowledge, al-Tirmidhī was the first to compose a dedicated volume on the characteristics of the prophet *shamā'il*, which will evolve into a genre, as will be seen later. Annemarie Schimmel also argued that al-Tirmidhī was the first to compose a work of this type, Schimmel, 32–33.

38 In Al-Dhahabī's view, citing multiple earlier ḥadīth scholars, al-Tirmidhī summarized all his legal opinions in his *jāmi'*, which, by al-Dhahabī's time, had become one of the Sunni canonical ḥadīth collections. Al-Dhahabī explained that, save for 2 out of 3,956, all traditions collected by al-Tirmidhī had legal import. See al-Dhahabī, 13: 275–6.

39 Schimmel, 32.

40 Al-Ṭabarī, *Tārikh al-Rusul wa al-Mulūk*, 2: 277–8.

41 On the physical signs of prophecy on Muḥammad's body, see Kister, " 'And He Was Born Circumcised.' "

42 Al-Ṭabarī, 2: 279.

43 Ibn Ḥibbān, *Al-Sīrah al-Nabawiyyah wa Akhbār al-Khulafā'*, 59–60.

44 Burge, "Reading Between the Lines," 184–5. Schimmel cites a famous passage from al-Ghazālī's *Iḥyā'ī*, "Know that the key to happiness is to follow the sunna and to imitate the Messenger of God in all his coming and going, his movements and rest, in his way of eating, his attitude, his sleep and his talk. I do not mean this in regard to religious observance, for there is no reason to neglect the traditions which were concerned

with this aspect. I rather mean all the problems of custom and usage, for only by following them unrestricted succession is possible" (Schimmel, 31). She argues, "But it was through this imitation of Muhammad's actions as transmitted through the ḥadīth that Islamic life assumed a unique uniformity in social behavior, a fact that has always impressed visitors to all parts of the Muslim world." (718–19). Although this attitude toward the prophet survives in a variety of ways, Schimmel's claim obfuscates how this deep interest in the minutiae of the prophet's life meant as well that their understanding, the reasoning behind them, and how they were to be followed changed significantly over time. Although Muḥammad remained a central discursive character, he was remodeled and refashioned by Muslims and Muslim life to the same degree that his words were meant to model and fashion Muslim life.

45 Al-Bukhārī, 1: 12. The same ḥadīth was also reported by Muslim ibn al-Ḥajjāj in a chapter entitled, "The Obligation to Love the Prophet." Loving the prophet was invariably understood by commentators to include obeying his orders and recommendations and following his ideal.

46 Al-Bukhārī included a tradition about loving *al-anṣār* being a sign of faith, "Loving al-Anṣār is the sign of faith, and hating al-Anṣār is the sign of hypocrisy [in belief]" (1:12). Muslim had a similar chapter as well. Ibn Ḥanbal discussed loving the companions and loving the Arabs in his *Sunna.*

47 Jones explained how the works of Ibn Isḥāq and al-Wāqidī relied on the traditions of *Qaṣṣ* (or story telling) in their sīra narratives. Such a connection was obviously at the heart of how sīra, maghazi, and ḥadīth were part of the overall adab literary traditions, as is explained later in the chapter. See Jones, "Ibn Isḥāq and al-Wāqidī."

48 Al-Shāfiʿī, *Al-Risālah*, 78. In his Jāmiʿ, al-Shāfiʿī argued for interpreting "wisdom" as referring to the sunna of the prophet by insisting that the two, "book" and "wisdom," referred to two different entities, and in response to the argument that "wisdom" might refer to the detailing of the book of God. Musa examined Quranic commentaries in this period and concluded that, apart from the commentary of ʿAbd al-Razzāq al-Ṣanʿānī (himself a scholar and compiler of ḥadīth), no other commentators used this interpretation (Musa, "Al-Shāfiʿī," 176). See also Musa, *Ḥadīth as Scripture*.

49 Al-Shāfiʿī, 97. Musa makes the same observations through analyzing Jāmiʿ al-ʿilm. See Musa, "Al-Shāfiʿī," 175.

50 Duderija used the term "Quranico-Sunnahic hermeneutic" to refer to the emerging authority of sunna in interpreting the Quran and understanding the legal and pietistic obligations that it creates. He argued that, with the work of al-Shāfiʿī, this method came to be more strictly connected to ḥadīth, Duderija, "Evolution in the Canonical Sunni Ḥadīth," 411.

51 Al-Shāfiʿī's argument was in part based on the reasoning behind *asbāb al-nuzūl* (occasions of revelation). See Rippin. "Asbāb al-Nuzūl." On tafsir, see Rippin, *The Qur'an and Its Interpretative Tradition.*

52 Al-Shāfiʿī, 106–9.

53 Ibid., 115. In choosing the example of prayers, al-Shāfiʿī avoided arguments about authenticity of ḥadīth or reliability of the sunna, as he chose what would be known as a *mutawātir* tradition – or tradition reported from multiple routes that avoids the possibility of falsification. Although the term and category would be consolidated in the following decades, the authenticity of a practice like the nature of prayer was seen as undoubtedly part of the sunna, therefore perfectly meeting al-Shāfiʿī's purpose. On debates about authenticity, see Hallaq, "Authenticity of Prophetic Ḥadîth" and Brown, "Did the Prophet Say It or Not?" On the uses of the sunna and prophetic traditions in interpreting the Quran in the late ninth century, see Brunelle, "From Text to Law."

54 Al-Shāfiʿī, 103.

55 El-Shamsy, *The Canonization of Islamic Law*, 49–50. Ahmad Khan argues that this view on the difference between the prophet's generation/century and the centuries

that followed reformulated the concept of 'testimony' (*shahādah*) and emphasized the importance of chains of transmission as the proof of the authenticity of specific practices, Ahmad Khan, " 'The People of My Generation Are Best.' " On the development of legal thought after al-Shāfiʿī, see Temel, "The Missing Link."

56 Burge, 185.
57 Kister, "The Sirah Literature," 356–8.
58 Sperl, "Man's 'Hollow Core,'" 463.
59 See, for instance, Muslim ibn al-Ḥajjāj, *Ṣaḥīḥ Muslim*.
60 Sperl, "Man's 'Hollow Core,'" 465.
61 Khalidi, *Arabic Historical Thought in the Classical Period*, 130.
62 Brown, "Critical Rigor vs. Juridical Pragmatism."
63 Brown, "Even If It's Not True It's True," 7.
64 Al-Dhahabī, 16: 74.
65 See some of the biographies of al-Rāmhurmuzī in al-Kutubī's *ʿUyūn al-Akhbār*, 12: 147; Ibn al-Nadīm's *Fihrist*, 1: 155; and Yāqūt's *Muʿjam al-Udabāʾ*, 9: 5–17.
66 Al-Nadim, *Al-Fihrist*, 1: 155.
67 Al-Rāmhurmuzī, *Al-Muḥaddith al-Fāṣil Bayna al-Rāwī wa al-Wāʿī*, 183.
68 Al-Dhahabī, 5: 245–9.
69 Al-Rāmhurmuzī, 182.
70 Ibid., 183.
71 On *niyyah* (intention), see Powers, "Interiors, Intentions, and the 'Spirituality' of Islamic Ritual Practice." The centrality of *niyyah* and interior in Islamic rituals and pronouncements of faith played an important role in the formulation of discourses around *taqiyya* (or hiding true faith for fear of persecution) in various contexts. See Bernabé-Pons, "Taqiyya, Niyya;" O'Banion, "They Will Know Our Hearts;" Kohlberg, "Some Imāmī-Shīʿī Views on Taqiyya."
72 Al-Rāmhurmuzī, 182.
73 On piety and ḥadīth, see Melchert, "Piety of the Ḥadīth Folk."
74 Sperl, "Man's 'Hollow Core,'" 464.
75 Burge, "Myth, Meaning and the Order of Words."
76 The importance of linguistic heritage from pre-Islamic and early Islamic Arabia rose during the early Abbasid period and became central to linguistic discussion. See Webb, "Creating Arab Origins;" Zakharia, "Imruʾ al-Qays;" Drory, "The Abbasid Construction of the Jahiliyya."
77 Robinson, "History and Heilsgeschichte."
78 Khalidi, *Images of Muhammad*.
79 Ibid.
80 See Rahman, *Health and Medicine in the Islamic Tradition*. Galenic medicine was not the only medical practice in ninth-and tenth-century caliphal centers. Evidence suggest that Indian and Persian physicians played an equally important role in creating an "Islamicate" medical tradition, Shefer-Mossensohn and Hershkovitz, "Early Muslim Medicine and the Indian Context."
81 Perho argued that narratives around the prophet's health and illness, or what will become later "prophetic medicine," acquired clear medical orientation after the work of ʿAbd al-Laṭīf al-Baghdādī (d. 1231) and Ibn Ṭarkhān (d. 1320), who were both trained as physicians and who wrote on prophetic medicine, Perho, *The Prophet's Medicine*, 56–7.
82 Al-Ṣanʿānī, 11: 151–3. On ʿAbd al-Razzāq al-Ṣanʿānī's *Muṣannaf*, see Motzki, "The Muṣannaf of ʿAbd al-Razzāq al-Ṣanʿānī."
83 Al-Ṣanʿānī, *Al-Amālī fī Āthār al-Saḥābah*, 101.
84 Al-Anṣārī, *Kitāb al-Āthār*.
85 Al-Shaybānī, *Kitāb al-Āthār*.
86 Al-Miṣrī, *Al-Kitāb al-Jāmiʿ*.
87 Ibn Rāshid, *Al-Jāmiʿ*, 404–6.

88 Ibid., 407.
89 Motzki, "The Muṣannaf of ʿAbd al-Razzāq al-Ṣanʿānī," 21.
90 Ibn Saʿd, *Al-Tabaqāt al-Kubrā*, 1: 342–7.
91 Ibn Abī Shaybah, *Al-Kitāb al-Muṣannaf fī al-Aḥādīth wa al-Āthār*, 5: 31–66.
92 Ibn Abī Shaybah, *Kitāb al-Adab*, 207–14.
93 Lucas, "Where Are the Legal Ḥadīth?" Lucas used the term "prophetic traditions" to refer to the traditions that reached back to the prophet. It is unclear whether this includes traditions about the prophet's deeds, which medieval scholars classified as *marfūʿ*, or not. In either case, a cursory examination of the *muṣannaf* shows that Lucas's calculations stand roughly at the same number in either case.
94 Al-Bukhārī, 7: 114–21.
95 Ibid., 7: 122–39.
96 Al-Bukhārī used rather restrictive selection criteria to classify the traditions in his compendium as "authentic *ṣaḥīḥ*." He also used *marfūʿ* traditions almost exclusively. These restrictive selection criteria caused a rather rough reception of his compendium by his contemporaries before it acquired the authority and reverence it enjoys among Sunni Muslims today. See Brown, *The Canonization of al-Bukhārī and Muslim*.
97 Muslim Ibn Al-Ḥajjāj, *Ṣaḥīḥ Muslim*. Kitāb al-Salām extends from 4: 1703–62. The chapters on medicine spread over 20 chapters from 4: 1718–52.
98 Al-Tirmidhī, *Al-Jāmiʿ al-Kabīr*, 3: 449–83.
99 Al-Tirmidhī, *Al-Shamā'il al-Muḥammadīyah wa al-Khaṣā'il al-Muṣṭafawwīyah*, 299–304.
100 On charms and amulets in learned Galenic medicine, see Olsan, "Charms and Prayers."
101 Compilations of ḥadīth, among others, contributed to the making of a landscape of emotions to be felt *fi allāh* (lit. *in God; for the sake of God*) that regulated how everyday emotions could be deployed pietistically. Chief among these emotions was the love of the prophet, as is later discussed in this chapter. Invariably, these emotions were experienced by the prophet himself in specific manners. They included love, anger, and sadness for reasons related to specific pietistic reasons. See, for instance, al-Bukhārī's chapter on "*al-ḥubb fī allāh*" (Love for God), al-Bukhārī, *Saḥīḥ*, 8:14.
102 Jews continued to represent a central enemy of Muḥammad in most writings about the prophet. See, for instance, Rose, "Muhammad, the Jews and the Constitution of Medina" and Arjomand, "The Constitution of Medina." Later narratives blamed Jews for altering or attempting to falsify reports about the prophet or about previous prophets, in what came to be known as *isrāʾiliyāt*. Tottoli has traced the use of *isrāʾiliyyāt* as a pejorative term used to describe fantastical stories to the early tenth century in the writings of al-Masʿūdī (d. 956). Tottoli, "Origin and Use of the Term Isrāʾīliyyāt." See also, McAuliffe and Diyari, "Assessing the Isra'iliyyat."
103 Al-Bukhārī, *Ṣaḥīḥ*, 7: 139; Ibn Abī Shaybah, *Al-Kitāb al-Muṣannaf fī al-Aḥādīth wa al-Āthār*, 5: 41; Muslim ibn al-Ḥajjāj, *Ṣaḥīḥ Muslim*, 4: 1721.
104 See, for instance, Faizer, "Muhammad and the Medinan Jews."
105 Al-Bukhārī, *Ṣaḥīḥ*, 7: 137; Ibn Abī Shaybah, *Al-Kitāb al-Muṣannaf fī al-Aḥādīth wa al-Āthār*, 5: 41; Muslim ibn al-Ḥajjāj, *Ṣaḥīḥ Muslim*, 4: 1719; Ibn Mājah, *Sunan Ibn Mājah*, 2: 1173.
106 Al-Bukhārī's chapter that included this tradition was entitled "On Magic" (Al-Bukhārī, *Ṣaḥīḥ*, 7: 136) and was followed by other chapters discussing magic and its treatment. Ibn Abī Shaybah included the accounts on magic and poison in the same section (Ibn Abī Shaybah, *Al-Kitāb al-Muṣannaf fī al-Aḥādīth wa al-Āthār*, 5: 41) and was followed by chapters on magic as well. Both Muslim ibn al-Ḥajjāj and Ibn Mājah entitled their chapters, "On Magic."
107 Al-Tirmidhī, *Al-Jāmiʿ al-Kabīr*, 3: 483; Al-Bukhārī, *Ṣaḥīḥ*, 7: 115.
108 For instance, Muslim ibn al-Ḥajjāj, *Ṣaḥīḥ Muslim*, 4: 1721; Ibn Abī Shaybah, *Al-Kitāb al-Muṣannaf fī al-Aḥādīth wa al-Āthār*, 5: 46; al-Bukhārī, *Ṣaḥīḥ*, 7: 134.

109 Muslim ibn al-Ḥajjāj, *Ṣaḥīḥ Muslim*, 4: 1721; Ibn Abī Shaybah, *Al-Kitāb al-Muṣannaf fī al-Aḥādīth wa al-Āthār*, 5:46.
110 On the battle of Badr, see Victor Bauhng, "Early Sīra Material and the Battle of Badr."
111 Ibn Mājah, *Sunan*, 2: 1147; Al-Bukhārī, *Ṣaḥīḥ*, 7: 122.
112 Ibn Sa'd, *Al-Ṭabaqāt al-Kubrā*, 1: 342.
113 Ibn Abī Shaybah, *Al-Kitāb al-Muṣannaf fī al-Aḥādīth wa al-Āthār*, 5: 33.
114 Al-Tirmidhī, *Al-Jāmi' al-Kabīr*, 3: 390.
115 Ibn Mājah, *Sunan*, 2: 1152.
116 Ibn Abī Shaybah, *Al-Kitāb al-Muṣannaf fī al-Aḥādīth wa al-Āthār*, 5: 39; Al-Bukhārī, *Ṣaḥīḥ*, 7: 125.
117 Ibn Sa'd, *Al-Ṭabaqāt al-Kubrā*, 1: 342.
118 Ibid., 1: 346.
119 For instance, Ibn Mājah reported three traditions rejecting (and even outlawing) cautery. He then reported three traditions, where the prophet accepted or applied cautery himself, Ibn Mājah, *Sunan*, 2: 1154–55. The same can be seen in al-Tirmidhī, al-Tirmidhī, *Al-Jāmi' al-Kabīr*, 3: 388–90.
120 Al-Tirmidhī, *Al-Jāmi' al-Kabīr*, 3: 381
121 Ibid., 3: 383.
122 Ibid., 3: 384.
123 Al-Bukhārī, *Ṣaḥīḥ*, 7: 123.
124 Al-Tirmidhī, *Al-Jāmi' al-Kabīr*, 3: 409.
125 Schimmel, 31.
126 Schimmel, 44–45.
127 Al-Bukhārī, *Ṣaḥīḥ*, 7: 132; Ibn Mājah, *Sunan*, 2: 1163; Al-Tirmidhī, *Al-Jāmi' al-Kabīr*, 3: 463.
128 In her history of prophetic medicine, Perho argues that there were two contradictory positions articulated by jurists and "ascetics": one that rejected treatment and considered it to be antithetical to *tawakkul* and another that accepted treatment. She observes that Aḥmad ibn Ḥanbal accepted both positions and explains the latter's position as directed to ascetics, on one hand, and regular believers, on the other, Perho, *The Prophet's Medicine*, 65–7.
129 Al-Tirmidhī, *Al-Jāmi' al-Kabīr*, 3: 393; Ibn Abī Shaybah, *Al-Kitāb al-Muṣannaf fī al-Aḥādīth wa al-Āthār*, 5: 42, 46, 49.
130 Al-Bukhārī, *Ṣaḥīḥ*, 7: 131–2; Muslim ibn al-Ḥajjāj, *Ṣaḥīḥ Muslim*, 4: 1721.
131 Al-Bukhārī, *Ṣaḥīḥ*, 7: 132.
132 Al-Tirmidhī, *Al-Jāmi' al-Kabīr*, 3: 395; Al-Bukhārī, *Ṣaḥīḥ*, 7: 132; Muslim ibn al-Ḥajjāj, *Ṣaḥīḥ Muslim*, 4: 1724.
133 Al-Tirmidhī, *Al-Jāmi' al-Kabīr*, 3: 397.
134 Ibn Abī Shaybah, *Al-Kitāb al-Muṣannaf fī al-Aḥādīth wa al-Āthār*, 5: 48.
135 Ibid., 5: 46.
136 Muslim ibn al-Ḥajjāj, *Ṣaḥīḥ Muslim*, 4: 1748; al-Bukhārī, *Ṣaḥīḥ*, 7: 135.
137 Ibn Mājah, *Sunan*, 2: 1166; Al-Tirmidhī, *Al-Jāmi' al-Kabīr*, 3: 471.
138 Ibn Abī Shaybah, *Al-Kitāb al-Muṣannaf fī al-Aḥādīth wa al-Āthār*, 5: 39.
139 Al-Tirmidhī, *Al-Jāmi' al-Kabīr*, 3: 456; Ibn Abī Shaybah reported a tradition where 'Ā'isha exhorted God not to heal anyone who used wine for treatment. He also reported that Ibn 'Umar, who was a known authority among Sunnis, disliked that animals be treated with wine, even if applied to their anuses, Ibn Abī Shaybah, *Al-Kitāb al-Muṣannaf fī al-Aḥādīth wa al-Āthār*, 5: 38–9.
140 Al-Bukhārī, *Ṣaḥīḥ*, 7: 139.
141 On camel urine, see Ibn Mājah, *Sunan*, 2: 1158. On asses' milk, see al-Bukhārī, *Ṣaḥīḥ*, 7: 140.
142 Khalidi, *Images of Muhammad*.

143 Sperl, "Man's 'Hollow Core.'"
144 Drory, "The Abbasid Construction of the Jahiliyya."
145 See Bosworth, "A Pioneer Arabic Encyclopedia of the Sciences;" Biesterfeldt, "Medieval Arabic Encyclopedias of Science and Philosophy;" Kilpatrick, "A Genre in Classical Arabic Literature;" Orfali, "Arabic Poetry up to the Fall of Baghdad."
146 Traveling to seek ḥadīth or *al-riḥlah fī ṭalab al-ʿilm* came to be a central part of the professionalization of ḥadīth scholars and was eventually shortened as *riḥlah* as it became a fixture in the biographies of ḥadīth scholars. See Duderija, "Evolution in the Canonical Sunni Ḥadīth," 405; Raisuddin, "Baqī b. Makhlad al-Qurṭubī," 264.
147 See, for instance, Ibn Abī Shaybah, *Kitāb al-Adab*. Within major ḥadīth *muṣannafāt*, the term adab was used to refer to the refinement of morals and to how one was supposed to deal with others. This emphasis on the original meaning of the term does not negate its operative use as a genre of intellectual activity, but emphasized how ḥadīth was instrumental in achieving these goals of such intellectual and linguistic activity.

2 From medical prophetics to prophetic medicine

As seen in the first chapter, the ninth century witnessed an increasing interest in the character of Muḥammad as a *beau ideal* or a model for divinely ordained behavior. Such interest was premised on a form of epistemic piety, whereby knowing about the prophet and an interest in his life was in itself a pietistic act. Studying ḥadīth, which was sometimes connected to the evolving and growing writings on adab, was premised in part on this particular form of piety. Aside from the importance of ḥadīth at the legal level, knowledge about the prophet was significant in itself. This pietistic impulse and the concurrent interest in the character of the prophet and the details of his life manifested across various genres constituting a body of literature which I have termed prophetics. This literature focused on the prophet's body, his habits, and various behaviors, many of which had little, if any, legal significance. Books on *shamā'il* (characters) of the prophet and those on *dalā'il* (proofs or signs) of prophecy, along with various chapters in different ḥadīth compilations, contributed to constructing a prophetics archive that included materials addressing various aspects of the prophet's life. As part of this growing prophetics literature, medical prophetics represented a subgenre that paid attention to questions of medical relevance – including the prophet's diseases, his injuries, and his medical recommendations, among other related issues. Similar to other prophetics writings, medical prophetics existed across various genres of writings from ḥadīth compilations to writings on adab, shamā'il, dalā'il, and others.

One of the main characteristics of medical prophetics was that it did not actually concern medicine. Emerging as a part of prophetics materials and couched within ḥadīth and sīra literature, medical prophetics operated under the same logic and within the same cosmology as other writings on prophetics. The emphasis of medical prophetics was not on medicine but rather on knowledge about the prophet, and the genre's internal logic and organization vividly represented this cosmology. This literature paid little attention to the composition of the body, the reasons behind diseases, or the manners of treating different diseases. Instead, it focused on the illnesses suffered by Muḥammad or by his companions and diligently followed the events of their lives. Although this literature intersected with medicine, the intersection was circumstantial. Its focus and logic of organization were linked to the life and habits of the prophet and companions.

Contemporary to this literature of medical prophetics, another dependent genre emerged to resemble what would be termed *prophetic medicine* (*al-ṭibb al-nabawī* or *ṭibb al-nabiyy*) in the twelfth and thirteenth centuries. In these volumes of prophetic medicine, the emphasis on the prophet, imams, and/or companions remained central. Their habits were diligently reported and their recommendations carefully recorded. However, the logic of organization and the cosmology that governed these texts was not coming from the lives of the prophet, imams, and/or companions but rather from medical literature. These texts were attentive to medical theories and descriptions of the composition of bodies. They actively engaged in conversations, whether in person or in the pages, with medical authorities and citing medical scholars whose names started to appear more frequently in the genre. The discussion of diseases, treatments, and manners of health preservation did not follow what was important in the prophet's and companions' lives; instead, it followed what was deemed medically more significant or perhaps more urgent from the viewpoint of readers interested in health and disease.

Many of the anecdotes and narratives that figured in the medical chapters of ḥadīth compendia continued to figure prominently in these volumes of prophetic medicine. Similarly, many of the central legal questions that scholars discussed in ḥadīth compilations were also discussed in these volumes. The central difference between these genres resided in two main areas: the organizational schema and epistemic priorities, which now came to be more aligned with medical knowledge; and the clear and pronounced self-awareness of the difference between these books and other ḥadīth or legal compendia often composed by the same authors. In both cases, medicine came to play a more central role. At the organizational and epistemic levels, these new writings of prophetic medicine followed the manner of organization of medical texts. Authors professed that their intention was indeed to follow such organization and to emulate the structures adopted by people of medicine while also filling this framework with a mixture of medical and prophetic materials.

The new organizational scheme posed distinct challenges. First and foremost, authors contended with new interests that did not map exactly onto the interests and priorities of the prophetic corpus. They needed to expand the prophetics archive to address new questions and to explain issues that were not addressed before. Second, they needed to engage with some potential contradictions between the medical and prophetic corpus that emerged as they engaged with various new issues related to medicine. At another level, this renewed engagement with medicine had significant effects on the production of pietistic discourses around health and disease. On one hand, the expansion of the prophetics archive to address new questions related to medicine provided even more texture and details to the pietistic narratives constructed around the prophet's character. On the other hand, having more freedom to deal with questions other than the prophet's illnesses and his own recipes, these texts came to engage with the production of a pious healthy body that represented the priorities of the learned elites in the ninth and tenth centuries. At another level, writing at the intersection of medical and religious knowledge allowed for the development of a certain form of piety that was conditioned on the care for a Galenic body. By this, I mean that these texts contributed to consolidating the Galenic understanding of the body and connected this understanding to the prophetic and Imami archive. As such, they allowed for renewed attention to caring for the body and for developing a new medicalized mode for attending to one's health that were also engulfed in a pietistic narrative.

In this chapter, I will trace the historical development of these new writings. First, I will start with the work of Ibn Ḥabīb al-Qurṭubī (d. 853), who was an important legal and ḥadīth scholar from al-Andalus and who composed perhaps the first text of this type. I will look at how his text was received and how it affected discussions around medicine and the prophetic literature. Then, I will move to the work of the two Twelver Shiite scholars Abū ʿAtab ʿAbd Allāh and al-Ḥusayn, the sons of Bisṭām ibn Sābūr (both fl. ca. 800) who produced one of the earliest texts on medicine in the Twelver Imami tradition. Following the development of this literature into the tenth and eleventh centuries, I will turn to the influential texts by Ibn al-Sunnī (d. 1003) and Abū Nuʿaym al-Isfahānī (d. 1038), whose texts on prophetic medicine constituted central moments in the development of the genre in the Sunnī context. Finally, in examining the Twelver Shiite text the *Golden Treatise*, which was attributed to Imām ʿAlī al-Riḍā but likely produced in the eleventh century, I will investigate the making of a pious healthy body. Throughout, this chapter investigates the production of the newly expanded archive of *prophetic medicine* that would continue to inform pietistic discussions about health and illness in the coming centuries.

Writing on the margins of ḥadīth

Perhaps the earliest volume that can be classified as "prophetic medicine" was composed by the Andalusian scholar ʿAbd al-Malik ibn Ḥabīb al-Qurṭubī (d. 853) and was entitled *Al-Mukhtasar fī al-Ṭibb* (The concise [treatise] in medicine). *Al-Mukhtaṣar* relied in its arrangement on the interests of medical sciences. The book contained a significant number of ḥadīths and paid special attention to the treatments preferred by the prophet. The book, however, read as a summary in medicine, not necessarily for physicians, but mainly for educated scholars and jurists who were interested in (and perhaps knowledgeable about) the subject. Ibn Ḥabīb was described by some of his biographers as a scholar, litterateur, and physician, among many other descriptions. However, Ibn Ḥabīb did not figure in the biographical dictionary of physicians composed by his compatriot, Ibn Juljul al-Qurtubī (d. 994).[1] The descriptive (of Ibn Ḥabīb as a physician [*ṭabīb*]) may indicate his knowledge or training in medicine and his evident interest in the topic. Because of his wide-ranging activities and interests and his large oeuvre, Ibn Ḥabīb was labeled the scholar of al-Andalus (*ʿālim al-Andalus*).

Ibn Ḥabīb's major contributions and his significance come from his works on ḥadīth and law. His summary and commentary on al-Muwaṭṭāʾ, known as *al-Wāḍiḥah*, was cited frequently and represented an important moment in the consolidation of the Malikī madhhab in al-Andalus.[2] Ibn Ḥabīb was one of the earliest scholars who introduced ḥadīth and ḥadīth sciences to al-Andalus, along with Muʿāwiyah ibn Ṣāliḥ al-Dimashqī (d. 774) and Ṣaʿṣaʿa ibn Sallām (d. before 817). Maribel Fierro has shown that no transmissions from Ṣaʿṣaʿa have survived either in al-Andalus or in the East. Muʿawiyah ibn Ṣāliḥ, on the other hand, was a well-known scholar of ḥadīth and respected by major ḥadīth authorities in the East. However, Fierro argued, his legacy in al-Andalus seemed to have been all but forgotten and was only recalled when Andalusi scholars were asked about his writings by their Eastern masters.[3] Ibn Ḥabīb, whose legacy in al-Andalus was more firmly established, went on a journey (riḥla) to learn ḥadīth in the East, mainly Egypt, Levant, and Medina but not Iraq, and studied with some of the more important scholars of ḥadīth at the time. His later works contained transmissions from Eastern luminaries like Wahb ibn Munabih, al-Wāqidī, al-Layth ibn Saʿd, and Asad ibn Musā.

However, later scholars, including Ibn Ḥabīb's own students, seemed skeptical of Ibn Ḥabīb's ḥadīth learning and accused him of faulty and unreliable transmissions. For instance, Ibn al-Faradī (d. 1012) reported an account in which Ibrāhīm ibn al-Mundhir al-Khuzāmī (d. 851) said to some of his students about Ibn Ḥabīb, "Your Andalusian friend, 'Abd al-Mālik ibn Ḥabīb, came to me with a sack full of books and said, 'This is your knowledge. Do you license me (tujīz) in it?' so I said, 'Yes!' And he never read with me a letter, nor have you read with him."[4] A similar incident took place with an equally important scholar of ḥadīth, Asad ibn Mūsā (d. 827). While in Egypt, Ibn Ḥabīb was staying with a scholar called Ibn Abī Maryam, who was a student of Asad's. Ibn Abī Maryam said:

> When he was in Egypt, Ibn Ḥabib stayed with us. I have never seen a man more interested in books. One day, it was very hot. I walked in [the house] and saw Ibn Ḥabīb wearing a cloak and intently studying [one of Asad's] books. I told him, "What is this! A cloak in this weather?!" He said, "It is our [customary] formal attire." I told him, "And what is this book! When were you [permitted] to read it?" Ibn Ḥabīb said, "The man [Asad ibn Mūsā] permitted me to study it." So I went to Asad and told him, "O shaykh! You refuse to allow us to read in your books and permit people other than us [your students]?!" Asad said, "But I do not believe in reading [from books]! How would I permit it?!" So I told him [about Ibn Ḥabīb]. He said, "He [Ibn Ḥabīb] just took my book to copy from it. It is not on me [meaning, I did not license him]".[5]

Ibn al-Farḍī also transmitted the opinion of other ḥadīth scholars about Ibn Ḥabīb, "ʿAbd al-Malik ibn Ḥabīb did not have knowledge of ḥadīth, and did not know which [ḥadīth] is correct (*ṣaḥīḥ*) and which is problematic (*saqīm*). It was said about him that he was lax in his judgment and reported most of his traditions relying on collective reporting [ʿalā sabīl al-ijāzah]."[6]

Despite these concerns about his ḥadīth training, Ibn Ḥabīb broke new ground in al-Andalus, where most of his contemporaries had little interest or knowledge in the discipline. His work, whether in ḥadīth, Maliki jurisprudence, or other topics, relied on ḥadīth and followed the patterns and intellectual habits of the ḥadīth scholars and litterateurs (*udabāʾ*) of the East. For instance, he wrote a book on "strange ḥadīth" (*gharīb al-ḥadīth*), another on the merits of companions, and another on the generations of companions and later companions. These books, and others showed his interest in many of the questions that scholars of ḥadīth were interested in. At the same time, and also similar to many of his contemporaries in the East, he wrote on a number of adab topics using ḥadīth as his main material. He wrote on "the battles of Islam," "[reports and anecdotes about] the two [Holy] Mosques," "the signs of the end of times," and "the adab of women." He also wrote about "proper manners," "piety," and "the description of paradise." Along with these, he also wrote a history of al-Andalus, in which he relied on the writings of Ibn ʿAbd al-Ḥakam. Similar to his work on ḥadīth, his work on history was equally criticized by largely the same scholars and for the same reasons mentioned earlier.[7]

In this view, his treatise "A Concise [Treatise] on Medicine" should be seen as part of his wide-ranging interests and in following some of the interests of Eastern scholars. Contributing to the emerging prophetics literature, which was growing in popularity in the East as explained before, Ibn Ḥabīb wrote about medicine, the manners of the prophet, and the prophet's battles. Although his book on medicine was one of the earliest on the topic, it resided at the margins of contemporary literature on prophetics. Ibn Ḥabīb did not follow the schematics used by his Eastern contemporaries like al-Ṣanʿānī (d. 826) or Ibn Abī Shaybah (d. 850). His choices of ḥadīths were also different from what was becoming a generally agreed upon corpus of medical prophetic traditions spreading across various compilations. Instead, he followed a narrative that is closer to the concerns of readers interested in and familiar with medicine and that catered to their questions and priorities.

Ibn Ḥabīb's *Al-Mukhtaṣar* is made up of two distinct parts. The first is concerned with legal questions related to medicine and is generally built around a number of ḥadīths, both *marfūʿ* (reaching back to the prophet) or *mawqūf* (ending with companions), that address legal and jurisprudential questions. Although the traditions mentioned there are arranged in a manner distinct from other books of ḥadīth from this period, as will be discussed later, the first part maintains a commitment to prophetic materials as its central backbone, with elaborations and explanations from different companions. Throughout, Ibn Ḥabīb's commitment to Malikism is evident. Mālik and a number of his students were cited often and quoted on the various legal questions related to the practice of medicine. Ibn Ḥabīb also followed Mālik's method by paying special attention to the works of many companions and to their different habits and traditions.[8] Often, Ibn Ḥabīb referred to the practice of the people of Medina as an indication of the law, or at least of specific preferred pietistic practices. For instance, in discussing the use of kohl, Ibn Ḥabīb referred to what specific materials for treating the eyes of the companions and later followers preferred.[9] He expressed a similar pattern in relation to enemas, which Ibn Ḥabīb considered to be 'hated' or not preferred based on the preference of many companions and scholars.[10] In addition to Mālik, Ibn Ḥabīb cited a number of figures who were commonly cited by other Mālikī scholars. These included Muḥammad ibn al-Munkadar (d. ca. 650)[11]; Ḥabīb ibn

Salamah (d. 662),[12] who was particularly favored by Levantine scholars but not by Iraqis; Khabbāb ibn al-Arat (d. 657); Al-Miqdād ibn al-Aswad (d. 653)[13]; Wahab ibn Munabbah (d. 732)[14]; and Makḥūl al-Shāmī (d. 718)[15] along with al-Ḥārith ibn Kaladah. Ibn Ḥabīb also cited the practice of a number of Umayyad caliphs, including Al-Walīd ibn ʿAbd al-Malik,[16] and Hishām ibn ʿAbd al-Malik[17] as well as Umar II, who was cited rather frequently. To make the book easier to read, Ibn Ḥabīb removed the chains of transmission (*isnād*) from the traditions that he reported, explaining, "This is a summary with clipped chains of transmissions [so that] it would be easier to uptake by the reader."[18] The second part of *Al-Mukhtaṣar*, on the other hand, takes a different approach and focuses primarily on medicine and medical practice. Starting with discussions of humors and complexions, it proceeds to provide information about foods and materia medica and then moves to address important medical questions that have little legal or pietistic significance. Not only is the second part deeply dependent on medical writings and largely devoted to medical knowledge, it is also almost entirely devoid of traditions and of mentions of the companions.

The selections that Ibn Ḥabīb included in his work were rather different from those found in other contemporary ḥadīth compilations like those of ʿAbd al-Razzāq al-Ṣanʿānī, Ibn Abī Shaybah, or al-Bukhārī, among others. Moreover, there is little evidence that Ibn Ḥabīb's work on medicine had a significant impact on other authors writing about the same topic – namely medical prophetics or prophetic medicine – whether in the East or the West. For instance, later authors like Ibn al-Sunnī (d. 1003) and Abū Nuʿaym al-Isfahānī (d. 1038), who wrote books also arranged in a way similar to Ibn Ḥabīb's, did not refer to Ibn Ḥabīb at all. Ibn Ḥabīb's *Al-Mukhtaṣar* did not fare much better in al-Andalus either. For instance, Ibn ʿAbd Rabbih (d. 940) included a chapter on medicine in his text, *al-ʿAqd al-Farīd*. In that chapter, he relied heavily on prophetic materials, which he drew from Ibn Abī Shaybah's *Musnad*. Ibn ʿAbd Rabbih followed Ibn Abī Shaybah's schema and arrangement, circulating the same canon of medical prophetics that was dominant in the East without reference to Ibn Ḥabīb.[19]

Law and prophetics in Ibn Ḥabīb's work

The first part of Ibn Ḥabīb's treatise was written with a clear emphasis on legal considerations. Although this section relied on prophetic materials and addressed a number of concerns that medical chapters in ḥadīth compilations addressed, the organization that Ibn Ḥabīb chose was rather different from these writings. Writing from the legal perspective and aiming at using the prophetic heritage to build a legal corpus around medicine, Ibn Ḥabīb privileged the priorities of medical practice itself, paying attention to the potential legal concerns that medical practitioners and patients encountered. The known and central stories in Muḥammad's life, which were central in the chapters of medical prophetics, took a backseat to illustrating and differentiating the legal and the illegal. In the same way, Ibn Ḥabīb avoided much of the contradictory materials that were included by some ḥadīth scholars, such as Ibn Abī Shaybah. Instead, he curated materials that provided evidence for specific positions and particular views that he believed were more valid.

In the beginning, Ibn Ḥabīb commenced with a discussion of the legality of medical practice and of the prophet's recommendation to consult physicians and to follow their recommendations. As explained before, commencing with this discussion was consistent with other writings on medicine, as it connected medicine to the prophetic corpus and ensured its place in the socioepistemic hierarchy. While keeping to this same narrative structure, Ibn Ḥabīb explored additional points of legal significance exceeding the mere placement of medicine within the pietistic or religious corpus. At the same time, this focus on specific legal questions led to Ibn Ḥabīb utilizing traditions that were different from the common corpus used to discuss this question. For instance, Ibn Ḥabīb opted to start with a tradition about an injured companion for whom the prophet sought a physician. When two men presented themselves as knowledgeable of medicine, the prophet asked them who was more knowledgeable and chose the more knowledgeable person to treat his injured companion. In this tradition, and along with illustrating that medical care was indeed legally permissible, Ibn Ḥabīb highlighted the importance of choosing the more experienced physician and underscored the legal significance of experience in relation to medical practice.[20]

Experience as a central point in the legal organization of medical practice was a question that Ibn Ḥabīb revisited in an independent chapter. There, and in discussing whether physicians were required or expected to guarantee cure (therefore, they would become liable to complaints, compensation, or other forms of legal censure should they fail to cure their patients or should their patients die), he cited the practice of Umar I and Umar II and the opinion of Mālik in arguing that experienced and well-known physicians were not required to guarantee cure, and should their patients die, they were not required to pay blood money or be punished in any way. Novices and those whose learning and experience could not be verified would be required to prove their capacity and that they had exerted all necessary efforts. If they could not prove their effort and knowledge, they would be required to pay blood money and could be punished for the death of their patients.[21] In this context, experience legitimized practice from a legal standpoint, giving experienced and well-known physicians the benefit of the doubt while demanding a higher degree of accountability from those who were less known.

This presumption of good intention and good practice in considering the practice of experienced physicians, Ibn Ḥabīb argued, should not be extended to non-Muslim physicians who should always be doubted when their Muslim patients died:

> If the physician was a Christian and gave a Muslim [a medication] and [the Muslim patient] died, the ruler (*al-sulṭān*) should investigate what [the physician] prescribed, even if he was a physician known for his [experience] and knowledge of medicine. [. . .] This is because [. . .] their physicians purposefully prescribe to well-regarded Muslims what kills them. [. . .] It was said that a Christian physician in the Levant gave Sulaymān ibn Musā a syrup, after which he [Sulaymān] died. [At that time,] Sulaymān was a notable

among the scholars of the Levant. This happened during the reign of Hishām ibn ʿAbd al-Malik. So Hishām [the caliph] sent for Sulayman's servant and asked him "Do you know from which bottle the physician took the syrup?" [The servant] said, "Yes". Hishām then brought the physician [. . .] and told him "Drink from what you gave [Sulaymān]" [The physician resisted but then] he drank from it and died.[22]

In Ibn Ḥabīb's view, the caliph or the ruler should act in this manner because a non-Muslim physician is to be suspected of attempting to kill notable Muslims.

Paying attention to the potential legal concerns of Galenic practitioners, Ibn Ḥabīb engaged with two iconic features of Galenic practice: urine examination and dieting. He started with a discussion of the permissibility of showing urine to doctors. It appears that the discussion had no materials that could be traced back to the prophet. Instead, Ibn Ḥabīb reported the practice of Umar II (d. 720) as well as the practice of Ibn Shahāb al-Zuhrī (d. 741) and Abī al-Zanād ʿAbd Allāh ibn Dhakwān (d. 747), along with Mālik (d. 795) and Sufyān al-Thawrī (d. 778) – choices that betray Ibn Ḥabīb's Maliki views and training.[23] In discussing dieting, Ibn Ḥabīb marshalled some prophetic materials as well as references to companions to indicate that dieting, broadly understood as choosing specific food with the knowledge that they influence the course of particular diseases or influence health, was accepted and even sometimes recommended by the prophet.[24] He commenced this section with a statement of a general rule of his own: "I heard them [physicians] say, 'Give the body what it is used to! The best of medicine is [gained] by experience. And the center of medicine is dieting."[25] He also cited the authority of al-Ḥārith ibn Kaladah (d. 635), a companion who was known to be a Galenic or humoral physician. For Ibn Ḥabīb, al-Ḥārith, although not an oft-cited legal authority, provided an ideal figure that had knowledge of medicine and belonged to the generations with referential legal authority. Ibn Ḥabīb cited al-Ḥārith frequently and centered many of the topics that he addressed on the latter's exchanges with Umar I, who seemed to have trusted al-Ḥārith as a physician. For instance, in addition to dieting, al-Ḥārith was cited in discussing the use of alcohol in treatment, leprosy, visiting, and managing lands known to be disease ridden, along with a number of other topics. The outsized role given to al-Ḥārith ibn Kaldah, who was not a reference of prophetic traditions otherwise, reveals how Ibn Ḥabīb centered his book around medical practice and the legal concerns of medical practitioners.

Even in his discussion of questions and issues that were rather common in prophetics literature, Ibn Ḥabīb showed more interest in the legal implications. For instance, and like other contemporary ḥadīth collections, Ibn Ḥabīb discussed cupping, a technique favored by the prophet, and fevers, a condition oft mentioned in the prophetic lore. Unlike contemporary ḥadīth compilers, Ibn Ḥabīb expanded on medical details presenting accounts of ten areas that the prophet had cupped most frequently and referencing their medical significance. He further explained that five of these were for general purposes of protection against diseases and for treatment of an assortment of general ailments. The other five were used for specific illnesses or conditions that affected the prophet, including when he was poisoned by a Jewish woman.[26] Ibn Ḥabīb added that one of these positions (*al-Naqra* or the top of the forehead) was thought by physicians to cause forgetfulness. However, he explained, there might be some benefits to using this spot because the prophet indeed used it.[27] The rest of the narrative was devoted to specific conditions, listing how the prophet and other companions and followers dealt with these conditions.

The peculiar nature of Ibn Ḥabīb's volume can be further illustrated in his discussion of leprosy. Although the topic was a fixture in medical prophetics literature, the discussion always revolved around contagion and was often linked to belief in omen (*al-ṭayarah*). The discussion often extended to include the question of escaping plague as it related to the discussion of contagion and omens.[28] The topics formed a closely knit unit in prophetic lore because they relied on a set of traditions that discussed contagion and God's will, instructing people to reject contagion and omens but also to distance themselves from the leper.[29] For Ibn Ḥabīb, the discussion took a different and a more medical turn as he embarked on a relatively detailed investigation of the causes of leprosy in daily practice, the signs of leprosy, and the way to protect oneself against the disease. This discussion included prophetic traditions that were not common in most contemporary compilations, including one that explained that nose hair is a sign of one's being safe against leprosy.[30] At the same time, Ibn Ḥabīb did not discuss contagion and did not mention plague at all. He also did not engage in any discussions about omens, fortunetelling, or other related questions, which other scholars often engaged in.

The second part of Ibn Ḥabīb's book had little to do with the literature on prophetics. Instead, it was entirely focused on medical questions showing Ibn Ḥabīb's familiarity with medical texts, terms, and knowledge. Rooted in an overall discussion of complexional properties of animals and plants, the humoral composition of the body, and the connections between the humors and the elements that form the sublunar world, Ibn Ḥabīb commenced with a discussion of plants and different food stuffs and their role in treating diseases or protecting against illnesses.[31] Throughout, he paid special attention to the making of the body, the balance of humors, and other issues that defined health and disease from a Galenic perspective. Although this portion of the book was based on medical knowledge, it did not read and was not organized in the same way that medical textbooks of the ninth century were organized. Instead, it resembled books written by physicians about foods and drinks and their qualities and other books directed to the learned elite and connected to the preservation of health. The most prominent example of this genre would be Abū Bakr al-Rāzī (d. 925) *Man Lā Yaḥdurhu Ṭabīb* (For when a physician is not available) or Ibn al-Jazzār's (d. 980) *Zād al-Musāfir* (Provisions for the traveler).

Ibn Ḥabīb's volume presented a different view on how to organize materials related to medicine and prophetics. He had a clear interest in legal questions, which was not as immediately pronounced in the works of his contemporaries. He also intended to write a book that would be of use to people seeking medical advice by summarizing existing knowledge about different plants, animals, and types of foods. As such, the book was a summary of medicine in that it helped the reader, who was neither a physician nor a scholar of law and ḥadīth, to understand the major legal questions related to medical practice and to place medicine within the legal and pietistic structures of the time. It also allowed the reader to acquire enough knowledge to manage their own bodies according to the traditions of Galenic medicine. However, Ibn Ḥabīb's career and his education and pedigree in ḥadīth did not help his book. Ibn Ḥabīb's book remains an historically important episode in the development of this literature; however, it did not produce much influence on Ibn Ḥabīb's contemporaries either in the East or the West.

Prophets and imams: Ṭibb al-Aʾimmah

Almost contemporary to the work of Ibn Ḥabīb al-Qurṭubī and to the gradual proliferation of writings on medical prophetics, *Ṭibb al-Aʾimmah* (The Medicine of the Imams) by Abū ʿAtab ʿAbd Allāh and al-Ḥusayn, the sons of Bisṭām ibn Sābūr (both fl. ca. 800), was one of the earliest Shiite writings dedicated to questions of medicine, piety, and prophetics. Most sources do not provide a clear date for the birth or death of either of the two brothers. Moreover, and apart from their Medicine of the Imāms, they had rather undistinguished careers, and not many details are known about them. However, their father, Bisṭam ibn Sābūr al-Zayyāt, whose dates of birth or death are also unknown with certainty, was a more recognized scholar and a companion of the Shiite Imām Jaʿfar al-Ṣādiq (d. 765) and his son Imām Mūsā al-Kāẓim (d. 799).[32] This places the two brothers at the turn of the eighth and ninth centuries and places their book in the early ninth century. The book might be one of the earliest texts on prophetic medicine in both Sunni and Shiite traditions, with other books adopting similar themes over the tenth and eleventh centuries and beyond.[33] Although the book seemed to have enjoyed some popularity, was listed in many Shiite biographical and bibliographical dictionaries, and was translated into Persian as late as the seventeenth century, indicating perhaps its survival in circulation, it was criticized for including accounts from suspicious reporters. For instance, Andrew Newman explained that figures like al-Mufaḍḍal ibn ʿUmar, al-Muʿallā ibn Khunays, and Muḥammad ibn Sinān, among others, had "problematic careers" and were seen as weak or untrustworthy reporters by Shiite ḥadīth scholars during this period and beyond.[34] This, however, appears to be similar to what one can observe in Sunni collections, as explained before, where requirements of trustworthiness and bars of authenticity were lower in traditions that did not include specific legal obligations but were rather part of the larger pietistic discourses.[35]

The introduction to *Tibb al-Aʾimmah* was simple and straightforward, explaining that the book was about the medicine of the People of the House (of Muḥammad) and starting with a discussion of the divine reward that believers reap when afflicted with illness. The book then proceeded to describe the treatment for a variety of conditions using the traditions of many imams. Similar to Sunni discussions of the prophet's habits, *Ṭibb al-ʾAimmah* produced narratives of Imami lore that described the habits of the imams, their episodes of illness, and their preferred methods of treatment. Following the structure and organization of adab works of the period, the text was iterative with repetitions that recalled specific central questions and that anchored the narratives around specific pronouncements. It also flowed through associations that arranged the "little narratives" of these traditions and anecdotes, linking them to one another through associations around meanings and specific issues or even body parts.

For instance, when discussing recipes and prayers to treat pain in the belly, the authors moved on to discussing general recommendations about food. The connection here was not related to the pain in particular, but rather to the relation between the belly and the consumed food and the potential role of food in causing stomach problems.[36] In the same manner, the discussion of the use of the *lā ḥawl walā quwat illā billāh* (no might or power except through God), which was a reported saying that protects against some ailments, provided the opportunity to present a few traditions by various imams about the value and divine reward associated with this saying, even though such reward had no relation to medicine or disease.[37] The discussion of cupping also led naturally to a discussion of bloodletting and of one's looking at his own blood during a bloodletting. These topics also presented an opportunity to discuss the signs and symptoms associated with blood-related disorders from a humoral theory point of view, although these conditions were not necessarily prescribed cupping.[38] Similarly, dieting led to a discussion of overeating and then to a discussion of pietistic manners of eating, including pronouncing the name of God on the food. Food discussion prompted a return to discussing belly pain and to even more recipes about it.[39] These associations provided the opportunity for repetition of traditions and for repeating and extending the discussion of certain disorders. The additional recipes mentioned during repeated discussions of particular conditions (such as belly pain, which was discussed first separately as a primary topic and then as an extension to discussing overeating) were often more specific and related to a given cause for the condition, with more general overarching recipes mentioned in the first discussion of a condition. This form of circuitous structure was quite different from medical books of the period.[40] However, they fit the more traditional adab style and permitted more liberal and iterative readings that did not demand a fixed or unchangeable order.[41] Although Ibnā Bisṭām's book relied on a medical rationale and arrangement, it stood in the middle between the more traditional prophetics literature, where the emphasis remained on prophetic and Imāmī logic and materials, and near-contemporary or later writings, such as the *Golden Treatise*, which was attributed to Imām ʿAlī al-Riḍā or al-Asfahānī's *al-Ṭibb al-Nabawī*, which followed a stricter Galenic narrative structure.

Ibnā Basṭām's text focused in the majority of cases on verses, prayers, and amulets with only few recipes; however, these amulets and prayers were placed within a medicalized narrative that paid attention to symptoms and signs of diseases, to how patients experienced ailments, to how they described their conditions, and to the various stages of the development of their conditions. For prayers, most anecdotes commenced with the reporter complaining to one of the imams about their condition. Their complaint either included the name of the disorder, such as constipation or leprosy, or described the symptoms that the person suffered from, such as itching, night terrors, etc. The imam would then recognize the condition (or diagnose it if not mentioned from the outset) and describe a particular prayer that should be recited to treat this condition.

The vast majority of these prayers were based on verses from the Quran that related to the condition or touched on the symptoms in one manner or another. For instance, a prayer to help ease delivery was derived from the story of Mary and her giving birth to Jesus.[42] Another to treat severe acne was based on a verse where God turns mountains into dust that simply disappears.[43] A prayer for Quartan Fever involved four different writings, the most important of which was a verse that explained that the people of heaven do not fear heat or extreme cold – in reference to fever's effect on the body.[44] In all these cases, the prayers seemed to work through their word structure and their direct physical connections to the condition at hand. Invoking Mary's birth helped women give birth easier, and invoking specific physical qualities allowed for the elimination of particular conditions. Although not all prayers were derived from Quranic verses, they were all connected to the condition in these terms, whether or not they came from the Quran.

Prayers were also physically applied to sites of illness. In most cases, the prayers would be recited while a hand is placed on the site of pain or problem. Prayers for women to have an easy birth would be "placed" on their bellies or close to their vaginas.[45] Prayers for fever would be recited while touching the forehead and those for leprosy, while touching the site of affliction.[46] The question of touching the site of illness was also raised in Sunni literature, as explained before. Compilers of ḥadīth took care to mention that the prophet indeed touched the places that hurt or placed his hand on the body of particular patients while praying for them. The ubiquitous mention of this touching in the literature could evidence the pervasive nature of the practice. In the same context, certain prayers (*ruqya*) were read over pieces of cloth or bandages before applying them to the body. People suffering from severe fever were recommended to recite a prayer inside a garment and then wear the garment itself. In other instances, a prayer would be recited over water or written on a piece of paper and washed by water. The water would then be consumed, delivering the prayer to the inside of the body. The physical touch seemed crucial to the proper delivery of the prayer. In treating migraines, for instance, Imam al-Bāqir explained that one should place a hand on the half of the head that hurts before reading the advised prayer.[47] This discussion of prayers and the manner by which they are to be delivered (including how many times, how often, using which physical medium to deliver their power) contributed to the naturalization of these prayers and procedures as ways of treating particular ills. They were described in the same manner that specific recipes and medications would be described and addressed as predictable forms of treatment.

Also in the style of medical narratives, anecdotes often ended with evidence of success as reported by the patient. Although the authority of the imams describing these prayers was never questioned and the wording in the prayers themselves provided forms of intrinsic evidence on their efficacy – namely, through their being verses of the Quran or otherwise known prayers and through their connection to the conditions they treated – the authors followed the medical structure of recipes, ending with a description of the efficacy of these recipes and prayers.[48] Such structure could not be seen in the chapters of medicine in other ḥadīth compilations, which had little concern for evidence of efficacy, as it did not follow these medical narrative structures. The same can be seen in specific prayers where Ibnā Bisṭām used the known formula "tried" or "experimented" (*mujarrab*) to describe both recipes and prayers.[49] Following the traditions of recipe books, such designation may have shown that the authors themselves tried these recipes or prayers and found them effective, as prescribed by the Imām. Here again, this designation cannot be seen as lending more authority to specific recipes or prayers over others or attempting to lend more weight to a given recipe in the manner seen in treatises of pharmacopeia.[50] Ibnā Bisṭām and their readers required no such confirmation of the imam's authority, as will be explained later. These notes of experimentation represented an argument of applicability (meaning that readers would find such prayers and recipes easy and accessible) and were in keeping with medical narratives.

Perhaps the central caveat to this process of naturalizing recipes is connected to the authors' realization that the book might be challenged by Sunnis questioning many of the traditions in the book and their efficacy. In one anecdote, the authors revealed as much:

> We were with Imam Ja'far al-Ṣādiq, when Ḥabbābah al-Walabiyyah entered and asked him various questions. We marveled at the value of these questions. The Imam asked, "Have you seen questions better than Ḥabbābah's?!" We said, "O our lord, never! She gained such respect in our eyes." [When hearing this,] Ḥabbābah cried so the Imām asked her why she cried. She said, "O son of the prophet, the Malignant Disease [leprosy] has shown on me. [. . .] My neighbors say, if her friend [meaning al-Ṣādiq] was truly [an Imam], she would not be afflicted with this. [. . .]" The Imam then said something quietly that we did not hear and told her, "Go to the women's quarters and look at your body now." She looked at her body and there was no sign of the disease. The Imam said, "Go tell your neighbors, this is the man whose obedience is an obligation [meaning he is the true imam]."[51]

The woman-companion of the imam was worried about her neighbors taunting her and insulting the imam because of her illness. Although she believed that the affliction was a trial from God and was willing to withstand it, she could not withstand doubting the imam. Here, the prayer was never mentioned, and the reporter only explained that the imam muttered something that could not be heard. The anecdote was one of immediate miraculous healing that reinforced the legitimacy of the imam rather than one about replicable recipes. It also revealed the anxiety surrounding the efficacy of these recipes and how their potential inefficacy might be used as a weapon against the imams; this anxiety was further demonstrated by the proviso following a number of recipes and prayers stating that they would not benefit those who do not believe in them. In these cases, the patient's belief in the imam and their conviction that the recipe and prayer would work served as the true guarantee of its effectiveness. This view, that efficacy is dependent on belief, should not be seen as simply a manner of shielding oneself from attack by claiming that those not healed were simply unbelievers. Instead, this position had roots in Quranic and prophetic practice and sīra where it was argued that God may delude unbelievers by vindicating them and extending His earthly favor to them to drive them further into His wrath.[52]

At the same time, this proposition that belief is necessary for efficacy helped to remind the believers that testing God, his prophets, and the imams was never appropriate. This, too, was recalling a known debate around 'testing God' by Abraham, who asked God to show him how he resurrects the dead. Exegetes in this period went to great lengths to explain that this was not an anecdote of Abraham testing God, and God's retort in the Quran, "Have you not believed [in me] yet?!" was not an indication of this test. Instead, this was an act of solidifying belief by demanding a personal miracle that would aid Abraham in his debates with the infidels.[53] As such, the proviso that belief is necessary for healing served as a reminder to the believers of the proper manner in approaching these recipes: with absolute and unwavering belief in their efficacy. Should the remedies not work, the problem would not lie with them but rather with the application, the process, or with the believers themselves. Of course, the failure to heal may very well show God's favor by testing the believer for better reward in the hereafter, as will be shown later. In this context, we can better understand the various implications behind the authors' testimony about the effectiveness of some recipes and prayers. Far from validating the imam's authority or providing proof for his divine inspiration, the testimony is at once an indication of the accessibility of these recipes and prayers to various readers as they were accessible to the author and also a testimony to the authors' dedication and ability to achieve the results that the imams promised.

This view and concern about efficacy was also demonstrated in the anecdotes reported about the prophet that both Shiite and Sunni scholars reported. In the oft-cited ḥadīth about honey, a man came to Muḥammad and complained that his brother's belly ached. Muḥammad prescribed honey, which made the pain worse and brought the man back two more times. On the third time, Muḥammad said, "God's word is true and your brother's belly lies. Give him honey." Here, Muḥammad was referring to the verse about honey being a source of healing or was referring to his own recommendation as being inspired by God. In either case, the recommendation of honey was seen as inspired and revealed, and the man and his brother needed to be patient. In some Sunni accounts, the brother was healed after the third time and the anecdote delivered a message about faith and patience.[54] Ibnā Bisṭām reported the same tradition, but added that the sick brother was in fact a hypocrite (*munāfiq*).[55] In doing so, the entire anecdote was cast in a different light, as the brother was either lying about the ache continuing despite the prophet's cure or the treatment with honey did not work because the brother did not truly believe in the prophet and his message. In either case, even the minor inefficacy of the prophet's recommendation was caused by the lack of belief on the part of the patient, further highlighting the importance of faith in this pietistic process of healing.

Recipes

Although the majority of the recommendations in *Ṭibb al-A'immah* were about prayers and specific readings from the Quran, Ibnā Bisṭām's volume included a number of recipes for the treatment of particular conditions. Two recipes stand out as particularly important: the "Comprehensive Medicine" and the "Healing Medicine." Each of these was a recipe reported by one of the imams and used by many others to treat a variety of conditions, with or without minor modifications. The "Comprehensive Medicine" was reported to have been the medicine of al-Imām 'Alī al-Riḍā, although one anecdote explained that it was not al-Riḍā who first used it but that he used it consistently and believed it was exceedingly useful.[56] The "Healing Medicine" was attributed to al-Riḍā's father, Imām Mūsā al-Kāẓim. For both recipes, Ibnā Bisṭām presented a series of conditions that they treated. For each condition, a small modification in the recipe may be recommended, such as the addition of a new substance, boiling, heating, or simply a particular form of application. The two medications seemed to present a basic infrastructure for different sets of recipes that would treat various diseases.

Similar to the Comprehensive Medicine, the Healing Medicine did not originate with the imam either. It was rather revealed by God to Moses so that the Israelites would survive poisoning:

> When the pharaoh wanted to poison the Children of Israel, he held a feast for them on a Sunday and prepared for them a lot of food, which was poisoned. Moses came with his people and looked at the food. He then sent the women and children away and told the Children of Israel, "Do not eat their food or drink their drinks." He then gave each of them some of that medication knowing that they will disobey him and will eat from the Pharaoh's food.[57]

The Children of Israel survived, thanks to this medication, whereas many of the pharaoh's soldiers perished because they ate from what was left after the feast. God then revealed this medication to Muḥammad, and it was transmitted among the imams. Ibnā Bisṭām included only one other example of a revealed recipe, which Imam Ja'far al-Ṣādiq used when he suffered from fever. The imam received inspiration that he should drink rice water to treat his fever and it cured him.[58] Although all the recipes and prayers in the book were in some way inspired or revealed, because the prophet and imams derived their knowledge from divine inspiration, only these recipes were explicitly cited as directly revealed by God.

The book included a series of other recipes, some of which were prepared or described by the imams, such as ones for cough,[59] headache,[60] spleen pain,[61] excess urine,[62] and nosebleed,[63] among others. Other recipes were prepared by physicians. For instance, in one anecdote, a person asked the imam about the famous Theriac and whether it was permissible. The premise of the question was based on the fact that the Theriac was prepared using snake meat, which the questioner thought might be prohibited or dangerous.[64] The imam assured him that it was permissible and that "it would not hurt us."[65] In another anecdote, a questioner asked Imam Ja'far al-Ṣādiq about a syrup that a physician prescribed for general pain. Here, the question was not related to a potential legal issue but rather an attempt to find out what the imam thought about the efficacy of this recipe. The imam did not seem to know the recipe but he concluded that it was "sweet," as it included honey and sugar. He asked, "Is it not sweet?" The questioner affirmed so the imam said, "Drink sweet [syrups] whenever prescribed and wherever found."[66] More significantly, a physician by the name of Aḥmad ibn Rabbāḥ dictated to the authors, Ibnā Bisṭām, a series of recipes that the former said were beneficial in conditions of black bile, yellow bile, phlegm, stomachache, vomiting, and fever, among others, if combined with prohibition of dates, fish, vinegar, and beans. The physician Ibn Rabbāḥ explained that he showed these recipes to the imam, whose name was not mentioned, and that the imam approved of the recipes and said they would be beneficial.[67]

In the series of recipes reported by Aḥmad ibn Rabbāḥ, we find the most explicit engagement with Galenic practitioners and their recipes.[68] It is not clear whether Ibn Rabbāḥ's practice of consulting the imam about recipes was a common one or whether Ibn Rabbāḥ himself did this again or with other recipes that he used. Few other physicians were featured in the book as part of the chain of transmission of some of the ḥadīth traditions and anecdotes. The presence of some physicians as reporters, the narration of recipes that were dictated by a physician, and the testimonies of trial and efficacy that resembled those found in recipe books and formularies suggest that Ibnā Bisṭām were in conversation with physicians and medical practitioners and that this book was composed with the help and collaboration of these practitioners.

Ṭibb al-A'immah in dialogue

Ibnā Bisṭām's book differed on several levels when compared to its Sunni contemporaries. At the outset, the book was invested in different structures of authority and different lines of reporting. It relied primarily on the writings and anecdotes of the imams, and when discussing Muḥammad, the imams' reports about the prophet. The text departed from Sunni medical prophetics in two distinct ways. First, the reliance on different authorities and different reporters, and the discrediting and the outright rejection of other reporters, gave rise to a different corpus of ḥadīth. The central stories and traditions that populated Sunni medical prophetics were not necessarily present or equally prominent in Shiite medical prophetics, and some are absent from Ibnā Bisṭām's and others' works. Similarly, other anecdotes and questions that seemed central to the lives of particular imams would not make their way into the Sunni literature. Second, Ibnā Bisṭām and Shiite reporters of ḥadīth traditions relied on sources of authority that were largely contemporaneous and deeply engaged with the medical and intellectual environment of the eighth and ninth centuries. For instance, Ibnā Bisṭām quoted most often the

Imam Jaʿfar al-Ṣādiq (d. 765), his father Muḥammad al-Bāqir (d. 733), his son Mūsā al-Kāẓim (d. 799), and his grandson ʿAlī al-Riḍā (d. 818), all of whom were important contributors to the intellectual environment during their lives. Jaʿfar al-Ṣādiq, who was cited most often, was a well-known and revered source of judicial knowledge for Sunnis and Shiites alike.[69] He also sponsored a circle of scholars, authors, literati, alchemists, and physicians on which he had a lasting impact. Imam ʿAlī al-Riḍā, who was cited almost as often, was also connected with the Abbasid educated elites in the ninth century, especially as he became the heir apparent of the Abbasid Caliph al-Maʾmūn (d. 830).[70] The connections that the imams had with educated physicians and scholars meant that their recommendations and their views were more in line with the Galenic views and more connected with the concerns of the medical profession.

Ibnā Bisṭām's book also addressed questions that seemed to have not concerned any of the contemporary Sunni scholars writing about medical prophetics. These issues may have been derived from specific views and preferences among the imams and Shiite scholars that were not necessarily shared with Sunni scholars and readers. For instance, Imam Jaʿfar al-Ṣādiq was reported to have appreciated pigeons and to have believed that they protect people against *jinn* and against the evil eye. When one of his companions killed two pigeons in a fit of anger, the imam asked him to repent and pay money in charity because killing these pigeons was a transgression.[71] Although the report did not consider killing pigeons to be unlawful, it was clearly an objectionable act. Ibnā Bisṭām also reported that the mud from al-Ḥusayn's grave had healing qualities because of the blessing of al-Ḥusayn.[72]

The reports also revealed a particular dynamic in which the imam stood as a reference authority on matters related to health and disease along with many other issues in life. In many anecdotes, people visited the imam to complain about diseases and ask for guidance. They also consulted the imam about medications that they had been prescribed by physicians. And as seen before, physicians seemed to have visited the imams and discussed their own preparations with them for guidance. This constant consultation with the imam, which was evidently available to companions physically close to where the imam lived, highlights the significance of this form of renewed authority who lived alongside their companions (until the Occultation for Twelver Shiites) and how the sources of this type of medical prophetics remained in direct contact with patients in manners unlike those in Sunni prophetics literature.

At the same time, Ibnā Bisṭām's reports and anecdotes also engaged with a number of topics and included versions of the traditions and anecdotes that were addressed in Sunni literature. For instance, and as explained before, Ibnā Bisṭām reported the anecdote of the prophet prescribing honey to a companion's ailing brother. The report repeated the same points explained in Sunni literature in relation to the healing qualities of honey. However, Ibnā Bisṭām's version attributed the presumed early inefficacy to the fact that the ailing brother was a hypocrite, who was either an unsuitable recipient of this cure or was intentionally denying its efficacy. Ibnā Bisṭām also reported the prophetic tradition discussing what a

Muslim should do if a fly falls in one's drink on the authority of Imam al-Bāqir.[73] In both Sunni and Shiite iterations of the traditions, one should immerse the fly completely in the food or drink because it carries poison under one wing and the antidote under the other.[74] Because it is impossible to know which of the two fell in the food or drink first, the safest practice would be to immerse both to ensure survival. Imam al-Bāqir added a gloss to the tradition, explaining that this helps people avoid leprosy, "If it were not for the flies that falls in people's food without their knowledge, they would have been ravaged by leprosy."[75]

Similarly, Ibnā Bisṭām reported traditions indicating the healing qualities of the black seed which was reported in many Sunni medical prophetics chapters.[76] Adding to the Sunni literature, Ibnā Bisṭām reported a few recipes where the black seed was used by the imams. In the same vein, the use of camel milk and urine in treatment was also discussed in this book as it was in Sunni sources.[77] Instead of the prophetic anecdotes that Sunni scholars used, Ibnā Bisṭām used the practice and traditions of the imams to indicate the legality of using camel urine and milk for treatment.[78] The question of using urine for treatment and in recipes was expanded upon by Ibnā Bisṭām, who reported traditions and anecdotes concerning the use of human urine in recipes. Here, the imams indicated that using one's own urine in treatment was acceptable but not anybody else's urine.[79]

The questions about amulets and about the legality of certain incantations or *ruqyas*, which were common in Sunni medical prophetics,[80] were also discussed in Ibnā Bisṭām's collection. In discussing amulets, the imams, particularly Jaʿfar al-Ṣādiq, accepted the legality of amulets and recommended them in the treatment of some conditions. Most amulets described by the imams included verses from the Quran or other prayers that invoked the Quran as well. In fact, Ja'far al-Ṣādiq was asked directly about the legality of amulets, including those containing verses from the Quran, and answered positively.[81] On the other hand, Imam Muḥammad al-Bāqir explained that some amulets, prayers, and spells, especially those that are not made of Quranic verses or similar invocations, might be illegal and even a sign of idolatry, which was a position similar to many scholars of Sunni ḥadīth. The use of prohibited materials, especially alcohol, in different recipes was a frequent topic for Sunni compilers, who were almost unanimous in their rejection of such practices and insisted that using such materials could not bring healing.[82] Ibnā Bisṭām reported traditions from Jaʿfar al-Ṣādiq indicating he shared a similar position and prohibiting his companions from using such materials in recipes.

Cupping, a preferred treatment of the prophet's, was also prominent in Ibnā Bisṭām's collection. The authors reported traditions and anecdotes that explained the best times of the year, of the week, and of the day for cupping and the main places in the body for cupping. Other anecdotes explained the different benefits of cupping based on Galenic reasoning.[83] Similarly, enemas, snuffs, and the use of the bath were all discussed in Ibnā Bisṭām's collection. Whereas some Sunni authors seemed to dislike enemas, though they stopped short of declaring them illegal or prohibited,[84] Ibnā Bisṭām's sources had no objections to enemas and considered them, along with snuffs, cupping, and baths, to be some of the more important treatments.[85] Violet pastes, which were mentioned by ʿAbd al-Malik ibn

Ḥabīb,[86] were also noted by Ibnā Bisṭām as a treatment preferred by the prophet and the imams. Ibnā Bisṭām reported the same tradition as Ibn Ḥabīb wherein the prophet compared his own worth in relation to other prophets to the efficacy of violet in relation to other medications.[87] Similarly, Ibnā Bisṭām discussed additional issues that one could find in Ibn Ḥabīb's *Al-Mukhtaṣar*, especially in the latter's discussion of leprosy.[88] For instance, Ibnā Bisṭām reported a tradition where Imām Ja'far al-Ṣādiq explained that every person has "a twig of leprosy," which could become active and lead to leprosy at any time. In this vein, people with excess nasal hair were safer from leprosy because this hair was a sign of the weakness of their leprosy twig.[89]

In addition to discussing various questions related to medicine, the literary style employed by Ibnā Bisṭām as adab authors allowed them to discuss a number of other issues that may not be directly related to medicine. For instance, and in the context of discussing a few prayers that protect against a variety of ailments, they reported a tradition that included prayers for each day of the week and which are intended to protect from all evils.[90] When discussing prayers and recipes to improve offspring, they included a tradition about the harms that could befall children if they saw adults (presumably their parents) having sex. The child was at risk of growing up with eschewed morality and no sense of shame.[91] In the same vein, Imam Ja'far explained that it was prohibited to have sex with a freewoman while another freewoman watched. This was legal if one of the two was a slave, however.[92] In the same manner, and while discussing some prayers to protect against magic, they reported a prayer by Imam Ja'far that he used to protect himself from the wrath of the Abbasid caliph, Abū Ja'far al-Manṣūr (r. 754–775). The caliph had summoned Imam Ja'far al-Ṣādiq intending to imprison, harm, and/or kill him because of certain reports that the imam was actively advocating against Abbasid rule. Soon after Ja'far al-Ṣādiq entered the court, the caliph admitted that he did not feel any ill feelings and that whatever intentions he had harbored disappeared. Ja'far al-Ṣādiq then revealed that he had recited a special prayer that led to this reaction from the caliph.[93]

Fazlur Rahman has argued that prophetic medicine in Shiite, as opposed to Sunni, traditions was less concerned with connections to learned Galenic medicine and that it instructed its readers to be more patient and to withstand illnesses except in the extreme.[94] Such characterization, which was criticized by Michael Dols and Andrew Newman,[95] overlooks the wealth of materials in Ibnā Bisṭām's collection alone that focused on treatments and provided for ways to achieve cure. At the same time, Sunni literature, as will be seen later in this chapter and beyond, placed importance on patience and provided its readers with pietistic meanings of illness that encouraged forbearance in the same way that Shiite literature did. Moreover, a closer look at Ibnā Bisṭām's writings show similarities with contemporary Sunni works, demonstrating that these authors drew on similar sources and addressed similar problems.

The Medicine of the Imams (*Ṭibb al-A'immah*) constituted an important moment in the development of prophetic medicine because of the authors' investment in the production of a medicalized narrative. Although the text was primarily composed of prophetic and Imami ḥadīth and included only few detailed recipes, it was organized in a manner reminiscent of medical texts and responded to many of the medical needs of its readers. The book also included important moments where medical practitioners came in direct contact with or consulted, the imams, imbuing their own practice with the imam's authority. At this intersection of medical knowledge and religious authority, a new body emerged. Here, the readers were to think about the health of their bodies and to attempt to treat the ailments that affected them. This care for the body and for health, which was at the heart of the medical paradigm the treatise drew from, was now rooted in the practice of the imams and the prophet. Although care for the body was part of the overall pietistic narratives, this text along with others discussed in this chapter served to medicalize this narrative of bodily care and root it within Galenic knowledge and practice.

The new prophetic medicine: Ibn al-Sunnī and Abū Nuʿaym al-Iṣfahānī

In the introduction to his book *Prophetic Medicine (al-Ṭibb al-Nabawiyy)*, Abū Nuʿaym al-Iṣfahānī (d. 1038) explained the impetus for his writing:

> When you [al-Isfahānī's students] showed me the book of medicine compiled by Abū Bakr [. . .] ibn Isḥāq al-Sunnī, and asked to hear it from me in order to receive a license [for transmitting its ḥadīths], I saw that his book was composed of seven treatises along the method of the physicians so that each treatise can be sought for a particular reason with ease. [Then,] I decided to follow [the example] of his book chapter by chapter and section by section so that my book may serve as an alternative for you to his book.[96]

Abū Nuʿaym (d. 1038) was addressing a group of ḥadīth students interested in the volume composed by Ibn al-Sunnī (d. 974), a respected scholar of ḥadīth like Abū Nuʿaym himself. The students who failed to meet Ibn al-Sunnī and who were interested in the traditions that he reported in his book wanted to establish a solid line of transmission by listening to and learning these traditions orally from their master: Abū Nuʿaym. Had the master assented to their request, the work may have amounted to a commentary on Ibn al-Sunnī's text that would trace the latter's traditions, critique them, and perhaps add few more traditions on the same topics. It appears that Abū Nuʿaym, who seemed impressed with Ibn al-Sunnī's novel composition, was not interested in commenting on Ibn al-Sunnī's work.[97] Instead, and in a fashion common enough in ḥadīth scholarship at the time, he decided to mirror the organization but provide ḥadīths with chains of transmission that ended with him. As such, and as he explained, his students would be able to learn these traditions arranged in the manner that they, and their master, so admired and with the proper chains that they could report on their own later.

Abū Nuʿaym was aware of how Ibn al-Sunnī's book differed from other compilations. Ibn al-Sunnī's book was arranged according to "the method of physicians" and followed the priorities of medical practice. Ibn al-Sunnī began his book with a section on medical theory and on the composition of the body, following that with a section on different diseases, and concluding with a section on treatments, including different foods and drinks. Although many of the traditions included in both books could still be found in the medical sections of earlier compilations, similar to *Ṭibb al-Aʾimmah* and ʿAbd al-Malik ibn Ḥabīb's book that preceded them, the new compilations were arranged to address the concerns and priorities of readers seeking medical knowledge and familiar with the arrangement of medical texts. In fact, Abū Nuʿaym's and Ibn al-Sunnī's texts seemed to be more attuned to the expectations of readers of medical texts than Ibn Ḥabīb's, who had a much more pronounced interest in legal questions. In later collections, the format of these books, beginning with theory and arranging diseases from head to toe, mirrored contemporary medical texts of the tenth and beginning of the eleventh centuries.

What primarily sets these two volumes apart from Ibn Ḥabīb's text is the identity of their authors. Whereas Ibn Ḥabīb was primarily a jurist from al-Andalus whose training and methods in ḥadīth came to be suspected, as explained before, Ibn al-Sunnī and Abū Nuʿaym were well-known scholars of ḥadīth with solid reputations and whose integrity, knowledge, and trustworthiness remained (and remain today) impeccable among scholars of ḥadīth and jurists.[98] Ibn al-Sunnī was a well-known scholar who traveled extensively in search of ḥadīth and who learned from some of the more important masters in the first and second generations of major compilers, including al-Jamḥī (d. 917) and the now-more-famous al-Nasāʾī (d. 915).[99] Ibn al-Sunnī gained the trust and the admiration of his peers, many of whom reported traditions solely on his authority. Abū Nuʿaym al-Isfahānī was a more prominent scholar and was considered the most knowledgeable scholar of ḥadīth in his time. It was reported that he first started learning ḥadīth when he was eight years old and that he traveled widely (although the details of his travels are not clear) learning from many scholars of his time. In the latter years of his life, he became "a man to whom trips are made," as many scholars of ḥadīth explained, referring to the fact that he was a destination for students who wanted to learn ḥadīth. The praise that Abū Nuʿaym earned from other scholars of ḥadīth extended over several generations, starting from his prominent student al-Khaṭīb al-Baghdādī (d. 1071), to Ibn Taymiyyah (d. 1328), and al-Dhahabī (d. 1348).[100]

The pedigree and the intellectual authority that both al-Sunnī and Abū Nuʿaym enjoyed allowed their texts to occupy an important position in writings about prophetic medicine. Their collections changed and rearranged the central components of medical prophetics, replacing and rearranging many of the traditions, anecdotes, objects, and recipes that were first arranged in the medical sections of the major ḥadīth collections. With such credibility and authority, Ibn al-Sunnī and Abū Nuʿaymah were able to reconstruct medical prophetics by including specific traditions and adding particular anecdotes and objects. They were also able to rearrange the literature around medical priorities in a manner that did not exist before. The new arrangement of materials in these books provided the infrastructure and the source materials for later writings that would be recognized as a new genre: prophetic medicine. Moreover, this emerging archive at the intersection of prophetics and Galenic medicine contributed significantly to the construction of a practice of medical piety where care for the body and treatment of its ills along the principles of Galenic knowledge acquired pietistic meaning and religious valence through its connection to the prophetic corpus.

In addition to Abū Nuʿaym's remarkable Sunni credentials, he had important connections to Shiite scholars and ḥadīth reporters.[101] Abū Nuʿaym grew up and spent the majority of his active years under Buyid rule and in communication with Sunni and Twelver scholars. His grandfather, who was the first to convert to Islam in his family, was a client of ʿAbd Allāh ibn Muʿāwiyah ibn Jaʿfar ibn Abī Ṭālib (fl. ca. 744), who came to lead a faction of the Kīsāniyyah ʿAlids in a revolt against the Umayyads.[102] Although the revolt was short lived and the Kīsāniyyah themselves soon disappeared as a Shiite faction, this early connection between Abū Nuʿaym's family and ʿAlid circles fueled some speculations about his being a Shiite. Abū Nuʿaym himself wrote a book on the qualities of ʿAlī ibn Abī Ṭālib that included significant number of traditions that circulated among Twelver Shiite scholars. The book was cited frequently by Shiite scholars afterward, some of whom claimed that Abū Nuʿaym had ʿAlid sympathies which he hid for fear of persecution.[103] Whether or not Abū Nuʿaym was indeed a Shiite or had ʿAlid sympathies is difficult to determine. In either case, these "rumors" and "accusations" never meaningfully affected his status among Sunni scholars. What is more relevant for the purposes of this discussion is that Abū Nuʿaym sustained intellectual connections with ʿAlid scholars and often cited traditions and anecdotes that were more common in ʿAlid literature. As will be seen later, many of these traditions could be found in his book on medicine as well as in his writings about saints. Abū Nuʿaym, and perhaps Ibn al-Sunnī as well, were inspired and influenced by Shiite writings of prophetic medicine and, perhaps, by the arrangements of works like *Ṭibb al-Aʾimmah* and *Al-Risālah al-Dhahabiyyah* or the *Golden Treatise* which circulated in Buyid Iraq and Fars during Abū Nuʿaym's lifetime.[104]

Ibn al-Sunnī, Abū Nuʿaym, and their medicine

In the introduction to his treatise, Ibn al-Sunnī referred to another longer volume he had composed on medicine where he included what he claimed to be all the traditions that related to medicine. He then decided to create this treatise as a summary that included the more authentic and more relevant ḥadīths.[105] He also explained that this book, and presumably the older larger version, were arranged according to what is customary to the "people of the art," meaning medicine.[106] He thus arranged the book into seven treatises. The first addressed the benefit and privilege (*faḍl*) of medicine. The second was on the composition of the body and regimens intended to preserve health; the third on the types of illnesses; the fourth on medications and their benefits; the fifth on management of convalescent patients; the sixth on healthy habits and protecting the body from the harms of drinks and foods; and the seventh focused on incantations, blessings, and omens. Outside of its mention in the introduction, there was no record of a larger volume on medicine or prophetic medicine composed by Ibn al-Sunnī. It is not clear whether Abū Nuʿaym and his students were interested in the shorter treatise (seventy-five folios) or the longer one, or if they were aware of the existence of two treatises. If Abū Nuʿaym was aware of the longer version, he would have realized that his treatise, which was of comparable size to Ibn al-Sunnī's short treatise, fell short of the longer version.[107] Although Abū Nuʿaym mentioned that he decided to follow the arrangement and the chapters of Ibn al-Sunnī's book, he, in fact, deviated somewhat from the arrangement of the manuscript that we have. Whether this was because he relied on a different text, perhaps the longer one, or because he decided to diverge from the overall structure remains unclear.

Abū Nuʿaym's book was divided into seven treatises as well. The first, and similar to Ibn al-Sunnī's, addressed the importance of learning medicine and discussed some of the major legal questions governing medical practice. This treatise included roughly all the traditions found in Ibn al-Sunnī's with a few additions and discussed the legality of seeking treatment and medical care, of going to physicians and paying them, of women treating men, and of using prohibited substances in treatment. Also, similar to Ibn al-Sunnī's, the second treatise was "on the composition of the body and [the conditions] of health." It started with a discussion of anatomy and of the composition of the body's different organs. This was followed with a discussion of general rules on health and disease, including some general practices like sitting in the sun, drinking cold water, overall harmful materials, etc. The third treatise, "On the names of ailments and on treating patients," addressed various kinds of diseases arranged by the organ they affect – mostly starting from head to toe – an arrangement that was common in medical literature. In each of Ibn al-Sunnī's and Abū Nuʿaym's books, the chapter on ailments commenced with a discussion of how sadness increased diseases and how loss of friends led to deteriorating health. Both authors then discussed different diseases and how these diseases could be cured. The fourth treatise addressed different cures and recipes and was divided into two main parts: plant and animal materials. In this treatise, Ibn al-Sunnī's text, but to a lesser extent than Abū Nuʿaym's, contained nonprophetic materials such as poetry and sayings of various known litterateurs or from Arabic lore. The fifth addressed dieting, with a particular focus on convalescent patients. The sixth discussed fruits, both as part of recipes and as part of a regular diet. The final treatise addressed meats, describing their different sources, types, and uses and the various organs of different edible animals. In each of these chapters discussing treatment and food matters, Abu Nu'aym explained the medical uses, benefits, and harms of each of these materials. Conversely, Ibn al-Sunni included most of the discussion of fruits and meats in a single treatise as opposed to dedicating one treatise to meats and one to fruits. In short, Abū Nuʿaym followed the overall structure of Ibn al-Sunnī's work with few organizational differences. This may be attributed to Abū Nuʿaym's interests or to the fact that he may have had access to a slightly different text of Ibn al-Sunnī's than the one that survived.

The new prophetic medical corpus

Along with a new structure and organizational priorities, Abū Nuʿaym's book provided new sources and a new corpus of prophetic medical knowledge. By corpus,

I refer to traditions, anecdotes, materials, and areas of concern that became available to other ḥadīth scholars and played an important role in constructing the literature on prophetic medicine. In addition to the reorganization of the materials in a manner similar to medical books, Abū Nuʿaym expanded the corpus in three main ways: the introduction of new, unique, or otherwise weak and unknown ḥadīths and anecdotes; the rearrangement and reinterpretation of known ḥadīths to serve medical purposes, which they did not before; and settling or shifting the discussion of central themes in previous medical prophetics literature. Throughout, the book was permeated with deep connections to Galenism and humoral theory. Although the four humors were not explicitly discussed, nor were any details of humoral physiology, the description of diseases and their treatments utilized humoral language and repurposed Galenic concepts, as will be seen later.

New traditions

As one of the more important scholars of ḥadīth in his time, Abū Nuʿaym surely knew how scholars classified each and every ḥadīth in his book and would have been able to expand on any of the (deliberately) brief chains of transmission. However, he still included traditions that were universally recognized as "strange (*gharīb*)" and "weak (*ḍaʿīf*)" and reported traditions from people who were generally classified as untrustworthy or even lying (*kadhūb*). Ibn al-Sunnī's more limited set of traditions seemed to have fared somewhat better. He explained in his introduction that he chose the more trustworthy traditions from the larger corpus that existed in his larger text. In the discussion of eye ailments for instance, both Ibn al-Sunnī and Abū Nuʿaym reported a tradition where the prophet said, "The only [real] concern is one about religion, and the only [real] pain is one affecting the eye."[108] The tradition was used to introduce the chapter and to signify how the eyes were precious organs. However, the tradition was categorized as "denied (*munkar*)" by the majority of scholars contemporaneous to Ibn al-Sunnī and Abū Nuʿaym – a fact that they no doubt knew. In another tradition in the same chapter, the prophet was reported to have rubbed ʿAlī ibn Abī Ṭālib's eyes with his own [the prophet's] saliva when ʿAlī complained of pain in his eyes.[109] This tradition was seen as *munkar* as well by Sunni scholars, especially because the reporter was known to be an avowed Shiite who was deemed a liar by Sunni reporters. Similarly, in another tradition, this time reported by Jaʿfar al-Ṣādiq through his father and grandfather up to ʿAlī ibn Abī Ṭālib, "A man complained to the prophet of his few offspring. The prophet ordered him to eat eggs. The man asked, 'what eggs, O prophet of God?' The prophet said, 'Eat any eggs even if ant eggs."[110] This tradition was also deemed *ḍaʿīf* or *munkar* by contemporaneous and later scholars of ḥadīth. Moreover, it relied on a traditionally Shiite chain of transmission (through multiple imams), which was hardly used by Sunni scholars.[111] The same applies to another tradition reported on the authority of Salmān al-Fārisī about toothache, in which the prophet instructed the patient to eat palm dates.[112]

In addition to these weak traditions and a number of similarly weak or weaker ones, Abū Nuʿaym introduced traditions that could not be found in any of the other known compilations at the time. In one of these traditions, the prophet's wife Umm Salamah reported that when one of the prophet's wives complained of her eyes, the prophet would not have sex with her until she recovered.[113] The practice of introducing new traditions was not limited to this one occasion but rather included a few other occasions across the book. In one tradition, ʿAlī reported that the prophet said, "Eat raisins! It treats [yellow] bile, dissolves phlegm, strengthens the nerves, treats fatigue, improves composition, sweetens the breath and treats worries."[114] The tradition, which was first reported by Abū Nuʿaym, included important medical information and connected raisins to specific humoral signifiers such as bile and phlegm. Another tradition that was recognized by other scholars as unique and unreported before was also from Umm Salamah, who described a recipe of flour and ghee that was used to treat different ailments.[115] A third tradition was also reported on the authority of ʿAlī ibn Abī Ṭālib and discussed the values of palm trees and of palm dates.[116]

Remarkably, the majority of the traditions deemed as weak by contemporaneous Sunni scholars and all of the traditions that were first reported by Abū Nuʾaym relied on chains of transmissions or originators that were more common in Shiite ḥadīth or were respected by Shiite scholars. For instance, the majority of these traditions originated with ʿAlī ibn Abī Ṭālib, the first imam. Others originated with Umm Salamah, one of Muḥammad's wives esteemed by Shiites, and Salmān al-Fārisi and Abū Dharr al-Ghaffārī,[117] among other companions who were particularly revered and trusted by Shiite scholars. The chains of transmissions in these traditions raise the possibility that they were known to some degree among Shiite scholars with whom Abū Nuʿaym was connected.

As mentioned before, the use of weak or untrustworthy traditions in topics related to piety or to other adab-related volumes was not an unknown practice. In fact, many scholars of ḥadīth, including Abū Nuʿaym and his illustrious student al-Khaṭīb al-Baghdādī, used these traditions frequently and believed it was legitimate to utilize them in pietistic writings and to address other nonlegal concerns.[118] Medicine appeared to have been part of these pietistic and adab-esque topics which demanded less scrutiny and allowed compilers to accept varieties of traditions that were known to be weak or even forged. Similarly, both Ibn al-Sunnī and Abū Nuʿaym were clear in their desire to trim the chains of transmission, a move that would be seen later as problematic because it permitted people to trust traditions that should not be trusted. As the literature adapted more medical priorities and organizational formats, the role of chains of transmission and the importance of selectivity in choosing traditions receded, giving more space for newer, weaker, and more "odd" traditions that fit the chapters better and responded to the pietistic needs of this emerging subgenre.

Repurposed ḥadīths

In addition to using these new or weak traditions, Ibn al-Sunnī and Abū Nuʿaym utilized traditions that earlier scholars classified in chapters other than medicine in their *muṣannaf* texts. These traditions were seen by scholars as serving other purposes and answering questions that were not directly related to medicine. By including them in medical discussions, Ibn al-Sunnī and Abū Nuʿaym expanded the sources from which later scholars of prophetic medicine could draw and changed the landscape of medical prophetics. Whereas previous literature had been driven by the prophet's history of health and illness and focused primarily on anecdotes of his sickness, the new literature introduced by Ibn al-Sunnī and Abū Nuʿaym was driven by medical concerns. Therefore, this new literature addressed issues that were not previously discussed by scholars of ḥadīth, which made selecting and reinterpreting traditions a necessity to fill gaps in the corpus of medical prophetics. This is not to say that the central stories animating chapters on medical prophetics disappeared or that information about the prophet's episodes of illness were no longer included. These materials continued in the writings of Ibn al-Sunnī and Abū Nuʿaym. However, the new arrangement and new organizational priorities shifted and dispersed these materials, allowing them to serve various purposes, including but not limited to discussing specific conditions, cures, or procedures and items of materia medica.

For instance, Abū Nuʿaym included a tradition that was commonly reported in chapters about ritual cleanliness in which the prophet advised a man with bandages to wipe over the bandages when cleaning himself; from this tradition, Abū Nuʿaym commenced a discussion on bandages, wounds, and broken bones.[119] One of the clearest and most important examples of this process of reinterpretation and rearrangement came in a number of chapters that addressed questions never discussed before in the medical prophetics literature: women's diseases, sexual desires, and sexual prowess. In the first group, Ibn al-Sunnī and Abū Nuʿaym attempted to address questions related to "ailments of the womb," "the difference between menstrual and non-menstrual bleeding," "the changing odor of blood, after menstruation," "tightening the vagina and drying it" (to enhance sexual pleasure), and "feeding mothers after they give birth." In these chapters, Ibn al-Sunnī and Abū Nu'aym relied primarily on traditions that were classified in chapters about ritual cleaning, about women, or about menstruation.[120] For instance, in one tradition, a woman asked the prophet about her obligations to pray while having continuous bleeding. He explained to her that only menstruation exempted her from prayer. Once menstruations ended, she should use cloth to control the bleeding and pray normally, "The prophet said: 'Menstrual blood is dark. If [your bleeding] was of that [color and variety], stop praying. If it was another [type of bleeding], perform the ablution and pray. It is only a vein.'"[121] The tradition was seen by other compilers as relevant, not in chapters of medicine, but rather on one related to prayer, ritual purity, or menstruation. To supplement these traditions, Abū Nu'aym also used anecdotes by companions such as ʿAlī ibn Abī Ṭālib and ʿUmar ibn al-Khaṭṭāb that addressed similar issues. In discussing tightening the vagina, Abū Nuʿaym reported an anecdote in which the Umayyad Caliph ʿAbd al-Malik ibn Marwān insulted his general, al-Ḥajjāj ibn Yūsuf, calling the latter's mother "a vagina-tightener," which Abū Nu'aym explained indicated her promiscuity.[122] The anecdote was unrelated to the prophet or any of his companions because ʿAbd al-Malik was not considered a trustworthy companion by either Sunnis or Shiites. Moreover, it had no medical relevance, and it was not even related to the desire or the recipes needed to tighten vaginas. True to the adab form, however, Abū Nuʿaym reported this anecdote to simply introduce the linguistic uses of the phrase and its various connotations.

A second group of chapters included discussions of male sexual prowess, enhancing sexual desires and improving erection. Although a number of the musannaf texts included chapters on sex, which focused mainly on male sexual desires and enhancement, these were not seen within the scope of medicine and were not included in medical chapters. Here, Ibn al-Sunnī and Abū Nuʿaym included traditions from these chapters on sex but also from chapters on cleanliness, prayers, and even from the para-Quranic and exegetical literature. For instance, in one tradition reported by Abū Nuʿaym, it was reported that the prophet used to bathe after having sex with each of his wives even if he was planning on having sex with another one in the same night. When one of his companions asked him why he would not bathe only once in a given night, the prophet explained that this was cleaner and helped him smell better. In a similar tradition reported by both Ibn al-Sunnī and Abū Nuʿaym, the prophet advised that one should wash between different acts of intercourse with his wife. The tradition was located in chapters on cleanliness. Ibn al-Sunnī and Abū Nuʿaym included the tradition in their discussion of sex, indicating that these baths may have enhanced the prophet's sexual prowess or were part of the prophet's sexual etiquette.[123] In another tradition, a man explained to the prophet that he stopped eating meat because it gave him strong and sustained erections that bothered him. A verse was revealed admonishing people for prohibiting what God allowed, and the prophet ordered the man not to categorically prohibit himself from meat.[124] The tradition was more common in exegetical literature in relation to the referenced verse, "O believers, forbid not such good things as God has permitted you; and transgress not; God loves not transgressors [Q5:87]."[125] Exegetes were not interested in the details of the man's claims about his erection but rather in his self-imposed prohibition and restriction. However, Abū Nuʿaym placed the tradition in a chapter that discussed ways to enhance erections, using the tradition to indicate that meat enhanced erections and sexual prowess.

Even some of the traditions that had existed in medical chapters in previous collections before were reinterpreted to serve multiple purposes and serve in various chapters. In one tradition, the angel Gabriel advised Muḥammad to eat harissa to strengthen his back so that he could pray through the night.[126] Although Abū Nuʿaym reported the tradition in the chapter related to back pain, he used the linguistic connection between the back and sex (in that seeds originated in the back in traditional Arabic writings) to explain the tradition as one related to increasing sexual powers and fertility.[127] In this case, repeating the tradition served to use it for the two different chapters.

In all these cases and others, Ibn al-Sunnī and Abū Nuʿaym were confronted by the need to fill important chapters that were posed by their organizational scheme and not by the sources that they derived their traditions from. Compilers and authors arranged the traditions they had in chapters that corresponded to them. As such, chapters did not aim to cover all aspects of a given question or attempt to address all legal or pietistic questions. Instead, they expressed the best and most reasonable way to arrange an existing corpus. For Abū Nuʿaym, the chapters were not built on the corpus, but rather, the corpus was being rearranged to fill empty chapters. Ostensibly, chapters were built around the priorities of medical writings and of the reading habits and interests of readers of medical texts. The compilers were left with the task of filling these preconstructed chapters which pushed him to use weak or largely unknown ḥadīth traditions and to repurpose and reinterpret other ḥadīth traditions to fill these gaps. The result was the construction of a new archive of ḥadīth materials that were now able to fill these various chapters.

Re-engaging the questions of medical prophetics

Ibn al-Sunnī's and Abū Nuʿaym's texts engaged with the common tropes in medical prophetics literature, including the legality of medical practice or of using prohibited materials like alcohol for treatment. However, their engagement with these common tropes was inconsistent, as they dropped or disregarded some other themes that were discussed consistently in previous writings but that did not seem to concern them as much. For instance, Ibn al-Sunnī and Abū Nuʿaym engaged with these issues in the beginning of their books, accepting the legality of seeking cure and noting that the prophet recommended curing different diseases.[128] They also engaged with the legality of using prohibited materials for treatment[129] and with the legality of women treating and tending to sick men.[130] In both cases, Ibn al-Sunnī and Abū Nuʿaym agreed with the majority of ḥadīth compilers in rejecting the former and accepting the latter. Moreover, their discussion of the prophet's favorite treatments, like cupping, honey, the black seed, dates, etc., were distributed across the texts and organized alongside similar plants and materials or in relation to specific diseases. Although these treatments were indeed discussed in Ibn al-Sunnī's and Abū Nuʿaym's texts similar to other medical prophetics chapters, their special organization schema led to a different presentation.

On the other hand, Ibn al-Sunnī's and Abū Nuʿaym's texts did not dedicate much space or engage directly with the central anecdotes concerning the prophet's sickness and health, which were central to medical prophetics as discussed in the first chapter. Similarly, Abū Nu'aym did not engage in any discussion of magic or of the evil eye, which were consistent themes in medical prophetics. This might be due to the fact that these topics did not figure in medical texts on which Abū Nuʿaym based the structure of his book. He also did not address ruqya or the legality of amulets, which were both consistent discussions in other texts.[131] The question of contagion, which was addressed at a number of levels in discussions of leprosy and plague, was among the more contentious issues in various compilations, with scholars recording traditions supporting different, and sometimes contradictory, views and positions.[132] In Ibn al-Sunnī's and Abū Nuʿaym's texts, plague disappeared almost completely and none of the traditions related to plague were mentioned or discussed. Similarly, contagion, which was often connected to discussions of superstition, prognostication, and fortunetelling, was not discussed explicitly by Ibn al-Sunnī or Abū Nuʿaym. Instead, Abū Nuʿaym placed few traditions that concern contagion in the context of his discussion of leprosy. Whereas most other chapters of medical prophetics in ḥadīth compilations combined traditions that recommended avoiding the leper with others that recommended eating with them, Abū Nuʿaym chose to report only traditions that recommended keeping a distance from them and avoiding looking at them directly.[133] The rest of the discussion on leprosy focused on its prevention and treatment, with the authors limiting their traditions to those that discussed how it was caused and how it could be treated.[134]

Similar to medical prophetics writings, Ibn al-Sunnī and Abū Nuʿaym paid attention to the divine rewards attached to diseases and to how patience and forbearance delivered rewards to the sick. They included references to divine rewards for the sick in a number of chapters, such as those on headache[135] and on eye ailments.[136] For instance, in discussing headache, Abū Nuʿaym reported a tradition where the prophet asked a Bedouin whether he ever suffered from headache. The man did not even know the meaning of the word and, after the prophet explained it, he denied ever having such condition. The prophet looked to his companions when the man left and said, "If one wants to observe a man who will reside in hellfire, here he is."[137] The tradition was meant to underscore how headaches and fevers, among other diseases, were ways by which a person can repent their sins. As such, the man who never suffered from such conditions may well be weighed down by his sins and end in hellfire. As will be seen in Chapter 3, different renditions of this tradition were central to various pietistic narratives about illness.

Throughout the text, Ibn al-Sunnī and Abū Nuʿaym made important connections to Galenic/humoral explanations of various conditions, further emphasizing the medical nature of the book and departing from previous literature. In addition to the previously mentioned examples, Abū Nuʿaym's discussions of various foods included descriptions of their complexion, where the author explained that they were cold, hot, dry, or humid.[138] With certain materials, he explained their effect on various humors, whether beneficial or harmful.[139] Sometimes, Ibn al-Sunnī's and Abū Nuʿaym's explanations seemed to be out of sync with the prophetic materials that they cited. For instance, when discussing animal fetal meat, they both reported a tradition where the prophet was asked, "O prophet of God, we slaughter a cow or a camel and find a fetus inside. Are we permitted to eat it?" The prophet said, "They [the fetuses] are ritually pure through the purification of their mothers' meat."[140] Similar to other traditions that Ibn al-Sunnī and Abū Nuʿaym included, this tradition did not have a specific medical significance and only indicated the legality and purity of fetal meat. Ibn al-Sunnī and Abū Nuʿaym used it to discuss fetal flesh, which they considered to be medically harmful, and advised against eating it.

Moreover, Ibn al-Sunnī and Abū Nuʿaym implied specific humoral explanations were embedded in the prophetic corpus. For instance, in discussing headache, they outlined two major types of headache in two subchapters: one caused by yellow bile or exhaustion and one caused by blood. For the first, they used traditions that described the prophet's suffering from headaches after encounters with Gabriel and after instances of revelation. In Ibn al-Sunnī's and Abū Nuʿaym's interpretation, these headaches, which were caused by exhaustion, were similar to headaches caused by yellow bile or exhaustion.[141] On the other hand, they assumed that any condition for which the prophet recommended cupping, including headache or toothache, was caused by blood.[142] As such, they included traditions about treating headaches with cupping in a section for blood-caused headaches.

In the beginning of their books, Ibn al-Sunnī and Abū Nuʿaym each explained that their books were structured along the lines and methods of physicians. To achieve this goal, Ibn al-Sunnī, followed by Abū Nuʿaym, created chapters that resembled those in medical textbooks which they proceeded to fill with traditions, most of which came from previous sources of medical prophetics, but some of which were entirely new. Still others were reinterpreted from other chapters of prophetics and other ḥadīth texts and given medical meanings and connotations. They also expanded the corpus by including traditions that were weak and even suspect in their accounts. Finally, the texts were imbued with Galenic/humoral signifiers, from how diseases were described and diagnosed to how food materials and recipes were understood. In this process, a lot of the traditional concerns of the medical prophetics literature disappeared or were displaced to the margins as ḥadīth traditions were rearranged in the new medicalized texts.

The influence of Ibn al-Sunnī's and Abū Nuʿaym's book could be seen for centuries to come. The texts were the earliest influential writings that engaged with the production of a new archive of prophetic materials that engaged concretely and consistently with medical knowledge by covering different topics on medicine that were not addressed in other writings of medical prophetics. As explained before, this level of engagement allowed for the construction of a new archive of prophetic materials, some of which were introduced anew, brought to Sunni writings from Shiite traditions, admitted and rehabilitated from suspicious sources, or repurposed from other chapters or other locations in the prophetic archive. At another level, this engagement engendered new perspectives on health and on the performance of healthy bodies. In these texts, the body was one that required care and attention, and the knowledge of the body, as well as of the different materials, foods, drinks, activities that influenced its health, were rooted not only in a medical narrative but also in a pietistic and prophetic one. Ibn al-Sunnī and Abū Nuʿaym produced these narratives of bodily care, treatment, and health preservation at the intersection of three bodies of knowledge: the Galenic textual tradition, which inspired the organization of the treatises, Galenic thought and practice, which informed much of the medical discussion of the treatises, and the prophetic archive, which supplied almost all of the "little narratives" in these treatises. As such, Ibn al-Sunnī's and Abū Nuʿaym's writings attempted to chart a pietistic performance of medical knowledge and a pietistic approach to the management of healthy bodies. The resulting new archive and the rich intersections, at which it was produced, would continue to inform the practice of this medical piety for centuries to come.

The piety of health: *The Golden Treatise* and Imām ʿAlī al-Riḍā

ʿAlī al-Riḍā (d. 818) was the reigning imam for Twelver Shiites and a respected figure among most ʻAlids of the time. A descendent of the lineage of al-Ḥusayn, Muḥammad's grandson, Alī al-Riḍā was the heir to the imamate after his father Mūsā al-Kāẓim and commanded the loyalty of large contingents of Shiites and Alids in Iraq and in many of the eastern regions of the Abbasid caliphate.[143] It is for these reasons that al-Maʾmūn's decision to appoint al-Riḍā as his heir to the caliphal throne was one of the more politically challenging moments of al-Maʾmūn's reign.[144] The reasons and motivations behind al-Maʾmūn's decision were usually colored by the religious and political sentiments of the commentators. Whereas many Sunni authors, who disliked al-Maʾmūn for his pro-Mutazilite views, accused him of assenting to Shiite demands, many Shiite authors considered his decision to be part of his political cunning and an attempt at subverting brewing Shiite mutinies and rebellions.[145] Their views are confirmed by what Shiite near-contemporary scholars argued: that al-Maʿmūn poisoned ʿAlī al-Riḍā to escape a toxic political situation in which he had put himself by appointing him and which led to significant discomfort, if not rebellion, among Abbasid emirs and in the Abbasid capital. Such in-house difficulties were as significant as an attempt to overthrow him in Baghdad; he was able to quash these efforts while he resided in Marv.

Regardless of the political circumstances around the appointment and the death of the heir to the caliphate, ʿAlī al-Riḍā became part of the Abbasid court and an active participant in al-Maʾmūn's circle of scholars and his court's intellectual activities. When he decided to appoint him, al-Ma'mūn summoned al-Riḍā from Medina, where he and his father before him had resided, to join al-Maʾmūn's court in Marv.[146] Although he presumably detested the move, al-Riḍā obeyed the caliph and honored his request, taking a long tortuous route that was designed by al-Maʾmūn and his entourage to avoid major ʿAlid centers like al-Kūfah and Qum, isolating the imam from his most ardent supporters, according to Shiite historians.[147] When he arrived and was finally appointed the heir to the caliphal throne, he joined the court and became well known for his contributions to various debates and discussions in the court. The most famous debates that the imam participated in were ones concerning the nature of the divine, the difference between God's identity and his attributes, and the doctrine of the infallibility of the prophets.[148] *The Golden Treatise* purported to report one of these discussions, which was related to medicine, and ended in al-Maʾmūn's requesting ʿAlī al-Riḍā to compose a treatise on the subject.[149] Some weeks later, when al-Maʿmūn was in Ṭūs, he sent a message to al-Riḍā, urging him to finish the treatise and asking him to send it as soon as it was finished. When the treatise was finally completed and received by al-Maʾmūn, the caliph was so delighted and impressed that he ordered the treatise to be written in gold water, and it was hence named *Al-Risālah al-Dhahabiyyah* (The Golden Treatise). Other reports claimed that al-Maʿmūn showed the treatise to a number of physicians who were equally impressed by Imam ʿAlī's knowledge.[150]

The authorship of the treatise is subject to doubts. Notably, a number of contemporary and near-contemporary sources did not mention the treatise nor discuss it, which is surprising considering the importance of its author.[151] This, however, may have been influenced by al-Maʾmūn's anti-ʿAlid policies following the death of ʿAlī al-Riḍā, which included his ordering the governors of different regions to wash and cleanse the pulpits from which ʿAlī al-Riḍā was pronounced heir to the throne.[152] Anti-ʿAlid sentiments further intensified under Maʾmūn's successors, which may explain why Ibn al-Nadīm did not mention this treatise in his *Fihrist*. Sunni sources aside, it is instructive that the treatise was never mentioned in the most authoritative hagiography of Imam ʿAlī al-Riḍā: al-Shaykh al-Ṣadūq's, Muḥammad ibn ʿAlī ibn Bābawayh al-Qummī (d. 991), *ʿUyūn akhbār al-Riḍā* (The most prominent anecdotes about al-Riḍā). Ibn Bābawayh was not only a hagiographer of the imam but also an author of one the most important Twelver ḥadīth collections. A son of a well-known scholar in his own right, Abū Jaʿfar ibn Bābawayh, he grew up in the city of Qum and then traveled to Baghdad to begin a long career of travel, learning, and writing that earned him the title *al-shaykh al-sadūq* (the truthful scholar).[153] Ibn Bābawayh's views on the centrality of ḥadīth matched the views of his contemporary, al-Kulaynī, who also argued for the absolute rejection of speculation in favor of the views of the imams.[154] This deep interest in ḥadīth and significant devotion to ʿAlī al-Riḍā in particular, being the only imam for which Ibn Bābawayh wrote a hagiography, further underscores the fact that *The Golden Treatise* was not mentioned and raises the possibility that Ibn Bābawayh had no knowledge of this treatise or that the treatise was not known when he composed his book before 991.

The earliest mention of this treatise could be found a century later in (yet another) *Fihrist* by the famous Shiite scholar, Abū Jaʿfar al-Ṭūsī (995–1067).[155] In al-Ṭūsī's account of Shiite authors and ḥadīth reporters, he mentioned Muḥammad ibn al-Ḥasan ibn Jamhūr al-Qummī al-Baṣrī, who reported *The Golden Treatise* on the authority of Imām Alī al-Riḍa himself.[156] Although Ibn Jamhūr was a relatively prolific author, we know little about his life and lack the precise dates of his birth and death. We know that he was a good writer, that he was friends with al-Qāḍī ʿAlī al-Tanūkhī's father, and taught the son some reading and writing as a child,[157] which means that Ibn Jamhūr was alive in the 940s, as al-Tanūkhī was born in 939. Also, al-Ṭūsī mentioned that Ibn Jamhūr's works and ḥadīths were transmitted by a number of people, including al-ʿAmrakī ibn ʿAlī (fl. Before 874) and ʿAlī ibn al-Ḥusayn ibn Saʿīd al-Ahwāzī (fl. Ca. 868). This places Ibn Jamhūr's activity in the period from 860s to 940s. Ibn Jamhūr mentioned that he heard about and reported *Al-Risālah al-Dhahabiyyah* or *The Golden Treatise* on the authority of his father, Muḥammad ibn Jamhūr, who was a respected Shiite reporter and a contemporary of ʿAlī al-Riḍā and reported many traditions on ʿAlī al-Riḍā's authority.[158]

The evidence from Ibn Bābawyah and al-Tūsī's writings suggest that the treatise came to be known sometime between ca. 990 and ca.1065. Although this suggested dating places the treatise more than a century after the death of ʿAlī al-Riḍā, it appears that it enjoyed the approval of the highest echelons of the

Twelver Shiite community, who did not seem bothered by this gap in its history. For one, al-Ṭūsī himself was the most prominent student of al-Sharīf al-Murtaḍā (965–1044), himself a descendant of Imam Mūsā al-Kāẓim and a grand-nephew of ʿAlī al-Riḍā. Al-Ṭūsī was in contact with many members of the ʿAlid household, who likely did not object to the attribution of the treatise, suggesting that it did not appear out of complete obscurity. The same is true about al-ʿAmrakī ibn ʿAlī, who reported from Ibn Jamhūr and who was a client of Imam al-ʿAskarī (d. 874), who was the eleventh imam and the direct descendent (great grandson) of ʿAlī al-Riḍa himself. It is difficult to suppose that al-ʿAmrakī would report from Ibn Jamhūr on his accounts about Imam Alī al-Riḍā without this being known to Imām al-ʿAskarī. Similarly, ʿAlī ibn al-Ḥusayn, the other reporter from Ibn Jamhūr, was the son, student, and heir of al-Ḥusayn al-Ahwāzī, who was a close companion of Alī al-Riḍā himself.[159] The fact that he reported from Ibn Jamhūr indicates that the latter's accounts were seen as truthful and were largely accepted by those closest to the heritage of ʿAlī al-Riḍā.

Although none of these connections provide evidence that ʿAlī al-Riḍā was the author of *The Golden Treatise*, they indicate that this treatise circulated among some of the more important and well-known Shiite scholars of the tenth and eleventh centuries, including direct descendants of Imam ʿAlī al-Riḍā himself and others who belonged to his family or were taught by his companions and students. As such, and despite the doubts on its authorship, it is clear that the contents of the treatise were perfectly acceptable and represented what could be the general consensus in these circles of high culture in major Abbasid centers.

The treatise's context

Regardless of the actual date and context of its appearance, the *Golden Treatise* created a unique internal context where the conditions of its composition were reported as part of the treatise itself. The self-reported setting for commissioning the treatise and the occasion for its composition were deeply important for its meaning, role, and significance. The narrator mentions some of the names in attendance in al-Maʿmūn's court, as they discussed questions of medicine, such as the harms and benefits of food and drink or, "How God has composed the [human] body and created it from these contradictory four natures?" The people in attendance included three famous physicians of the ninth and tenth centuries: Yūḥannā ibn Masāwayh, the famous physician and the appointed chief of the House of Wisdom; Jibrīl ibn Bakhtishūʿ, the patriarch of the famous medical dynasty and a prominent physician in the Abbasid court following his father and brother; and Ṣāliḥ ibn Bahlah al-Hindī, who was an Indian physician and possibly the son of another Indian physician who served Hārūn al-Rashīd, al-Maʿmūn's father.[160] Witnessing this discussion, ʿAlī al-Riḍā remained silent as the caliph and his physicians discussed questions of medicine until the caliph asked about his opinion. The reported silence of the imam plays an important rhetorical and discursive function in the text, indicating his reliance on a knowledge and a tradition superior to those propagated by the physicians. Unlike al-Maʾmūn, who was quite concerned and somewhat perplexed by these questions, ʿAlī al-Riḍā explained,

> In this matter [of medicine and healing], I know what I have tried and asserted its correctness by experiment over time, along with what I have learned from my ancestors, that which man cannot be ignorant of and cannot be excused for casting away.[161]

The sources that al-Riḍā cites served to further the authority of his statements. Instead of referencing physicians and medical authorities, he emphasized his own experience and the experiences and traditions of his ancestors – those of Muḥammad's lineage. The statement emphasized the normative sources of the imam's knowledge[162] and his own thinking and experience and the traditions of his ancestors and imbued the treatise with the power and authority of the imam himself.[163] The difference between al-Riḍā and al-Maʾmūn in needing this information is equally revealing of their varying statuses in the minds of the authors and readers of the treatise. The first was the imam, the source of divine and divinely inspired knowledge on earth, and the second was an educated Abbasid caliph, who came to recognize the truth of ʿAlid claims – hence appointing al-Riḍā as his heir – but remained short of the knowledge of the imam. Even the caliph needed the imam's knowledge and experience, underlined by the fact that al-Maʾmūn asked ʿAlī al-Riḍā to write this treatise. In fact, al-Maʾmūn seemed insistent on having this treatise, as he sent a second request after he journeyed to Balkh.[164]

Yet, despite the imam's insistence on this knowledge being based on his inherited knowledge and acquired experience, the treatise proceeds in very familiar Galenic terms. In the introduction, the four humors are mentioned as the basis for the making of the human body. As we move through the treatise, we find more evidence for the treatise's complete reliance on Galenic ideas and recommendations about the human body despite the presence of the Indian physician, Ṣāliḥ ibn Bahlah, at Maʾmūn's court according to the treatise. The treatise, as the work not of a physician but of a litterateur, composed by or attributed to a figure of tremendous knowledge, culture, and authority, stands to describe this body, what it meant, what it required and how it was understood in this period. Imbued with the authority of the imam, the treatise eloquently showed how the tenth-century pietistic body emerged in the context of the Abbasid intellectual milieu, Arabicized from various Greek, Persian, Indian, and Arab origins, to form the Islamic body that would serve as the subject of medical knowledge and practice for centuries to come. In the subsequent pages, we will trace how the treatise understood and described the body and how this body resonated with other authors in the period.

The pious galenic body

The treatise begins with the prophetic tradition that remains central to all literature on prophetic medicine: God has not created an illness without also creating a cure for it. Here, however, the tradition was not cited from the Prophet but rather mentioned as part of what the imam thought himself.[165] The formulation served as a form of pietistic basis for medical practice. It was the legal justification for seeking treatment as well as the legal and pietistic grounding for the development and study of the science of medicine. Medicine and treatment was not seen as defying God's will, but rather as acting on His plans. The formulation stops short of proclaiming treatment or learning medicine a religious obligation and leaves space for patience and forbearance as responses to illness.[166] Although the treatise says that the body is created healthy, the body was portrayed in the treatise as fragile, and in need of constant care. The treatise proclaimed:

> The body is like a fertile, uncultivated land. If it is cared for with cultivation and irrigation, not given too much water so that it drowns or too little so that it grows desiccated, it will flourish, its profit will increase and its produce will grow. If one ignores it, it will become corrupted and grass will claim it. The Body is like that. And management of food and drink benefits it and provides it with health and wellness.[167]

In the treatise's view, the body was healthy and fertile, but it could not survive except by careful consideration of everything that it consumed and encountered.

In the same way, the body was also deeply connected to its environment and could be influenced by the slightest change in the environment that surrounds it. Travelers needed to be careful about their food, as they should not travel while full or while hungry and should strive to be always satisfied without fullness.[168] Strange and unusual water could cause problems to travelers, because the body was not able to adjust to sudden changes:

> The traveler should not drink from each place where he stops, except after mixing this place's water with the water of the place that preceded it, or with a single drink that is not different and that would mix with the different waters. The traveler should also carry [some] of the soil of his home so that he would throw some of that soil in the water of each new places he descends to.[169]

In the same way, this connection to the environment was also evident in the different measures required for each season and each month of the year in order to protect the body from seasonal dangers.

The treatise went through each of the four seasons and each of the twelve months of the solar calendar (using Greek months), explaining the nature of their weather; the potential problems; and the necessary foods, drinks, and sexual habits for each of these times.[170] The effect of the different seasons could be understood by understanding the composition of the body,

> Because God has built [human] bodies on four natures: blood, phlegm, yellow bile and black bile. Two are hot and two are cold. They were conversely

> matched so that they are hot and dry, hot and soft (*layyin*), cold and dry, and cold and soft.[171]

Although the treatise conforms to the traditional Galenic discourse, which associated the four humors with the specific organs that produced them, the treatise deviated significantly from the Galenic narrative, as it enumerated the head, the chest, the omentum, and the bottom of the belly as the four areas in which these humors reside,

> [God] had then divided these on four parts of the body: the head, the chest, the omentum and the bottom of the belly. Know, O Prince of the Believers, that the head, ears, eyes, nose, nostrils and mouth are of blood; that the chest is of phlegm and wind, the omentum of yellow bile and the bottom of the belly of black bile.[172]

Importantly, the organs and body parts that are described here are far from the Galenic views on the matter, despite the prevalence of a humoral description on the body's composition among many scholars writing in the period. These descriptions rely more on visual resemblance and connection based on function and name, such as the chest with phlegm and air and the omentum with yellow bile.

The four humors structure lent itself to further elaboration on the virtue of moderation, one that permeated the entire text and was repeated frequently as the central rationale behind all advice given in the treatise. As it was made of four humors delicately balanced, this balance was always subject to disturbance, requiring constant care. As seen before, changes in the environment could lead to unforeseen problems, and bad habits, bad foods, or even inopportune activities could also disturb this balance. Even the temperature and the environment of the bathhouse needed to be managed to suit the nature of the body, the season and the month of the year, and the needs of the bather.[173] One rule governed all: moderation is key in all activities involving the body. The treatise warns the caliph:

> Never say "I have always done so and so and ate so and so and it never harmed me; or I have drunk so and so and it did not hurt me; or I have done so and so and I have not been ill." Those who say so, my lord the Prince of Believers, are like a beast that does not know what harms and what benefits it. [Consider that] if a thief is caught the first time he steals, was punished and never stole again, his punishment would be easier. However, [God] gives him time and power so he [steals] again, until he is caught with the biggest of thefts so he is mutilated, is severely humiliated; a result of his greed.[174]

The fact that one could be used to bad habits but that these bad habits should never be indulged emphasized the necessity of self-reflection that was guided by overall principles and laws and not just by previous experience. In this context, the narrative of preserving health acquired the characters of a pietistic narrative about self-reflection and self-care.

The unique and fragile balance on which the body is built is further evidenced in the changes that occur in the body because of age. Again, life could be divided into four main states, each of which is under the control of one of the four humors, where its nature dominates. From birth to fifteen years of age, the body is under the control of blood, showing vigor and constant growth. The reign of the yellow bile follows, from ages fifteen to thirty-five, which is the best, most active and balanced stage of life. The third stage, which is under the reign of black bile, extends from ages thirty-five to sixty years of age. Here, the person is at their wisest, most knowledgeable, and most trustworthy. The fourth stage, which extends from age sixty to the time of death, is under the rein of phlegm and is the worst of the four, featuring forgetfulness, estrangement, and difficulties in sleep and speech.[175]

Although the body is said to be composed of four humors in some form of balance, it is not a single whole, nor are each of its parts of equal importance. The body is like a kingdom, the treatise explained, in which the heart is king and the vessels are its workers and servants. The head is the house of the king, and the whole body is his land, "His servants are his hands, legs, eyes, lips, tongue and ears; his treasures are his stomach and his belly, his chest and his diaphragm"[176] The metaphor of the kingdom was repeated many times, for centuries to come, to describe the hierarchy of different parts of the body as well as the value of each of these parts. The metaphor showed the confusion and hesitation related to the relative positions of the heart and the head: Which of the two reigned over the rest of the body? Ultimately, the treatise opted for the heart over the head, a choice consistent with previous accounts from prophetic traditions and Quranic heritage. The metaphor emphasized the connections between different parts of the body, underscoring the need for care and vigilance but also explaining how drugs taken in one vein or in one part of the body can affect the rest of it.

The treatise paid significant attention to healthy habits for eating, drinking, sleeping, having sex, etc. The idea that one should strive to develop correct and healthy habits was mentioned a few times in the treatise, where the caliph was advised to pay attention to what he did. The notion of the habit was embedded in the idea that repeating small violations or wrongdoings would lead to serious problems, many of which might not result from one single instance of wrong behavior. For instance, drinking cold water after soft fish resulted, over time, in hemiplegia,[177] eating pears at night led to squint,[178] and sex with menstruating women led to leprosy in the child. Similarly, eating figs "to the extent of addiction" resulted in lice infestation[179] and eating raw meat generated worms in the stomach.[180] The treatise used the verb *yuwarrith* (lit. bequeath) to describe most of these conditions. The verb indicated the gradual process of the development of these conditions and how the effects might appear after the actual causing acts had ceased. This insistence on habits and repetition highlighted the importance of vigilance in relation to health and of the importance of habits, bad or good, in the making of health and disease. The idea of habits and the development of these habits is central to the view that the body was similar to a land requiring constant care and attention. As will be seen in Chapter 4, the question of habits played an important role in instilling spiritual health as well.

Following the overarching theme of moderation, the treatise advised that the caliph should eat cold foods in the summer and hot or warm foods in the winter and moderate food in all seasons.[181] One should prefer eating lighter foods, using local foods that the body is used to, which are suitable to the activity and the time of day. But in general, one should eat eight hours after the beginning of the day or eat three times every two days,

> You would eat lunch early in the first day and then eat dinner. In the second day, you eat eight hours after the beginning of daytime and you would not need dinner. In all cases, [you] should eat specific amounts, that do not increase or decrease, leave food while still desiring it, and have aged, pure drink, that is legally permissible, after food.[182]

Finally, some foods were better avoided altogether, as they could cause specific problems if consumed regularly or excessively. For instance, eggs could cause problems in the spleen and gases in the stomach, and boiled eggs caused asthma. Also, raw meat could lead to worms in the intestine and, as mentioned before, "addicting consumption of figs leads to lice infestation."[183]

Water, in general, seemed to be an undesirable drink. If it could be replaced with other, aged drinks, including some syrups or wines, that would always be best for one's health. The treatise included a recipe for a specific aged drink made of raisins, meant to replace water after each meal.[184] "Have three glasses of this drink after your food [. . .]. If you still desire water after that, drink half the amount that you would have had before."[185] More importantly, and as explained before, water seems to carry specific qualities based on its location and the direction of its flow. If traveling, one should carry water from one's home or from one station to the next, mixing old and new waters to acclimate the body to new waters. Also, rainwater was preferred to other types of water, followed by spring water flowing from the east.[186] Water flowing from or through mud mountains or hills was seen as very useful because it was warm in the winter and cold in the summer, and it acted as, "a laxative. It is also useful for fevers."[187] Salty heavy water was seen as bad for the stomach as well as ice or snow water, which caused several problems in the body. Well water could be very good, as it was "light, clear and very useful to bodies, as long as it was not stored long underground." Pond waters, especially those on salty soil, caused yellow bile diseases and enlarged the spleen.[188]

In discussing sex, the treatise was clear on the importance of cleanliness, which included the prohibition against sex with menstruating women or women before they bathed after the end of their menses, as this might lead to leprosy in the offspring.[189] Holding in the seed after orgasm was also advised against, as it might lead to bladder stones and difficult urination.[190] Finally, the treatise explained that one should not have sex at the beginning of the night or just before sleeping. Rather, it advised having sex at the end of the night, as one woke up, just before light.[191] This matched the advice related to sleep, as the caliph was advised to sleep only two-thirds of the night and to wake up early to relieve himself and to have sex, if he so desired.

It is not possible for us to determine whether these recommended habits were actually observed or followed by elite individuals in the ninth and tenth centuries. The recommendations seem quite extensive with significant restrictions and recommendations on what one should and should not do to guarantee good health. However, the presence of a form of literature invested in regulating life according to healthy habits reveals an important layer in the making of medico-pietistic culture during this period. Members of the elite, who now had access to the new translations and compilations made by the Abbasid translators and who had become more and more connected to learned physicians, were adopting an image of the body rooted in self-care and attention to the details of one's life. Part of elite living, it appears from this treatise, would be to adopt specific habits of healthy living or at least to continually aspire to following these habits. The extent and the reach of these recommendations to all aspects of life emphasize the medicalized nature of the body, which could not be seen outside of the medical framework and outside of the reference points of health and disease. There is no behavior that is neutral or unconcerned with medicine, and there is no experience that is devoid of implications for health and illness. Good living, which is part of virtuous living, as will be explained later, is conditioned on the ability to know the body and to adopt a healthy, pious lifestyle. Violating these recommendations or, worse, disregarding and ignoring this knowledge, is only a sign of ignorance and decadence that makes a person comparable to a beast that does not understand what is good and what is bad.[192]

The Golden Treatise drew a particular body that was based on both medical and pietistic knowledge. On one hand, and similar to the other contemporary texts discussed in this chapter, *The Golden Treatise* relied heavily on Galenic medical knowledge. It utilized Galenic ideas about health and diseases, the Galenic organization of the body and of humors, and the overall view on the values of different foods and drinks and of different activities. Although there were differences between Galenic texts and the views and recommendations expressed in *The Golden Treatise*, the overall scheme of organization and the conceptual framework that characterized the discussions and recommendations were decidedly Galenic. On the other hand, and also similar to the other texts discussed in this chapter, *The Golden Treatise* was deeply rooted in a prophetic/Imami pietistic narrative. It was premised on the authority of Imam ʿAlī al-Riḍā and reported through a lineage of Shiite ḥadīth reporters. Although it did not include many direct traditions reported from the prophet or previous imams, it was in itself a long single ḥadīth by Imām ʿAlī al-Riḍā himself. In that sense, the recommendations that the treatise included were imbued with the same pietistic authority that other collections of ḥadīth exhibited. Thus, *The Golden Treatise's* body was drawn at the intersection of medical and pietistic discourses.

In *The Golden Treatise*, the attention to details about health preservation and the recipes that were described there created a pietistic environment whereby caring for the body, preserving health, and treating diseases were part of a person's pietistic performance. This medico-pietistic performance was rooted in some of the same virtues that governed pietistic performances in other areas of a person's life and also intersected with the virtues that governed the life of the urban learned elites. In all these cases, one needed to pay attention to their own bodies and their various activities. This attention to one's body and soul, as will be seen later, was part of the virtues of the urban elite life. Similar to other forms of pietistic performances, this medical piety was based on self-reflection and constant observance and was rooted in the practice of moderation and balance. The new writings of prophetic medicine, now structured around the traditions of medical literature, were constructing a space of medical piety that conditioned the healthy bodies of their readers.

Conclusion

In a way, the task of the majority of ḥadīth scholars was to construct an archive – a task that involved collecting specific objects that matched the archive's criteria and arranging them properly according to preset rules and in accessible formats. This task involved criticizing the collected materials and arranging them in categories and spaces that can be easily recalled and collected. As explained before, medical prophetics emerged as a textual genre and a heading under which certain traditions were classified. By definition, this arrangement was one that is built on and rooted in the logic of the ḥadīth archive itself. As seen in the first chapter, even the word *ṭibb* was used to mean medicine, magic, and prognostication, all of which were part of the linguistic origins of the word in Arabic. Although the majority of the scholars writing in the ninth century and beyond were using the term to mean medicine in the vast majority of instances, the term recaptured its linguistic heritage to include what it might have meant in the prophetic corpus. The arrangement and organization were based on what seemed important in the prophetic corpus and not what seemed important for medical practitioners or readers interested in medicine. These were not chapters on medicine. They were chapters of prophetics that happened to touch on medicine.

Alongside this literature, a new genre started to emerge that adopted a different logic of interpretation and arrangement, despite relying on similar materials. In these volumes, the central logic of arrangement was one that relied on medicine and that addressed the main concerns of medical practice and of consumers of medical knowledge. The earliest example of this nature was probably ʿAbd al-Malik ibn Ḥabīb al-Qurṭubī's volume, *The Concise in Medicine* (al-Mukhtaṣar fī al-Ṭibb). Ibn Ḥabīb was a scholar, adīb (litterateur), jurist, and a pioneer of ḥadīth in al-Andalus.[193] However, his work on ḥadīth came under scrutiny and was gradually sidelined even by some of his own students, who became more familiar with the developing ḥadīth sciences. As such, Ibn Ḥabīb's influence and the significance of his book was rather limited even among Andalusi scholars. Ibn Ḥabīb's attention to some details of medical practice and his desire to arrange a book that adopted their methods may have stemmed from his legal interests and training. After all, the book did not address the basics of medical theory, but rather was interested in the most legally relevant questions that could be encountered in medical practice.

In the century after Ibn Ḥabīb's work, some of the more prominent examples of this same approach came to be produced by more influential scholars, and therefore, had more lasting impact. Unlike Ibn Ḥabīb, ʿAbd Allāh and al-Hussayn ibn Bisṭām, Ibn al-Sunnī, and Abū Nuʿaym al-Iṣfahānī were better positioned in the genres and in the communities of Twelver Shiite (for the first two) and Sunni (for the last two) ḥadīth. They all descended from important and dignified ḥadīth genealogies and came to be recognized as major authorities in their fields. In the same way, the attribution and the lines of transmission for *The Golden Treatise*, which was attributed to Imām ʿAlī al-Riḍā, gave it important influence. Abū Nuʿaym was the more prominent figure of these four scholars and had a large number of students (al-Dhahabī counted close to eighty who reported from him) that would further affect the ḥadīth landscape. In the works of all these scholars, a new archive (or rather subarchive) emerged to address questions of medicine. Traditions were collected and arranged not to portray the major intellectual and epistemic priorities of prophetics literature, but rather to answer to the concerns of medical practitioners and consumers of medical knowledge.

In her periodization of prophetic medicine, Irmeli Perho correctly identifies significant differences between the medical chapters in early and central ḥadīth compilations such as those of al-Bukhārī and Muslim and later writings such as those of Ibn Qayyim al-Jawziyah, Ibn Mufliḥ, and al-Dhahabī. She explains that the later texts showed clear attention to the details of Galenic medicine and were more attuned to the interests of medical literature and practice. Perho attributes these changes to the work of physicians such as ʿAbd al-Laṭīf al-Baghdādī (d. 1231) and Ibn Ṭarkhān (d. 1320), who wrote books in prophetic medicine and presumably provided religious scholars with a template to address medical questions in a more direct fashion. This periodization, however, is based on authors' attention to the medical questions and the engagement with the details of medical theory and practice. It neglects the changes that occur in the ḥadīth archive that provided the materials for later writings on prophetic medicine. This archive, which relied on but was also more expansive than the writings in chapters of medicine in ḥadīth compilations, started to take shape in the work of these scholars, who first attempted to organize their texts according to the method of the people of medicine. Moreover, these works provided a new coding for this archive of "little narratives," along with adding or repurposing more narratives that would come to populate later texts.

In following Perho's argument that the new literature of prophetic medicine emerged from an increased interest in medicine among ḥadīth scholars, the works of Ibn al-Sunnī and Abū Nuʿaym figure prominently. Soon after, Ibn al-Jawzī (d. 1201), who followed Abū Nuʿaym's work diligently, composed a treatise in medicine entitled *Luqat al-Manāfiʿ* (the selected benefits). In that treatise, Ibn al-Jawzī attempted to produce a volume on medicine and not on prophetic medicine. Although his book contained numerous prophetic materials, it was proposed as a summary of medicine directed to the literate public and not necessarily a book of ḥadīth. In fact, as will be later demonstrated, ʿAbd al-Laṭīf al-Baghdādī and Ibn Ṭarkhān came to copy extensively from Ibn al-Jawzī's *Luqat al-Manafiʿ*. Taken as a whole, the works of Ibn al-Jawzī, ʿAbd al-Laṭif al-Baghdādī, Ibn Ṭarkhān, and later Ibn Mufliḥ, Ibn al-Qayyim, al-Dhahabī, and many others relied extensively on the new archive and organizational framework constructed by Ibn al-Sunnī and Abū Nuʿaym, citing them frequently and relying on their arrangement and organization.

At another level, these works presented an important moment of encounter between the pietistic and medical making of the learned body in the tenth and eleventh centuries. Steeped in both pietistic ḥadīth writings and in medical knowledge, these texts engaged with the production of a medico-pietistic understanding of the body and of health. In these works, the body emerged as an endowment from God that required care. It was built on balanced humors, which further emphasized the importance of moderation as a virtue for the learned urban elites at the time. Caring for the body required constant attention to what one ate and drank and how one moved, slept, had sex, etc. This attention required some knowledge of medical theory and practice, including knowledge about the medical qualities of foods and drinks and access to trusted recipes and tried medications, as well as to incantations and prayers that helped preserve health and treat diseases. This view of the body and the need for constant care and diligence mirrored other pietistic narratives, which will be explored in the coming chapters and which focused primarily on the need for self-reflection and for attention to one's various deeds and thoughts. Similar to how a person needed to monitor their activities and their thoughts to ensure that they conformed with religious law and various pietistic expectations, one also needed to monitor their food and drink and to pay attention to their bodies. This particular form of care engendered a form of medical piety – one that resembled and was derived from the main virtues and principles of various pietistic discourses but that was directly connected to the body and its care.

Notes

1 Ibn Juljul and Sayyid, *Ṭabaqāt al-Aṭibbāʾ wa-al-Ḥukamāʾ*. On Ibn Juljul and his biographical dictionary, see Millán's excellent study where she discusses many of the limitations of the dictionary, Millán, "Medical Anecdotes." Although Ibn Juljul did not include all physicians in al-Andalus, it is reasonable to expect a reference to a scholar of Ibn Ḥabīb's stature and importance if he was indeed a physician or a medical author.

2 Eastern biographers credited Ibn Ḥabīb with introducing the Maliki madhhab to al-Andalus, Al-Dhahabī, *Siyar Aʿlām al-Nubalāʾ*, 103–5. Modern studies have shown that Malikism was introduced to al-Andalus before Ibn Ḥabīb's time. Although he played an important role in the consolidation of the Madhhab, Malikism had replaced al-Awzaʿī's madhhab in al-Andalus by the first half of the ninth century. On Malikism and its spread in al-Andalus, see Idris, "Réflexions sûr le Malikisme"; Aguadé, "Sectarian Movements in al-Andalus"; Fierro, "Proto-malikis, Malikis and Reformed Malikis"; Fierro, "Islamic Law in al-Andalus"; Fierro, "History of Maliki Hadīth" and Fierro, "Local and Global in Hadīth."

3 Fierro, "Local and Global in Hadith," 71–2.

4 Ibn Al-Farḍī, *Tārīkh ʿUlamāʾ al-Andalus*, 1: 313.

5 Ibid., 1: 313–14.
6 Ibid., 1: 313. The same can be found in Ibn Ḥabīb's biography by Ibn ʿUmayrah, who wrote that "[Ibn Ḥabīb's] traditions [in his *al-Wāḍiḥah*] have many strange [reports]." (Ibn ʿUmayrah, *Bughyat al-Multamis fī Tārīkh Ahl al-Andalus*, 1: 377. Ibn ʿAbd al-Barr agreed with these criticisms and explained that Ibn Ḥabīb, whom he credited with the introduction of ḥadīth to al-Andalus, did not know the methods of ḥadīth and confused copying from writing with actual *samā* (cited in Fierro, "Local and Global in Hadith," 76).
7 Ibn Al-Farḍī, *Tārīkh ʿUlamāʾ al-Andalus*, 1: 313; Al-Dhahabī, *Siyar Aʿlām al-Nubalāʾ*, 12: 104. Ibn al-Farḍī considered Ibn Ḥabīb to be "a grammarian (*naḥawiyyan*), a poet, a reporter of anecdotes, genealogies and poetry (*ḥāfizan lil-akhbār wa al-nasāb wa al-ashʿār*), eloquent and knowledgeable of various sciences" (1: 315).
8 On the role of ḥadīth and companions' practice in the making of Islamic law, especially Maliki and Medinan schools of law, see Dutton, *The Origins of Islamic Law*. As an example, see also Dutton, "ʿAmal v. Ḥadīth in Islamic Law."
9 Ibn Ḥabīb Al-Qurṭubī, *Al-Mukhtaṣar fī al-Ṭibb*, 22.
10 Ibid., 35.
11 Ibid., 22 and 42.
12 Ibid.
13 Ibid., 29.
14 Ibid., 95.
15 Ibid., 20.
16 Ibid., 22.
17 Ibid., 32.
18 Ibid., 121.
19 Ibn ʿAbd Rabbih, *Al-ʿAqd al-Farīd*, 7: 299.
20 Ibn Ḥabīb Al-Qurṭubī, *Al-Mukhtaṣar fī al-Ṭibb*, 9–10.
21 Ibid., 30–1.
22 Ibid., 32.
23 Ibid., 12.
24 Ibid., 12.
25 Ibid., 12.
26 Ibid., 16.
27 Ibid., 17.
28 This is the case for ʿAbd al-Razzāq al-Ṣanʿānī, Ibn Abī Shaybah, al-Bukhārī, and others. Even in the earliest chapters on medicine found in Muʿammir ibn Rāshid's compendium, contagion, leprosy, and plague were combined in the same context along with omens.
29 For instance, one of the oft-cited prophetic traditions, which al-Bukhārī cited in his treatise on medicine, is one where the prophet is reported to have said, "There is contagion and no omens [in Islam]. And flee from the leper as you flee from a lion." This tradition and others cemented the connections between leprosy, contagion (and hence plague), and omens in prophetic lore. On contagion in later medical and religious writings, see Stearns, *Infectious Ideas*.
30 Ibn Ḥabīb Al-Qurṭubī, *Al-Mukhtaṣar fī al-Ṭibb*, 27.
31 Ibid., 62.
32 Newman, "Islamic Medical Wisdom;" Al-Ṭihrānī, *Al-Dhariʿah ilā Taṣānīf al-Shiʿah*, 15: 139–40. According to al-Ṭihrānī, the book was first translated into Persian by Fayḍ Allāh al-Tusturī in 1678. Al-Tusturī was a scholar of medicine and astrology and was also asked to translate *Ṭibb al-Imām al-Riḍā*, also known as *The Golden Treatise*, which will be discussed later, by the same patron, Ibid., 4: 114.
33 Al-Ṭihrānī, *Al-Dhariʿah ilā Taṣānīf al-Shiʿah*, 15: 903–61. Al-Ṭihrānī listed a total of fifty-eight texts on medicine, with few repetitions, in this section. This does not include

other texts that may have been also about medicine but their titles started with words other than *ṭibb* or did not include the term *ṭibb* at all. Al-Ṭihrānī also classified Abū Nuʿaym al-Isfahānī's *Ṭibb al-Nabiyy*, which will be discussed later in this chapter, as a Shiite book with no explanation. Along with Abū Nuʿaym's book, only two other texts carried the title *Ṭibb al-Nabiyy* indicating that they focused on traditions from the prophet, perhaps with less emphasis on, or to the exclusion of, the imams. On medical texts in the Twelver Shiite tradition, see Newman, "Islamic Medical Wisdom." Newman has also shown how al-Majlisī recovered medical (or seemingly medically related materials) from the various collections produced by Ibn Bābawayh (Newman, "The Recovery of the Past"). Al-Majlisī cited also other authors of prophetic and Imami medicine, including Abū al-Wazīr ibn Aḥmad al-Abharī and al-Mustaghfirī, both of whom produced texts of *Ṭibb al-Nabiyy* and did not include traditions from the imams in their works (Al-Ṭihrānī, *Al-Dhariʿah ilā Taṣānīf al-Shiʿah*, 15: 143–4).

34 Newman, "Islamic Medical Wisdom," XXI-XXII.

35 On this question in Sunni ḥadīth, see Brown, "Even If It's Not True It's True," 7. Al-Majlisī, who cited Ibnā Bisṭām's *Ṭibb al-Aʾimmah*, was clearly aware of the problems in some of their transmitted reports but explained that it was fine to cite these traditions because they did not include legal pronouncements (Al-Ṭihrānī, *Al-Dhariʿah ilā Taṣānīf al-Shiʿah*, 15: 140).

36 Ibn Basṭām, *Ṭibb al-aʾImmah*, 29.

37 Ibid., 39.

38 Ibid., 55.

39 Ibid., 60.

40 Most Kunnāsh (see al-Kashkarī, *Kunnāsh fī al-Ṭibb*; and *Man Lam Yaḥḍuruhu Ṭabīb* volumes; see also Abū Bakr al-Rāzī & Rashīdī, *Ṭabīb Man lā Ṭabīb la-hu, aw, Man Lā Yaḥduruhu al-Ṭabīb*) focused on a head-to-toe structure that addressed conditions affecting different parts of the body. Books on food stuffs (Israeli & Ṣabbāḥ, *Kitāb al-Aghdhiyah wa-al-Adwiyah*) focused on specific materials starting with single drugs followed by more complex preparations.

41 See Bonebakker, "Adab and the Concept of Belles-Lettres." See also Sánchez, "Reading Adab as Fiqh."

42 Ibn Basṭām & Ibn Basṭām, *Ṭibb al-Aʾimmah*, 69.

43 Ibid., 51.

44 Ibid.

45 Ibid., 69.

46 Ibid., 51 and also 18, 20.

47 Ibid., 20.

48 See for instance, Ibid., 25, 73.

49 Ibid., 53.

50 On the use of the term *mujarrab*, see Forcada, "Ibn Bājja;" Millán, "Case History."

51 Ibn Basṭām and Ibn Basṭām, *Ṭibb al-Aʾimmah*, 103–4.

52 For instance, various exegetes agreed that the verse [2: 15], "God shall mock them, and shall lead them on blindly wandering in their insolence," referred to God deluding and extending favor to unbelievers, ending with their eventual demise. See Al-Ṭabarī, *Tafsīr al-Ṭabarī*; Al-Qurtubi and Bewley, *Tafsir al-Qurtubi*; Al-Ṭūsī, *Al-Tibyān fī Tafsīr al-Qurʾān*.

53 Al-Ṭūsī, *Al-Tibyān fī Tafsīr al-Qurʾān*.

54 See Al-Bukhārī, *Ṣaḥīḥ al-Bukhārī*, 7: 123.

55 On 'hypocrites' in the sīra lore, see Rose, "Constitution of Medina."

56 Ibn Basṭām and Ibn Basṭām, *Ṭibb al-Aʾimmah*, 88–91.

57 Ibid., 125.

58 Ibid., 104.

59 Ibid., 19.

60 Ibid., 22.
61 Ibid., 30.
62 Ibid., 68.
63 Ibid., 65.
64 There might be a parallel here to the discussion of using poisons in recipes that was a fixture in Sunni ḥadīth compilations, although there was no direct mention of the Theriac there. See Al-Bukhārī, *Ṣaḥīḥ al-Bukhārī*, 7: 139.
65 Ibn Basṭām and Ibn Basṭām, *Ṭibb al-A'immah*, 63.
66 Ibid., 61.
67 Ibid., 75–8.
68 On the connection between Galenic medicine and Shiite prophetic medicine during this period and after, see Newman, "Baqir al-Majlisi and Islamicate Medicine;" Newman, "Recovery of the Past."
69 Sunni scholars revered and respected Ja'far al-Ṣādiq but attributed to him anecdotes where he rejected the claims of Shiites, see Al-Dhahabī, *Siyar A'lām al-Nubalā'*, 6: 255; see also M.G.S. Hodgson, "D̲ja'far al-Ṣādiḳ."
70 Al-Qummī, *'Uyūn Akhbār al-Riḍā*.
71 Ibn Basṭām and Ibn Basṭām, *Ṭibb al-A'immah*, 111.
72 Ibid., 52.
73 Ibid., 106.
74 See Al-Bukhārī, *Ṣaḥīḥ al-Bukhārī*, 7: 140. On this tradition and how different Sunni scholars dealt with it, see Zinger, "Tradition and Medicine."
75 Ibn Basṭām and Ibn Basṭām, *Ṭibb al-A'immah*, 106.
76 Ibid., 28. For examples of discussion of Black Seed in Sunni compilations, see Al-Bukhārī, *Ṣaḥīḥ al-Bukhārī*, 7: 124; Al-Tirmidhī, *Al-Jāmi' al-Kabīr*, 4: 385.
77 See Al-Tirmidhī, *Al-Jāmi' al-Kabīr*, 4: 385–86; Al-Bukhārī, *Ṣaḥīḥ al-Bukhārī*, 7: 123.
78 Ibn Basṭām and Ibn Basṭām, *Ṭibb al-A'immah*, 102.
79 Ibid., 61.
80 See Al-Bukhārī, *Ṣaḥīḥ al-Bukhārī*, 7: 131–2, 7: 135–6; Al-Tirmidhī, *Al-Jāmi' al-Kabīr*, 4: 393–7; Ibn Abī Shaybah, *Al-Kitāb al-Muṣannaf fī al-Aḥādīth wa al-Āthār*, 5: 35.
81 Ibn Basṭām and Ibn Basṭām, *Ṭibb al-A'immah*, 49.
82 Al-Tirmidhī, *Al-Jāmi' al-Kabīr*, 4: 387.
83 Ibn Basṭām and Ibn Basṭām, *Ṭibb al-A'immah*, 55–7.
84 Ibn Abī Shaybah, *Al-Kitāb al-Muṣannaf fī al-Aḥādīth wa al-Āthār*, 5: 34.
85 Ibn Basṭām and Ibn Basṭām, *Ṭibb al-A'immah*, 54.
86 Ibn Ḥabīb Al-Qurṭubī, *Al-Mukhtaṣar fī al-Ṭibb*, 40.
87 Ibn Basṭām and Ibn Basṭām, *Ṭibb al-A'immah*, 93.
88 Ibn Ḥabīb Al-Qurṭubī, *Al-Mukhtaṣar fī al-Ṭibb*, 27.
89 Ibn Basṭām and Ibn Basṭām, *Ṭibb al-A'immah*, 105. Ibn Ḥabīb reported the tradition as a saying by the prophet on the authority of Mujāhid.
90 Ibid., 41–5.
91 Ibid., 133.
92 Ibid., 133.
93 Ibid.
94 Rahman, *Health and Medicine in the Islamic Tradition.*
95 Newman, "Islamic Medical Wisdom."
96 Al-Aṣbahānī, *Al-Ṭibb al-Nabawiyy*, 171.
97 According to *ṭabaqāt* or the Generations of al-Dhahabī, al-Sunnī belonged to the twentieth *ṭabaqah*, and al-Aṣbahānī belonged to the twenty-third, making al-Sunnī an older scholar and placing him at a higher order in chains of transmission. However, the relative stature and importance of each was similar, with Abū Nu'aym seemingly more important than al-Sunnī. See, for Abū Nu'aym and Al-Dhahabī, *Siyar A'lām al-Nubalā'*, 17: 454–64; and for Ibn al-Sunnī, 16: 256–8.

98 This is not to say that Abū Nuʿaym, in particular, was not criticized by later scholars. For instance, Ibn al-Jawzī objected to Abū Nuʿaym's use of suspect and weak traditions in his famous book on saints *Ḥulyat al-Awliyāʾ*, which Ibn al-Jawzī railed against in the introduction of his own book on saints *Ṣifat al-Ṣafwa*, enumerating ten problems, two of which were related to the authenticity of traditions used by Abū Nuʿaym (Ibn Al-Jawzī, *Ṣifat al-Ṣafwah*, 9–12 especially 10). Similarly, al-Dhahabī criticized Abū Nuʿaym, along with other important scholars of his generation such as al-Khaṭīb al-Baghdādī, for using weak and forged traditions in their writings on *raqāʾiq* or *adāb* (writings that touch on piety and other similar topics but not on legal questions). This was part of a later trend among ḥadīth scholars that featured less tolerance for use of weak or forged materials in pietistic writings – a practice rather common among the early titans of ḥadīth, including Aḥmad ibn Ḥanbal, al-Khaṭib al-Baghdādī, and also Abū Nuʿaym (see Brown, "Even If It's Not True It's True," 24).

99 Al-Dhahabī, *Siyar Aʿlām al-Nubalāʾ*, 16: 257.

100 Al-Dhahabī, *Siyar Aʿlām al-Nubalāʾ*.

101 In fact, Abū Nuʿaym's book was listed by al-Ṭihrānī as one of the Shiite books on prophetic medicine (only one of two entitled *prophet's medicine* and focused on traditions from the prophet, not the imams). It appears that al-Ṭihrānī included the text on account of Abū Nuʿaym's Shiite connections and the fact that some of its traditions were cited by other Shiite scholars such as al-Majlisī. See Al-Ṭihrānī, *Al-Dhariʿah ilā Taṣānīf al-Shiʿah*, 15: 140.

102 Ibn Al-Athīr, *Al-Kāmil fī al-Tārīkh*.

103 Al-Aṣbahānī, *Rawḍāt al-Jannāt fī Aḥwāl al-ʿUlamāʾ wa al-Sādāt*.

104 Abū Nuʿaym's works have been mainly studied in the context of his work on saints, which constituted an important source for accounts of Sufi saints. On this aspect of his work, see Frank, " 'Taṣawwuf is. . . ' ", Melchert, "Transition from Asceticism to Mysticism."

105 Ibn Al-Sunnī, "Al-Ṭibb al-Nabawī."

106 Ibid., 3v.

107 Al-Aṣbahānī, *Al-Ṭibb al-Nabawiyy*, 1: 171.

108 Ibid., 1: 332; Ibn Al-Sunnī, "Al-Ṭibb al-Nabawī," 22v. Scholars like al-Bayhaqī and Ibn Ḥibbān considered this tradition to be *munkar*. Ibn al-Jawzī included this tradition among few others in his book on forged traditions *al-mawḍūʿāt*.

109 Al-Aṣbahānī, *Al-Ṭibb al-Nabawiyy*, 1: 342; Ibn Al-Sunnī, "Al-Ṭibb al-Nabawī," 24r.

110 Al-Aṣbahānī, *Al-Ṭibb al-Nabawiyy*, 1: 465; Ibn Al-Sunnī, "Al-Ṭibb al-Nabawī," 38r. Abū Nuʿaym reported two versions of this tradition, only one of which was in Ibn al-Sunnī's.

111 Although the majority of Sunnī ḥadīth reporters stopped short of condemning or explicitly doubting Shiite imams or most other members of Muḥammad's family, they hardly used these chains of transmission. A famous example is al-Bukhārī's refraining from using any ḥadīth reported by Jaʿfar al-Ṣādiq in his *Ṣaḥīḥ*, despite the latter being a respected figure by Sunnis as well as Shiites. Al-Bukhārī reported ḥadīths on the authority of Jaʿfar al-Ṣādiq in his *adab*. See Al-Dhahabī, *Siyar Aʿlām al-Nubalāʾ*, 6: 270.

112 Al-Aṣbahānī, *Al-Ṭibb al-Nabawiyy*, 1: 382; Ibn Al-Sunnī, "Al-Ṭibb al-Nabawī," 29r.

113 Al-Aṣbahānī, *Al-Ṭibb al-Nabawiyy*, 1: 346. The tradition was not included in Ibn al-Sunnī's.

114 Ibid., 1: 379.

115 Ibid., 1: 435.

116 Ibid., 1: 477.

117 Al-Najāshī, *Rijāl al-Najāshī*.

118 For instance, Daaif traced some ḥadīth forgeries to a number of known ascetics and explained that forging ḥadīths for purposes of pietistic instructions was not severely

condemned. See Daaïf, "Dévots et Renonçants". See also Brown, "Even If It's Not True It's True," 7. In his typology of pietistic discourses, Melchert argued that the works of Ibn Abī al-Dunyā and, to some extent, Abū Nuʿaym were criticized by *ahl al-ḥadīth* (or Hadith Folk) because they resembled adab works, contrasted their austere pieties, and relied on less authentic materials. As shown before and as explained by Brown and others, evidence suggest these criticisms were levied rather late and after the predominance of texts like the ṣaḥīḥ books of al-Bukhārī and Muslim, which entrenched views around authenticity of ḥadīth and its importance. See Melchert, "Piety of the Hadith Folk," 433–4.

119 Al-Aṣbahānī, *Al-Ṭibb al-Nabawiyy*, 2: 447; Ibn Al-Sunnī, "Al-Ṭibb al-Nabawī," 36r. For instance, Ibn Mājah reported the same tradition in his treatise on ritual cleanliness (*al-ṭahārah*). Ibn Mājah, *Sunan Ibn Mājah*, 1: 215.

120 Al-Aṣbahānī, *Al-Ṭibb al-Nabawiyy*, 2: 465–70. Ibn Al-Sunnī, "Al-Ṭibb al-Nabawī," 37r-39v.

121 Al-Aṣbahānī, *Al-Ṭibb al-Nabawiyy*, 2: 459; Ibn Al-Sunnī, "Al-Ṭibb al-Nabawī," 37v.

122 Al-Aṣbahānī, *Al-Ṭibb al-Nabawiyy*, 2: 463–4; Ibn Al-Sunnī, "Al-Ṭibb al-Nabawī," 38r.

123 Al-Aṣbahānī, *Al-Ṭibb al-Nabawiyy*, 2: 470–1; Ibn Al-Sunnī, "Al-Ṭibb al-Nabawī," 39r. See, for instance, Ibn Mājah, *Sunan Ibn Mājah*, 1: 194.

124 Al-Aṣbahānī, *Al-Ṭibb al-Nabawiyy*, 2: 466–7; Ibn Al-Sunnī, "Al-Ṭibb al-Nabawī," 38r. In this and many other occasions, Abū Nuʿaym included more than one version of the same or similar traditions while only one was reported in Ibn al-Sunnī's.

125 Al-Ṭabarī, *Tafsīr al-Ṭabarī*, 7: 11.

126 Al-Aṣbahānī, *Al-Ṭibb al-Nabawiyy*, 1: 410; Ibn Al-Sunnī, "Al-Ṭibb al-Nabawī," 32v.

127 Al-Aṣbahānī, *Al-Ṭibb al-Nabawiyy*, 2: 468; Ibn Al-Sunnī, "Al-Ṭibb al-Nabawī," 38r. In the second iteration of this tradition in the sex-related chapter, Both Ibn al-Sunnī and Abū Nuʿaym added other narrations (only one in the case of Ibn al-Sunnī) of the traditions that included direct reference to sexual prowess. Ibn al-Sunnī included only the single version.

128 Al-Aṣbahānī, *Al-Ṭibb al-Nabawiyy*, 1: 173–86; Ibn Al-Sunnī, "Al-Ṭibb al-Nabawī," 4r, 4v. Unlike most other compilers, Abū Nuʿaym included twenty-seven traditions on this note alone.

129 Al-Aṣbahānī, *Al-Ṭibb al-Nabawiyy*, 1: 199–201; Ibn Al-Sunnī, "Al-Ṭibb al-Nabawī," 6v.

130 Al-Aṣbahānī, *Al-Ṭibb al-Nabawiyy*, 1: 196–7; Ibn Al-Sunnī, "Al-Ṭibb al-Nabawī," 6r.

131 The missing treatises in Ibn al-Sunnī's text may have included discussions of these topics.

132 On contagion, see Stearns, *Infectious Ideas*.

133 Al-Aṣbahānī, *Al-Ṭibb al-Nabawiyy*, 1: 353–5; Ibn Al-Sunnī, "Al-Ṭibb al-Nabawī," 26r.

134 Al-Aṣbahānī, *Al-Ṭibb al-Nabawiyy*, 1: 353–69; Ibn Al-Sunnī, "Al-Ṭibb al-Nabawī," 26r-27v. Ibn al-Sunnī and Abū Nuʿaym discussed the causes of leprosy, its different treatments, the use of cupping to treat leprosy, signs of being free or safe from leprosy, the age in which one can be safe from the disease, and which lands are better for treating leprosy.

135 Al-Aṣbahānī, *Al-Ṭibb al-Nabawiyy*, 1: 322–23; Ibn Al-Sunnī, "Al-Ṭibb al-Nabawī," 21v.

136 Al-Aṣbahānī, *Al-Ṭibb al-Nabawiyy*, 1: 331; Ibn Al-Sunnī, "Al-Ṭibb al-Nabawī," 21v.

137 Al-Aṣbahānī, *Al-Ṭibb al-Nabawiyy*, 1: 322; Ibn Al-Sunnī, "Al-Ṭibb al-Nabawī," 22v.

138 See, for instance, Al-Aṣbahānī, *Al-Ṭibb al-Nabawiyy*, 2: 719, 722, 723.

139 See, for example, ibid., 2: 750.

140 Ibid., 741. Ibn Al-Sunnī, "Al-Ṭibb al-Nabawī," 69v. Both Ibn al-Sunnī and Abū Nuʿaym explained the disadvantages of fetal meat in a single sentence that preceded the ḥadīth.

141 Al-Aṣbahānī, *Al-Ṭibb al-Nabawiyy*, 1: 325; Ibn Al-Sunnī, "Al-Ṭibb al-Nabawī," 22r.

142 Al-Aṣbahānī, *Al-Ṭibb al-Nabawiyy*, 1: 326; Ibn Al-Sunnī, "Al-Ṭibb al-Nabawī," 22r.

143 Yūsuf, *Al-ImāM ʿalī Al-Riḍā Waliy ʿahd Al-Maʾmūn.*

144 See Tor, "Appointment and Death of Ali Al-Riḍā." See also Crone and Hinds, *God's Caliph*, 94–8.
145 Tor, "Appointment and Death of Ali Al-Riḍā."
146 Yūsuf, *Al-ImāM 'alī Al-Riḍā Waliy 'ahd Al-Ma'mūN*.
147 Ibn Bābawayh al-Qummī, *'Uyūn Akhbār Al-Riḍā*.
148 Ibid.
149 Al-Riḍā, *Al-Risālah Al-Dhahabiyya*, 5–7.
150 Ibid., 67.
151 Most significantly, al-Shaykh al-Ṣadūq, Muḥammad ibn Alī al-Bābawayh al-Qummī, who wrote a celebratory biography of 'Alī al-Riḍā, did not mention this treatise or the conversations about medicine (See Ibn Bābawayh al-Qummī, *'Uyūn Akhbār Al-Riḍā*). This, however, could be explained by al-Shaykh al-Ṣadūq's interest in theological matters more than anything else.
152 Tor, " Appointment and Death of Ali Al-Riḍā."
153 Ibn al-Nadim, *Al-Fihrist*, 196; al-Ṭūsī, *Rijāl Al-Ṭūsī*.
154 Al-Rāzī, *Al-Kāfī*, 1: 56.
155 On al-Shaykh al-Ṭūsī, see Amir-Moezzi "al-Ṭūsī."
156 Al-Ṭūsī, *Al-Fihrist*, 146.
157 Al-Ḥamawī, *Irshād Al-Arīb Ilá Ma'rifat Al-Adīb*, 2502–3.
158 Al-Riḍā, *Al-Risālah Al-Dhahabiyya*, 4–5.
159 Al-Najāshī, *Rijāl Al-Najāshī*.
160 Al-Riḍā, *Al-Risālah Al-Dhahabiyya*, 6. On Ibn Bahla, see Shefer-Mossensohm and Hershkovitz, "Early Muslim Medicine," 278. Considering the previous discussion of the treatise's date of composition, the reference to an Indian physician indicates that Indian physicians were part of elite medical practice well into the tenth century.
161 Al-Riḍā, *Al-Risālah Al-Dhahabiyy*, 7.
162 See Bayhom-Daou, "Imam's Knowledge and the Quran."
163 The same sources of knowledge and the emphasis on how the Imām follows the traditions of his ancestors are also emphasized in al-Riḍā's biography: Ibn Bābawayh al-Qumm, *'Uyūn Akhbār Al-Riḍā*.
164 Al-Riḍā, *Al-Risālah Al-Dhahabiyy*, 8.
165 Ibid., 10.
166 On ṣabr or forbearance, see for instance, Behnamafar and Bakhshaee-zadeh, "Tolerance and Forbearance." The question of forbearance in relation to sickness continues to be relevant today. See Hamdy, "Islam, Fatalism, and Medical Intervention."
167 Al-Riḍā, *Al-Risālah Al-Dhahabiyya*, 13–14.
168 Ibid., 43.
169 Ibid., 44–5.
170 Ibid., 17–20.
171 Ibid., 48. Note the use of the word soft [layyin] as opposed to humid [raṭib], which is more common in Galenic writings.
172 Ibid., 48.
173 Ibid., 30.
174 Ibid., 66.
175 Ibid., 52–3.
176 Ibid., 11.
177 Ibid., 26–7.
178 Ibid., 27.
179 Ibid., 29.
180 Ibid., 26.
181 Ibid., 15.
182 Ibid., 15–16.
183 Ibid., 28–9.

184 Ibid., 21–5.
185 Ibid., 26.
186 Ibid., 22.
187 Ibid., 45.
188 Ibid., 45–6.
189 Ibid., 27.
190 Ibid., 35.
191 Ibid., 64.
192 Ibid., 66.
193 Fierro, "Local and Global in Hadīth."

3 Piety and illness

As seen in the previous chapters, the ninth and tenth centuries witnessed the emergence of writings on medical prophetics focusing on questions of health and disease in the prophet's life. Starting from chapters in different ḥadīth compilations (*muṣannafāt*), this literature developed into independent volumes that took a more decidedly medical approach. Whereas the medical chapters in the *muṣannafāt* maintained an organization that privileged the prophetic narrative and placed the prophet's encounter with health and illness in the center, the new medically oriented writings, such as those produced by Ibn al-Sunnī and Abū Nuʿaym al-Isfahānī, organized different traditions in manners similar to books on medicine and addressed some of the more important concerns related to medical practice. Sickness, as the object of medicine and the antithesis of health, figured prominently throughout the different stages of this literature. As previously noted, in the prophetics literature, the prophet's episodes of sickness or injury came to dominate the organizational structure and were given a prominent place in these different compilations. These accounts of the prophet's sickness did not simply aim at discussing his consultation of physicians or his attempt to seek cure, but also focused – sometimes in the same spaces and other times in separate chapters – on the prophet's behavior when sick, how he understood the causes of his illness, and how he modeled a pietistic behavior during illness. At a deeper level, some of these reports and traditions engaged with questions about the causality of illness and with the role of diseases in the pietistic cosmology that pious Muslim patients inhabited.

Although sickness continued to figure in the more medically oriented texts of prophetic medicine, such as those of Ibn al-Sunnī or Abū Nuʿaym al-Isfahānī, it was also given special attention by other scholars who investigated sickness more deliberately. These writings addressed questions that ranged from the reasons behind diseases, why diseases and other calamities affected Muslims and non-Muslims equally, whether a Muslim should indeed seek medical care or look for physicians to help them, and the specific pietistic behaviors and attitudes that a pious Muslim should adopt during these times of distress. In the same vein, sickness figured in writings about zuhd, or renunciation of earthly life, which aimed to constitute and provide instructions for specific forms of piety and asceticism.[1] In these writings, the sensorium of sickness was remodeled in a pietistic space. Patients were taught through the words and examples of the prophet and his companion how to feel the pain that affected them and understand the calamities that befell their bodies.[2] They were provided with tools, from thoughts to ritual practices and words, that aimed to produce a specific space in which sickness was modified into a form of pietistic practice and in which calamity was transformed into divine reward. Although these writings did not engage with medical practice or provide recipes or modes of treatment, and they certainly did not engage in any discussion of medical theory, they imparted a pietistic meaning to the experience of illness – as an object of medical practice. In these accounts, illness was understood as an affliction of the body that could often be treated by medical knowledge. Afflictions of the soul were also a topic of interest, but these were discussed in different spaces, as will be seen in the following chapter.

In the context of illness, Ibn Abī al-Dunyā (d. 894), known for his multiple books on a variety of questions concerning piety, composed an entire treatise entitled *Al-Maraḍ wa al-Kaffārāt* (Illness and Penance).[3] In it, he discussed how Muslims needed to address the experience of illness in a pietistic manner with an emphasis on the role of diseases as penance. Ibn Abī al-Dunyā's treatise was primarily a work of ḥadīth in that it was entirely composed of prophetic traditions listed one after the other with varying lengths of *isnād* (chains of transmission). Although the treatise contained a few Qur'anic verses and some verses of poetry, traditions formed the heart of the text. Ibn Abī al-Dunyā's text continued to be used and cited by scholars in the following centuries. Before Ibn Abī al-Dunyā's volume, al-Bukhārī dedicated a chapter in his collection of ḥadīth (*Ṣaḥīḥ al-Bukhārī*) to sickness. Many of the traditions in this chapter were similar to traditions placed by other compilers in chapters on medicine, patience, or renunciation; however, al-Bukhārī's (d. 870) dedicated chapter constructed a more concrete space for illness, ordering and organizing the various materials pertaining to this question. Both al-Bukhārī and Ibn Abī al-Dunyā relied in their writings about illness on a growing wealth of prophetic traditions that belonged to the genre of zuhd (asceticism) and *raqāʾiq* (exhortations),[4] which addressed various pietistic issues.[5] Some of the earliest surviving texts of this genre were composed by important figures in the emerging group of ḥadīth scholars, such as Ibn al-Mubārak (d. 798), who was a known scholar of ḥadīth and a reporter and a teacher of many important scholars of the ninth century.[6] Similarly, Wakīʿ ibn al-Jarrāḥ (d. 813), who was also a central figure in reporting ḥadīth, composed a volume on zuhd, which followed some of the structure of his contemporary Ibn al-Mubārak. Other books of the same title were attributed to Ibn Wahb (d. 813), who was a Maliki jurist in Egypt. Aḥmad ibn Ḥanbal (d. 855) also composed a book under the same title.[7] Perhaps one of the more voluminous and detailed texts on the topic came from Hannād ibn al-Sarī al-Kūfī (d. 858), a contemporary of Ibn Ḥanbal, whom the latter respected and appreciated and a student of Wakīʿ and Ibn al-Mubārak. Hannād was also a scholar of ḥadīth whose students included all the authors of the six Sunni compilations of ḥadīth, which would become the canonical books of Sunni ḥadīth: al-Bukhārī, Muslim ibn al-Ḥajjāj, Abū Dawūd, al-Tirmidhī, al-Nasāʾī, and Ibn Mājah. His students also included Ibn Abī al-Dunyā, who borrowed significantly from Hannād's *zuhd* in his own writings. Similarly, another volume on zuhd was attributed to the known ḥadīth critic, Abū Ḥātim al-Rāzī (d. 891), who was also in contact with Hannād and may have studied with him. Abū Ḥātim's son, Ibn Abī Ḥātim (d. 939), who was a scholar of ḥadīth in his own right, edited a book attributed to the famous follower and ascetic Ibn Marthad (d. 738) and entitled *Zuhd al-Thamāniyah* (The Renunciation of the Eight [Followers]) that focused on traditions by eight prominent followers.[8]

Focusing on the discussion of illness in these texts, with particular attention to the more detailed texts of Hannād, al-Bukhārī, and Ibn Abī al-Dunyā, this chapter explores the pietistic space of illness. Specifically, it examines how these texts aimed to produce a pietistic cosmology that provided meaning to the experiences of illness and that influenced the sensoria characterizing these experiences. I begin by looking at the authorial voice in these compilations. From there, I move to discuss the question of diseases and their connection to sins and reward. Then, I turn to consider the behavior that was recommended of pious Muslims when sick. Finally, I look at the social dimension of sickness and how this pietistic discourse arranged questions of visiting patients and caring for them with an eye towards the community at large.

Ḥadīth collections and the authorial voice

Ibn Abī al-Dunyā's treatise on illnesses, similar to most of his other works, is devoid of almost any editorial comments. Instead, it proceeds with different ḥadīths either *elevated* to the prophet (*marfū'*) or *stopping* with one of his companions (*mawqūf*). The title *Al-Maraḍ wa al-Kaffārāt* (Illness and Penance) under which Ibn Abī al-Dunyā's text circulated, reveals a central message that the text was perceived to discuss: the connection between diseases, sins, and penance. The different traditions that Ibn Abī al-Dunyā included explored in depth the question of whether diseases and afflictions indicated sins, were related to penance, or affected a person's fate in the afterlife. Ostensibly, the treatise was not interested in various types of diseases, their symptoms, or their treatments. Although the physical experience of illness and its impact on a person's life and their ability to engage in various social and religious activities were sometimes discussed, physical experience was not the epistemic locus of the treatise or its area of exploration. What Ibn Abī al-Dunyā set out to explore was an epistemology in which the physical was imparted on the relationship, social and individual, between the sick person and God. At the same time, this pietistic epistemology of sickness relied precisely on the physical as its key infrastructure. Sickness here was not to include "sickness of the heart" (*amrāḍ al-qulūb*), which denoted doubts and sins and was discussed in a variety of other contexts, or "sickness of the soul" (*amrāḍ al-nufūs*), which was also discussed in other contexts, as will be seen later. Sickness here included only the diseases of the body as physically and sensually understood by both Ibn Abī al-Dunyā and his readers. This understanding of sickness as a type of pain located within the physical body and, in part, a construct of medical knowledge and practice, contributed to a shared sensorium of illness.

Ibn Abī al-Dunyā's text built on this shared sensorium to investigate the pietistic epistemology that framed it and provided it with additional meanings.[9]

Although Ibn Abī al-Dunyā's authorial voice is difficult to detect, the arrangement and choices – whether novel or connected to previous texts that discuss the same matter – reveal much about Ibn Abī al-Dunyā's interests and areas of focus. In the treatise, three main themes seem to organize much of the materials collected. The first and most dominant theme is the place of diseases within a pietistic cosmology where traditions are used to explore the connection between sin and disease and how diseases could result in reward. The second theme focused on the proper pietistic behavior during sickness. This meant discussions concerning what one should or should not say, whether or how one should complain, how and when one needs to visit sick people, and what to say during these occasions. In this context, Ibn Abī al-Dunyā paid a lot of attention to how one needed to behave before and after sickness and whether one's pietistic behavior and observance had an impact on the rewards that they might receive while sick. Finally, and as a third theme, the treatise devoted a brief space for discussions of certain prayers that were reported from the prophet or from important companions that were meant to help cure certain conditions or to improve one's health. Ibn Abī al-Dunyā repeated certain traditions several times to address what appears to be a variety of concepts or ideas. At points, he seemed to follow tangents that emerged from one ḥadīth by engaging other traditions that address this seemingly side point before returning to the original issue. Such a return might be signaled by repeating the original traditions or by invoking another tradition that addresses the initial question.[10]

Ibn Abī al-Dunyā's education and training mirrored many of his contemporaries in the ninth century: he was trained in ḥadīth, adab (*belles lettres*), and a number of other linguistic and religious sciences. He was able to secure a position as a teacher of Abbasid princes and was said to have been the teacher of the Abbasid caliph al-Muʿtaḍid (r. 892–902), among other members of the Abbasid household.[11] A look at Ibn Abī al-Dunyā's bibliography shows his deep interest in many questions related to adab, ḥadīth, and piety. Using the adab format of short topical treatises, he collected and catalogued many prophetic traditions and used them to explore a variety of topics that touched on piety and belief, along with history and other related issues. He wrote on repentance, forgiveness, reliance on God, certain belief, silence, hosting guests, contemplation, charity, and reclusion from people, among many other topics that were related to piety.[12]

The treatises of Hannād, Wakīʿ, Ibn al-Mubārak, Aḥmad ibn Ḥanbal, or Abū Ḥātim al-Rāzī were similar to Ibn Abī al-Dunyā. All these treatises were entirely composed of prophetic traditions and anecdotes about companions listed one after the other. As explained before, compilers of these treatises exercised their authorial voice through selecting and curating these little narratives and utilized the flexibility of these narratives to deploy them, often at multiple times, to indicate or impress different points.[13] The sizes of the different compendia, however, allowed for different organizational techniques. Although Ibn Abī al-Dunyā did not arrange his treatise into chapters due to its smaller size and clear singular focus, other scholars, such as Hannād and Ibn al-Mubārak, whose compendium was one of the largest, arranged theirs in chapters that discussed specific questions.

Wakīʿ, Ibn al-Mubārak, Ibn Ḥanbal, and al-Rāzī did not have dedicated chapters to questions of illness. However, they addressed some of the main questions that concern illness and piety at several different points that ranged from questions of calamity and patience to discussing the piety of the prophet Job, as in the case of Ibn Ḥanbal.[14] Hannād's text had a few chapters that were either fully or mostly dedicated to addressing illness. These included a chapter on visiting patients and one on asking God for good health. Other chapters on patience in the face of calamity, the severity of calamities affecting Muslims, the forgiveness of sins, and punishment in the earthly world were mostly about illness but also made mention of other forms of calamity.

Similarly, al-Bukhārī's treatise on diseases found in his compilation *al-Ṣaḥīḥ* was composed almost entirely of prophetic materials, following the structure of the rest of his ṣaḥīḥ. However, al-Bukhārī's text differed from the previously mentioned texts in two main ways. First, and consistent with his overall selection criteria for the ṣaḥīḥ, al-Bukhārī attempted to include traditions that he deemed 'authentic' and that were almost all elevated to the prophet. Second, al-Bukhārī showed more focus on legal questions.[15] Al-Bukhārī's authorial voice was similarly visible through his selections and the arrangement of his materials.[16] Moreover, al-Bukhārī organized his materials in short chapters with headings that explained what he thought a given grouping of ḥadīths indicated. He also often added specific verses in the beginning of some of these chapters that would further elaborate the intended meaning of his selections. In the treatise on illness, al-Bukhārī started with a chapter on illness and penance, followed by one dedicated to discussing the relationship between the severity of illness and divine reward. The following chapters discussed specific diseases and the rewards attached to them. Finally, a few chapters included questions about behavior during visiting the sick and about what sick people should do or say when they are sick.

As expected, many traditions and anecdotes repeated in these different texts, and even within the same text. In this way, these works animated a web of references that created meanings and conceptions of piety and illness, showing less interest in legal questions and implications, with some minor exceptions in al-Bukhārī. In this iterative web of references, texts, particularly those by Hannād and Ibn Abī al-Dunyā, were equally invested in anecdotes and traditions that included behaviors readers should attempt to emulate and other anecdotes and traditions that showed the extraordinary or transcendent behavior of the prophet or some of his companions and followers. Whereas the first group of reports and anecdotes aimed to provide a list of actions to be taken, beliefs to be held, and prayers to be recited, the second group, which were not suitable for emulating, contributed to creating a pietistic space that conditioned how pious Muslims understood their experiences with illness.

Diseases, sins, and rewards

The connection between illness and sin was at the heart of all pietistic writings about diseases. In the collections where no chapters were dedicated to illness, authors dispersed illness-related materials in chapters on patience and penance, emphasizing the centrality of this connection. Of course, in Ibn Abī al-Dunyā's case, the entire text was entitled "Illness and Penance." In this section, I will begin by investigating the concept and usage of 'penance *kaffārah*' in the cosmology of illness. I will then move to questions related to the severity of illness and to whether all diseases were seen as equal in terms of reward. Then, I will address the question of seeking cure or medical care from a pietistic perspective.

"Whomever does evil shall be recompensed for it"

The iterative nature of these ḥadīth compilations, especially in Hannād's and Ibn Abī al-Dunyā's texts, and Ibn Abī al-Dunyā's text's lack of strict organization provided the textual resources for creating sets of urtexts. Such texts were repeated several times, creating specific narrative units flowing from such texts to explore a variety of directions or questions. In discussing the question of illness and sin, the central urtext appeared to be a Quranic verse, which reads, "It is not your fancies, nor the fancies of the People of the Book. Whosoever does evil shall be recompensed for it, and will not find for him, apart from God, a friend or helper" [Q4:123]. Al-Ṭabarī (d. 923) explained that the verse was revealed when groups of Muslims, Jews, and Christians were debating who was more favored by God, each of whom enumerated specific advantages that they had over the others – such as having the first or the last of the religions and being more faithful to the heritage of Abraham, among others.[17] The verse then presented a rebuke to all these competing groups, explaining that whoever does evil will be recompensed for it. This was confirmed by the following verses, which also provided clearer indications of the superiority of Muslims over the people of the Book:

> And whosoever does deeds of righteousness, be it male or female, believing – they shall enter Paradise, and not be wronged a single date-spot. And who is there that has a fairer religion than he who submits his will to God being a good-doer, and who follows the creed of Abraham, a man of pure faith? And God took Abraham for a friend.
>
> [Q4:124–125]

In Ibn Abī al-Dunyā's narrative, however, these concerns were nowhere to be found. Instead, the various traditions reported to be engaging with this verse focused only on its second part, "Whosoever does evil shall be recompensed for it," which appeared to have caused much anxiety and generated many questions among the companions. In a version of the tradition attributed to ʿĀʾisha, she exclaimed that this verse was the most serious and worrisome verse in the Quran. It appears that she was not the only one who felt the severity of this verse.[18] Other companions, in the different iterations of the tradition reported by Ibn Abī al-Dunyā, wondered about its meaning or expressed their despair of salvation on account of this verse. For all of them, the notion of one's being punished for every bad deed removed the chance of mercy and made it virtually impossible for Muslims to survive the wrath of God. In all of these accounts, the prophet explained that Muslims are recompensed for their evil deeds not only in the afterlife, but more importantly, through illnesses and other forms of calamities that befall them during their lives. In some of the responses, the prophet mentioned illness specifically. In other responses, he explained that these afflictions and calamities might be as little as a prick by a thorn[19] or even a fleeting worry, as if one misplaced money and then found it.[20] In this context, the verse provided the opportunity to frame diseases within a narrative of atonement and to create a space in which afflictions were to be welcomed and accepted with hope and joy because they allowed a person to be cleansed of their errors and evils.

Hannād also addressed this verse in two different chapters – the chapter on patience in the face of calamity and the one on punishment for sins in earthly life. In the chapter on patience, one of the followers was asked about the meaning of the verse and explained, "for a believer, whatever calamity befalls him and he [faces it with] patience, [it is the recompense for the sins.] He then meets God with no sins."[21] Hannād also began his chapter on punishment in the earthly world with a tradition about this verse. In this tradition, Abū Bakr al-Ṣiddīq[22] was saddened when this verse was revealed for fear that it meant he would never survive the wrath of God. The prophet responded to him, explaining that such recompense happened through earthly suffering.[23] Similar traditions were also cited by Ibn Abī Ḥātim al-Rāzī (d. 939) in his tafsir (Quranic exegesis). There, he explained that the verse could be understood in two different ways. The first, to which Ibn Abī Ḥātim paid more attention and dedicated more space, recounted sickness and other calamities as ways to punish believers for their bad deeds. He cited the tradition by ʿĀʾisha, which Ibn Abī al-Dunyā mentioned. In another tradition, the prophet heard that some of his companions were distressed by the verse so he explained, "Yes. Believers are recompensed by afflictions in their bodies and other things that hurt them."[24] Ibn Abī Ḥātim also cited a version of the tradition reported by Hannād about Abū Bakr. In Ibn Abī Ḥātim's narrative, Abū Bakr was worried about his previous deeds before Islam, but was assured by the prophet in the same manner. Abū Bakr also reported that the prophet read the verse, "Whomever does evil shall be recompensed for in this life," thereby adding "in this life" to the verse to further clarify it.[25] In a second way to understand the verse, Ibn Abī Ḥātim cited al-Ḥasan al-Baṣrī, who explained that this applied only to the unbelievers citing another verse, "Punish we ever save the unbelievers?" [Q34:17][26]

The first chapter in al-Bukhārī's treatise, which was entitled, "The Penance [achieved by] Illness (*kaffārāt al-maraḍ*)," also started with the same verse, "whomever does evil shall be recompensed for it." Although none of the traditions that al-Bukhārī selected addressed this verse directly in the manner explained by Hannād or Ibn Abī al-Dunya, the presence of the verse at the beginning of the chapter further demonstrates its importance in pietistic discourses around sickness. The first two traditions in this chapter explained how each calamity that affects a Muslim could be a cause for reward. The third and fourth traditions explained the difference between believers and nonbelievers in relation to sickness. In this tradition, the prophet said:

> The believer is like a soft plant that is bent back and forth by the wind, (whenever it stands straight, it is then bent by calamities). The hypocrite is like a tree that stands straight to the wind until it is broken once and for all.[27]

For Ibn Baṭṭāl (d. 1058), the author of one of the earliest detailed commentary on *Ṣaḥīḥ al-Bukhārī*, the connection between diseases, sins, and reward required further elaboration.[28] Ibn Baṭṭāl (d. 1058) explored whether diseases and other calamities allowed for just redemption from sin or also increased the reward for believers. In this context, he cited the famous companion Ibn Masʿūd as saying, "No reward is earned by pain. But sins are forgiven by it."[29] Ibn Baṭṭāl recalled another tradition reported by al-Bukhārī in his chapter on jihad where the prophet said, "[I]f a servant falls sick or travels, whatever he did of good while resident or healthy will be counted for him." He explained that these traditions were not contradictory, "This is not a contradiction but rather an increase on top of what was mentioned in this chapter [of al-Bukhārī] in relation to forgiving sins based on pain and suffering." He then proceeded to explain, citing Abū Mūsā al-Ashʿarī, that if a person had a good habit that was interrupted by sickness or travel, God will continue his reward even while sick or traveling.[30]

Ibn Baṭṭāl then proceeded to give more attention to the last tradition in al-Bukhārī's chapter, which likened a Muslim to a small plant and the unbeliever to a solid tree. In this context, Ibn Baṭṭāl explained, citing al-Muhallab, "[A] Muslim is like a plant that bends back and forth following God's will; accepting God's orders as they come to him and accepting the calamities and distress hoping for God's reward in them."[31] Here, "standing back up" when affected with calamity referred to gratitude to God for afflicting the believer with pain and distress and responding with prayer and devotion.[32] Moreover, a believer awaits God's will and wishes that God would choose for him the best outcome – be it the continuation of distress and pain to earn forgiveness or the removal of pain and the blessing of good living. In contrast to this, the unbeliever is spared the pains and distress and awarded strength and power similar to a solid tree; however, as a solid tree that is capable of breaking, the unbeliever would be punished more in the afterlife, "So when God wills his [the unbeliever's] demise, he would break him like a solid tree is broken so his death is more painful as a punishment for the sins that were not repented."[33] Here, proper behavior is seen to center around accepting God's will and receiving it with patience and promise, which results in the acceptance of disease and illness, or "standing back up" in the face of calamity. In contrast, the continuation of health is seen as a foreboding sign of a worse outcome at death and in the afterlife.

"I suffer like two of you combined"

Although connecting diseases with penance and earthly (more tolerable and finite) punishment served to locate diseases within a pietistic narrative, it also posed important questions of causality: Are diseases caused by sins? The prophet, as sinless and infallible, but also commonly affected with diseases, was naturally located at the center of this question, and his diseases remained an anchoring point to narratives of medicine and disease in the prophetic heritage. Ibn Abī al-Dunyā started his book with a number of traditions about the prophet's illness. In the first tradition, the companion Abū Saʿīd al-Khudariyy said, "I visited the prophet while he was feverish. I put my hand over his clothes and found them to be very hot. So I said, "How severe your fever is! O prophet of God!" He said: "This is how it is for us prophets. Pain is doubled for us as is reward."[34] This tradition focused on the accrual of reward because of illness and pain while sidestepping the question of sins and their forgiveness altogether.

Similarly, Hannād reported two traditions in his chapter on "Forgiveness of Sins (*ḥaṭṭ al-khaṭāyā*)," where the prophet explained that he suffered twice as much as other people.[35] In another tradition, and similar to Ibn Abī al-Dunyā's, the prophet explained that prophets suffered more than other people and were also rewarded more.[36] In the same vein, the second chapter in al-Bukhārī's treatise discussed the question of the severity of illness starting with a tradition where ʿĀʾisha explained, "I have never seen a person who suffered in illness more than the prophet."[37] In another tradition, the prophet explained that he suffered twice as much as any other Muslims. Citing ʿAbd al-Razzāq al-Ṣanʿānī's (d. 826) *muṣannaf*, Ibn Baṭṭāl recalled a tradition about a companion who went to visit the prophet when the latter was sick:

> When [the companion] approached the prophet, he exclaimed, "I cannot even touch your skin from the severity of fever," to which the prophet replied, "We, prophets, are awarded twice the calamity as we are awarded twice the reward. Some prophets were afflicted with lice until lice killed them [. . .], and prophets used to rejoice when afflicted as you rejoice with your wellbeing."[38]

In this context, piety and closeness to God often meant one experienced even more severe calamities and more strenuous suffering that one must always receive with patience and belief. In the case of the prophet, diseases did not only remove sins but increased his favor with God and were conduits of reward in the afterlife. This idea, that diseases atone for sins but also add to the reward, played an important role in constructing the pietistic landscape in these narratives. Here, diseases are not seen as signs of sins but rather as conduits of God's favor, either through the forgiveness of past sins or for augmenting one's place in the afterlife.

In fact, this understanding of illness as a conduit of mercy and favor is emphasized in various occasions, underwriting layers of suspicion of health and of people who do not suffer from diseases. In one tradition, the prophet was reported as saying, "On the day of Judgement, the people of health (*ahl al-ʿāfiyah*) wish if their skins were peeled with peelers [during their lives]."[39] Here, people who did not suffer are shown to wish for suffering to deliver them from their sins and to provide them with more favor with God. In another account, a Bedouin visited the prophet to ask about a number of issues. When the question of illness and suffering was brought up (in one account in relation to headaches and migraines, from which the prophet seemed to have suffered frequently, and in another in relation to fevers), the Bedouin explained that he never suffered from any diseases. As he left, the prophet commented that this was a man who belonged to hellfire.[40] Although it was not clear whether this prophetic pronouncement did indeed seal this man's fate, the immediate point that the tradition discussed was the difficulty that a person would have in the afterlife if they were spared all diseases in their earthly life. To further discuss this point, Ibn Abī al-Dunya reported several times an account of Khālid ibn al-Walīd, the famous companion and military commander. In this account, Khālid divorced one of his wives who was known to be good to him and good to other people as well. When asked by his friends about the reasons for divorcing her, Khālid explained that "she never got sick in my home." In this view, the fact that she was always healthy was seen as potential evidence for her being impious or for her possible suffering in the afterlife. For Khālid, such an observation was a reason to divorce her despite her seemingly good behavior and their good companionship.[41]

This cosmology of illness, which saw diseases as a sign of God's favor, also presented a narrative that further underscored the differences between the pious and impious. Whereas the pious were afflicted with diseases and emerged with reward and forgiveness, the impious remained shackled with their sins.[42] Moreover, the pietistic discourse framing sickness, as articulated in Ibn Abī al-Dunyā's work and which entailed specific prescriptions for self-discipline and recommendations for behavior, was also a mode of distinction and differentiation along the same lines. In this context, and as will be seen later, the pious responded to illness with patience and delight, whereas the impious exhibited panic and desperation. Finally, this disease cosmology also differentiated between Muslims and non-Muslims. Diseases affecting Muslims were different and had different meanings, and Muslims were expected to deal with them differently from non-Muslims. Whereas Muslims benefitted from illness and emerged forgiven or blessed, non-Muslims and hypocrites were likened to beasts of burden that are loaded with heavy loads and demanded to carry them but without benefitting from them in any manner,[43] or likened to stiff trees that diseases broke and delivered to hellfire.

Piety in this context was also self-reflexive. The afflicted believer was to rejoice in their affliction as a sign of God's favor, but also recognize that this affliction was partly incurred by their own sins. In this mixture of delight and joy with God's mercy and regret for one's own shortcoming, the self-reflexive nature of this piety underwrote acceptance and patience.[44] This was demonstrated in a tradition originating with one of the companions and reported by Wakīʿ ibn al-Jarrāḥ where the companion bit his tongue during an episode of illness, exclaiming, "[I]t is you [the tongue] that delivered me to this."[45] Similarly, Ibn al-Mubārak reported a tradition where the prophet said that a man's health or wealth can be afflicted because of sin.[46] Ibn Abī al-Dunyā also reported that when the companion ʿImrān ibn Ḥuṣayn was afflicted by illness, he said, "I reckon this is incurred by my sins, and God pardons many more [sins]. He then recited, 'Whatever affliction may visit you is for what your own hands have earned.'"[47] The verse that ʿImrān used to conclude his words weaved his illness within a Quranic narrative that emphasized the connection between deeds and afflictions. Together, these traditions drew a narrative of pietistic self-reflexivity whereby the companion, known for his piety and his good deeds, admitted and reflected on his own sins and on God's mercy. Whether the afflictions that befell him ended up cleansing his sins or increasing his rewards would be impossible to know, but his disposition needed to be one of repentance and regret. In this context, diseases became occasions for self-reflection and for placing oneself within a narrative of pietistic performances.

Specific diseases have specific rewards

Ibn al-Mubārak, Hannād, and other authors of zuhd (renunciation of earthly life) were also interested in discussing specific diseases. For instance, in relation to fever, Hannād reported traditions that explained the significant rewards that came to those who endured fever, and Ibn Abī al-Dunyā mentioned a number of traditions that explained how fever was indeed a taste of hellfire.[48] Fever, a common and rather serious condition in this period,[49] played an important role at the physical and metaphorical levels. Physically, the debilitating nature of the disease, the potential mortality, and also the commonality of the condition underscored its place in this pietistic epistemology. At the same time, fever provided a perfect metaphor in relation to cleansing and purification as it was described to be similar to the fire that purifies iron. In these authors' narrative, when a Muslim suffers from fever, they encounter their share of hellfire for some past sins and emerge purer, much like iron emerges purer and stronger after being subjected to fire.[50] In one *mawqūf* tradition reported by Abī Hurayrah, the latter explained that fever enters every joint and every organ in the body, cleansing each of them from the sins that they have incurred.[51] Hannād reported three consecutive traditions on fever in his chapter on "enduring calamity." In the first:

> Fever sought permission to see the prophet. The prophet said, "Who is this?" She said "Umm maldam (a common moniker for fever)" The prophet said, "Go to the people of *qibā*ʾ [a town close to Medina]" When they suffered from it what only God knows, they came to the prophet and complained. He said, "If you wish, I will ask God to remove it from you. If you wish, it can be a cleansing for you." They said, "O prophet of God! Would you do [whatever we ask]?" He said, "Yes." They said, "[Then,] leave it. Let it be a cleansing."[52]

In this tradition, the prophet codified this description of fever as a form of cleansing (*ṭahur*). In Hannād's tradition, which was also cited in Ibn Abī al-Dunyā, the prophet explained to a feverish man that he was visiting, "God says, '[Fever] is my fire. I send it to my believing servant in this life to be his share of hellfire in the hereafter."[53] Connecting fever to hellfire further highlighted the original message of these narratives: diseases are recompenses and punishments of sins. The seemingly different physical and metaphorical natures of fever were eventually collapsed in Abū Hurayra's narrative, where the sprawling nature of the disease exhumed and removed traces of embodied sins left in each joint.

In two different chapters, al-Bukhārī, similar to Hannād and Ibn Abī al-Dunyā, focused on particular conditions specifying the promised rewards for them. In one chapter entitled, "The privilege of those who seizure (*faḍl man yuṣra*ʿ)," al-Bukhārī reported a tradition where a woman complained to the prophet about her epilepsy. Similar to the previously mentioned tradition concerning fevers, the prophet gave her the choice: he could pray for her cure, or she could withstand and earn heaven. She opted to withstand and the prophet promised her heaven.[54] His following chapter followed the same style when discussing blindness. Entitled, "The privilege of those who lost their eyesight (*faḍl man dhahaba baṣaruh*)," the chapter had one tradition where the prophet was reported as saying, "God says if I afflict my servant with his two darlings (meaning the eyes) and he was patient, I will recompense him with heaven."[55] In both cases, the specific nature of these diseases was connected to reward, thus creating a narrative linking the severity of the suffering a sick person experiences to receiving a divine reward. Ibn Baṭṭāl further explained that these two afflictions, among few others that were not explicitly mentioned, were particularly difficult diseases. In his comment on the woman afflicted with epilepsy, he explained that the tradition showed that "choosing calamity and hardship leads to paradise, and that choosing hardship is better than going with the license [meaning seeking relief] for whoever sees himself capable of withstanding difficulty and would not be weakened by it."[56] In relation to blindness, he explained that this was because eyesight is one of God's most important blessings and that withstanding such calamity leads to significant reward, "God recompenses a person for the loss of their eyesight with heaven, which is better because the duration of enjoyment of this bless (eyesight) in the earthly world is limited and, in the afterlife, it is unlimited."[57]

In these different works and narratives addressing illness, reward and forgiveness were conditioned in part on the knowledge of such rewards and forgiveness. Patience that was required and rewarded was one deeply rooted in the pious Muslim's knowledge and awareness that such patience is religiously recommended and pietistically favored. The pious Muslim's knowledge of this reward and their desire to achieve it were necessary to position this patience as a pietistic exercise and, therefore, were necessary to the achievement of the reward itself.[58] As a result, this knowledge placed diseases, or rather the experience of patienthood, in a varying cosmology with a particular form of action and agency emanating from it. In this context, seeking cure needed to be situated within this particular pietistic cosmology and the epistemologies that it stimulated. In Ibn Baṭṭāl's synthesis among others, seeking cure was characterized as the utilization of a license granted by God to the believers rather than opting for more difficulty and hardship in exchange for bigger reward. Yet, seeking cure, from a pietistic perspective, emanated still from patience and acceptance of God's will and operated within the licenses that God had granted to those who could not withstand.

At the same time, this pietistic cosmology was tethered to the embodied experience of illness. Not all illnesses were equal, and a new valuation of physical experiences of illness flowed from the relative sociocultural and professional values of organs, functions, and physiologies. In this view, blindness, as well as epilepsy, stood out as some of the more significant embodied experiences that rendered the most reward. Embodiment did not stop at the level of valuation and hierarchical worth of organs and faculties, but extended to render the disease process legible within the constructed pietistic epistemology. Here, fever, which could be placed within a hierarchical cosmology based on its severity, was also recalled experientially to refer to hellfire or to the purification of iron. The generalized experience that it generated was broken down into effects that engaged specific organs and particular spaces, purifying the body joint by joint. In other words, this emerging cosmology of illness was not in contradiction or even in competition with a physical cosmology that retrieved its components from medical discourses. Instead, the pietistic cosmology drew its resources and lexicon from the physical and experiential.

Seeking cure

The role of illness in this spiritual economy posed important questions about the legality of seeking cure and the pietistic implications of wishing a disease away – either through prayer to God or medical care.[59] To commence the exploration of this question, Ibn Abī al-Dunyā recalled the urtext centered around the verse, "Whosoever does evil shall be recompensed for it." In this account, the companion, who inquired about this verse and was answered by the prophet, explained that, since knowing the true meaning of this verse, he wished never to have a healthy day in his life.[60] In this context, the previously mentioned anecdote about the epileptic woman, which al-Bukhārī cited in a chapter about the reward for epilepsy, was one of the central narratives about seeking cure. In the anecdote, which Ibn Abī al-Dunyā repeated a few times, an epileptic woman came to the prophet to complain of her epilepsy. She suffered from convulsions and fainting that made her fall down in public and be exposed. When she asked the prophet to pray for her cure, he replied, "I can pray for you and you will be cured, or you can withstand your ailment patiently and I promise you heaven." With no hesitation, the woman opted to suffer and withstand her ailment with the prophetic promise of heaven. After a moment, she asked the prophet if he could pray for her not to be exposed in public, which he granted her.[61] In this case, the woman showed an example of opting for suffering to attain divine reward, turning down the prophetic offer for immediate and miraculous cure through his prayer. Her second request was not one of cure and healing, but rather, one focused on helping her to further perform her religious duties by not being exposed in public. Hannād reported a version of this tradition, which did not explain the condition from which the woman suffered (mentioning *lamam*, a generic term for illness or discomfort). In Hannād's version, the prophet promised the woman that, should she opt to endure, she would not be judged by God and thus would be delivered to heaven without judgement (*bilā ḥisāb*).[62]

In this context, Ibn Abī al-Dunyā's narrative betrayed an ambivalence toward seeking care. On one hand, he repeated the various traditions that explained how God has created cures for all illnesses. He also explained how the prophet sought cure and how he advised people to do the same or to benefit one another by providing care and cure for one another.[63] On the other hand, the pietistic impulse and the weight of the pietistic discourse was always centered on how one needed to be patient and to accept sickness with promise and joy.[64] This ambivalence ran deep throughout Ibn Abī al-Dunyā's text, with various traditions recommending patience and others recommending seeking a cure. Hannād's selections showed the same ambivalence. In a tradition that was also cited by Ibn Ḥanbal in his *zuhd*, Hannād described a scene by Abū Bakr's deathbed. There, when his family members asked whether he needed to see a physician, he remarked that he saw one and that he said, "I do what I want," referencing God. There was no use in seeking medical care when God would do what he had destined from the beginning.[65] Similarly, Ibn al-Mubārak in his *zuhd*, as well as Hannād and Ibn Abī Ḥātim al-Rāzī in his recension of Ibn Marthad's (d. 738) *Zuhd al-Thamāniyah* (The Renunciation of the Eight [Followers]), cited a tradition in which the follower al-Rabīʿ ibn Khuthaym was advised to see a physician when he was sick (or in Ibn al-Mubārak's version, when he was afflicted by paralysis). Ibn Khuthaym refused and cited the ruined nations of ʿĀd and Thamūd, who "had sick people and had physicians. Neither the sick survived [the wrath of God] nor the physicians."[66] In the same vein, asking God for healing could also indicate a lack of patience and a desire to escape the calamity destined by God himself. This point was emphasized in Ibn Ḥanbal's retelling of Job's story in his *zuhd*. There, Ibn Ḥanbal explained, through traditions reported from companions, that Job refused his wife's request to ask God for cure. Instead, he opted to withstand without complaint.[67]

While exhibiting similar ambivalence towards seeking cure, al-Bukhārī and Ibn Baṭṭāl attempted to resolve the potential legal quandary seeking cure posed. For Ibn Baṭṭāl, the preference of abstaining from seeking cure seemed to contradict the prophet praying for cures for his companions – a point on which al-Bukhārī reported a number of traditions in another chapter. Ibn Baṭṭāl quoted al-Ṭabarī, "These traditions mean, from a jurisprudential view, that wishing cure is better for the servant than wishing to stay in illness."[68] Ibn Baṭṭāl followed with a tradition where the prophet asked his companions, "Who would like to remain healthy and never to get sick?" When the companions said, "We do, O messenger of God," the prophet replied, "Do you wish to be like wild asses?!!" The prophet's face showed anger as he added, "Don't you wish to be people of sickness and of repentance?!"[69] The prophet then explained that God sends hardship on the believers to test them, forgive their sins, and award them with his favor. A seemingly contradicting tradition was reported in Wakīʿ, Hannād's, and Ibn Ḥanbal's *zuhd* books, where the follower Muṭrif said "It is more pleasing to me to be healthy and thank God than to be sick and endure."[70] Ibn Baṭṭāl explained:

> None of these traditions contradict another [. . .]. This is because illnesses and calamities are penance for the people of faith, and punishment, with which God removes sins from whom he desires [. . .]. Since illnesses and pains are punishment for sins, it is reported that the prophet prayed for health for only those who did not commit cardinal sins (*kabāʾir*), and only for those who were free from sins that mandate punishment and from injustices committed against the servants [of God]. [The prophet] hated to choose health over sickness for those who committed sins [. . .] and disliked that they choose to meet God with their sins unrepented.[71]

Ibn Baṭṭāl seemed to indicate that some people should choose to remain sick if they believe or know that they committed cardinal sins. For others, wishing for health was acceptable.

These different traditions show the different registers in discussing illness between jurisprudential views, cited by al-Ṭabarī and Ibn Baṭṭāl, and pietistic discourses. At the jurisprudential level, Ibn Baṭṭāl, following al-Bukhārī's narrative as well as al-Ṭabarī and others, emphasized the permissibility of seeking cure, citing traditions that showed the prophet seeking cure for some of his companions. At the pietistic level, as represented in the various books of zuhd, the overwhelming majority of traditions emphasized the primacy of accepting God's punishment and the desire for illness to be a penance, a conduit for forgiveness or for reward. In this context, Ibn Baṭṭāl seemed to suggest that those who committed cardinal sins should not seek cure, as they would benefit the most from the penance that came with illness. For others with lesser sins, like all believers, the choice and tension between the permissible and more pious remained. In all cases, believers were expected to accept the calamities sent by God and to understand that the best course would be to ask God to choose for them in the absence of the prophet's choice. The emphasis on how a believer receives calamity is highlighted in a gloss by Ibn Baṭṭāl, where he reported a tradition:

> The prophet said: "Great reward comes with great calamity. When God favors some people, he tests them with calamities. Whoever [receives the calamities] with gratitude, will receive gratitude [from God], and whoever receives them with anger, will receive anger."[72]

In this context, those who committed cardinal sins stood to benefit from calamities but also needed to receive these calamities with gratitude as they delivered them from sins and punishment.

Within narratives of illness and healing, death was presented as another possible end that both indicated further calamity (entailed in diseases not cured) as well as salvation from the pain of failing health. In one tradition reported by Ibn Abī al-Dunyā, a companion was warned against wishing for death to escape a severe illness.[73] Instead, he was advised to be patient and to count on God for rewarding his patience. These traditions located death within narratives of calamity and piety. One was not to wish for death as wishing represented a desire to escape God's will or a false understanding of the role of illness in this pietistic cosmology. Similar to Ibn Abī al-Dunyā's narrative, al-Bukhārī's discussion of withstanding illness was also connected to the prohibition of wishing death. Al-Bukhārī included a chapter entitled "On a sick person wishing for death. (*tamannī al-marīḍ al-mawt*)." The chapter started with a tradition where the prophet said, "No one of you should wish for death. If he has to, let him say 'God, keep me alive as long as life is best for me and take me to you if death is better for me.'"[74] For both al-Bukhārī and Ibn Baṭṭāl, this tradition was connected to illness and calamity, and death was seen as a form of relief from earthly pain. In this view, wishing for death was condemned because life – although burdened with its pain and suffering – would allow the believer to repent and have a better fate in the afterlife. Ibn Baṭṭāl was aware that ʿUmar ibn al-Khaṭṭāb (one of Muḥammad's closest companions and the second caliph) was reported to have wished for death and that he died only few days after. Similarly, ʿAlī ibn Abī Ṭālib (Muḥammad's cousin and the fourth caliph) also wished for death saying, "Oh God, I have grown weary of my people and they have grown weary of me." It was even reported that the prophet himself asked for death during his final illness, "ʿĀʾisha said, 'The prophet said, while leaning on me, O God, forgive me, have mercy on me and take me to your company.'"[75] Ibn Baṭṭāl commented, "The prophet has prohibited his nation from wishing for death when they are afflicted by calamity and ordered them to wish for death if death was good for them." As for the prophet's wishing for death, or rather saying "take me to your company," Ibn Baṭṭāl explained that this occurred after the prophet knew that he was going to die, as all prophets are informed of their death. For both ʿUmar and ʿAlī, Ibn Baṭṭāl reasoned, they wished for death when they felt that they would not be able to fulfill God's orders and their responsibilities as caliphs. In this context, a believer is to ask for death only if they fear that they could not fulfill religious obligations. Here, the calamity that would justify wishing for death is one that affects believers' religious obligations, threatening their ability to fulfill their God-given roles.

Reward is not for everyone: pietistic behavior when sick

Although these authors affirmed the connection between diseases, penance, and reward for Muslims, they also explained that such penance and reward relied on certain behaviors and specific acts. As such, these texts provided a template of correct or pious behavior that pious Muslim needed to follow to achieve reward. In this section, I start by discussing patience and its importance. I then look at how pious Muslims were instructed to place illness within the context of divine blessings.

Patience and complaining

In Ibn Abī al-Dunyā's narrative around sickness, divine reward was not just a consequence of diseases or a compensation for suffering, but rather a framework through which pietistic acts were constructed. Reward was based not merely on the connection to illness but also on the pietistic behaviors, thoughts, and intentions one performed to deal with illness. Selections in his treatise paid attention to how one should behave when sick, what sorts of thoughts, and intentions conformed with the practice and advice of the prophet, and how reward was adjudicated. Importantly, the connection between illness and reward motivated a discussion about the reasons behind reward and its connection to suffering. In addition to forgiving sins on account of patience in the face of calamity, Ibn Abī al-Dunya reported a number of traditions that presented a more vivid picture of God's connection to illness and reward:

> [The prophet] smiled and looked at [heaven]. We said, "O prophet of God, what made you smile and look up?" He said, "I was amused by two angels

> that descended from heaven looking for a servant where they used to see him pray but did not find him. So they ascended to God and told him, 'O Lord! We used to record so-and-so of good deeds for your servant (*fulān*) in a given day or night. We have found that you have tied him in your chains [by sickness] so we did not record any deeds for him [today]'. God told them, 'Record for my servant whatever he used to do in his day or night and do not take away any of it. I guarantee his reward because it is I who chained him, and he earns the rewards of what he used to do.'"[76]

Prior worship and devoutness became a conduit for further reward. Piety is emphasized as a rather constant state of observance and dedication that could only be interrupted by divine intervention – through sickness. Hannād reported a similar tradition, where God told his angels, "[R]ecord for my servant all that he used to do in his health so long as he is in my bondage." The prophet commented, "If God takes him, He takes him in goodness. And if He heals him, he changes his flesh with better flesh and his blood with better blood."[77] Hannād's and Ibn Abī al-Dunyā's narratives, which were also echoed by Wakīʿ and others, emphasized consistency, reliability, and maintenance of a constant state of devotion rather than 'discovering' God during times of illness. This particular characterization was not isolated to a single tradition; it was repeated in three other occasions in Hannād's and seven in Ibn Abī al-Dunyā's. In these narratives, sickness was woven within a larger discourse on piety and devotion that extended before and after the period of affliction.

In addition to piety before sickness, one's behavior while sick was central to receiving divine reward. In one tradition, the proper attitude toward sickness was directly linked to divine reward:

> Umm Salamah said, I heard the prophet say: "Whenever God befalls a servant with a calamity, He makes this calamity a penance and cleansing, as long as [the servant] does not reckon this calamity as caused by anyone but God, and [does not] ask anyone but God for relief."[78]

The reward attached to diseases or calamities is conditional on how one behaves and thinks during the affliction. Not only is one required to be patient and to accept God's will, they are also asked to fully believe that God was the cause of such calamity and that He is the only one able to remove it.[79] This conditional relationship is further demonstrated in an anecdote about a companion named Khālid al-Rabʿī who suffered from pleurisy that led to severe pain and cough. Ibn Abī al-Dunyā relates that Khālid coughed blood and moaned in pain, "and he had never moaned of pain before. [. . .] Khālid said: 'O Lord, it is not worthy of you that I moan because of a pain you have afflicted me with.'"[80] In this anecdote, Khālid showed his belief that it was God who caused him this pain and calamity. At the same time, he exhibited patience and endured the suffering, believing that even an involuntary moan was an affront to God and, perhaps, a sign of his impatience or his anger. In Khālid's regret of his moan, Ibn Abī al-Dunyā showed how complaining of illnesses might be a sign of impatience and anger with God. In another tradition, the prophet was reported to have said,

> If one hides a fever that afflicted him for a day, God will deliver him from his sins [so that he is like] the day he was born, will guarantee him deliverance from hellfire, and will hide [his sins and shortcomings (*satara ʿalayh*)] like he hid God's affliction in the earthly world (*kamā satara balāʾ Allāh ʿalayhi fī al-dunyā*).[81]

Thus, hiding illness and refraining from complaining was portrayed as akin to God's hiding the servant's own mistakes and sins – both using the verb *satara* (lit. to cover a defect).

In the same way, Al-Bukhārī dedicated a chapter in his treatise on illness to complaining and to what a person might say while sick. He entitled his chapter, "A chapter on a patient's saying 'I'm pained' or 'O my head!' or 'pain has tired me' and Job's saying '[A]ffliction has visited me, and Thou art the most merciful of the merciful'" (*Bāb qawl al-marīḍ innī wajiʿ aw wā rāʾsāh aw ishtadd biya al-wajaʿ wa qawl Ayyūb masaniya al-ḍurr wa anta arḥam al-rāḥimīn*). The mention of Job in the title of the chapter refers to the Quranic story:

> And Job – when he called unto his Lord, "Behold, affliction has visited me, and Thou art the most merciful of the merciful." So We answered him, and removed the affliction that was upon him, and We gave his people, and the like of them with them, mercy from Us, and a reminder to those who serve.
> [Q21:83–84]

The traditions that al-Bukhārī included in this chapter did not include any mention of Job and his story. It is clear, however, that al-Bukhārī understood this verse and Job's prayer for his healing to be connected to discussion about patient's complaining. In his *zuhd*, Ibn Ḥanbal addressed this verse directly in a chapter dedicated to Job's renunciation of earthly comforts and piety:

> A group of the Israelites passed by Job [while he was sick] and said, "He would not have been afflicted with this except for a grave sin that he has committed." Job heard [what they said.] He then said, "O Lord, affliction has visited me, and Thou art the most merciful of the merciful." and he [Job] had never prayed [for his healing] before.[82]

In Ibn Ḥanbal's view, Job's prayer was not motivated by his sickness but rather by what he deemed as even more intolerable: a doubt in his devotion to God.

In his chapter on complaining, al-Bukhārī included four traditions that addressed various aspects of the issue of complaining about illness and what one should say when sick. In the first, the prophet passed by a man who had a lice infestation and asked him whether the lice hurt him. When the man said yes, the prophet advised him to shave his head. The tradition was cited here to indicate that asking about pain and answering affirmatively were legally permissible. The prophet here used the verb *yu'dhī* (hurt) to inquire about his companion.[83] In the second tradition, ʿĀʾisha cried, "O my head!" which the prophet did not condemn; instead, the two engaged in a rather long and elaborate joke about whether or not he would be sad if she died. Here again, the importance lay in the specific words ʿĀʾisha used ("O my head!") that were sanctioned by the prophet. In the third tradition, the prophet is the one who was asked about his pain and who answered affirmatively. This was the same tradition that al-Bukhārī had used in an earlier chapter to indicate how the prophet suffered more than anyone else. Here, too, the tradition served to indicate the permissibility of asking and answering, as well as of explaining and describing one's pain following the example of the prophet, who had described his pain as being twice as much of any of his companions'. The final tradition was one often cited in issues related to the writing of wills and to questions of inheritance. A companion said:

> The prophet came to visit me when I was sick after his pilgrimage. I said, "I have been afflicted with what you see, and I have money and only one daughter to inherit me. Should I give two thirds of my money in charity?" He said no. I said, "then a half?" He said no. I said, "then a third?" He said, "a third is too much. To leave your heirs self-sufficient is better than leaving them a burden asking people [for money]. Whatever you spend of your money hoping for God, you will be rewarded for, including what you spend on your wife."[84]

Although the seeming core of this tradition addressed questions unrelated to health and disease, al-Bukhārī's interest in this chapter was related to the first lines of the tradition where the companion explained or complained to the prophet about his sickness by way of asking about his money after death.

In his commentary on this chapter, Ibn Baṭṭāl was aware of the various legal and pietistic issues at stake. First, he cited al-Ṭabarī as saying that it was permissible for people to complain about illnesses and to moan and groan out of pain, "because the souls of the children of Adam are naturally created to complain and to feel pain." However, "a servant was demanded [by God] to abstain from [as much complaining as] he could, [especially] crying in case of calamity or moaning in case of pain."[85] For Ibn Baṭṭāl, this obligation not to complain was wide-reaching. He cited a number of companions who said that complaining was not permissible and some who never moaned of pain throughout their disease-ridden lives. He concluded:

> It is the consensus of all on disliking a servant's complaining about his Lord because of a calamity or hardship [. . .]. This is because [complaining entails] one's mentioning to people what his Lord has tested him with by way of annoyance. [Therefore,] a person who moans and groans is in the same position as one telling people [about his hardship] with annoyance and impatience.[86]

Ibn Baṭṭāl differentiated two categories of those who complain. The first, discussed earlier, were those who complain about diseases with annoyance and impatience and show disrespect toward God. Another category included those who mention illness to their brethren in faith, hoping that they may pray for their recovery, which is similar to what the prophet and his companions did. Similarly, those who moan or cry because pain has overcome them were not to be blamed either. Job's statement, which Ibn Baṭṭāl reported that al-Ḥasan al-Baṣrī had repeated when suffering toothache, represented the perfect manner in which a person can complain or talk about illness with utmost acceptance and respect to God.

For Ibn Abī al-Dunyā, al-Bukhārī, and others, speech's declarative function was regulated to create a pietistic space, where performance did not assume epistemic relevance. Explaining the severity of illness to a questioner or, perhaps, to a physician, or mentioning illness by way of discussing other issues was permissible as such speech acts carried epistemic relevance. Yet when such acts did not carry this relevance and did not convey knowledge that is needed or required, speech acts came to be strictly regulated. For instance, although God knew how a person was hurting, and other people may have also been able to understand his or her pain and suffering, speech acts that defined, explained, or complained about this pain were deemed impious as they showed impatience with divine trials. In this case, speech acts were epistemically irrelevant and were strictly regulated. At the same time, when speech acts intervened or influenced people's epistemic access to one's condition, abstaining from complaining was further rewarded. When the prophet advised that hiding fever for even a day would yield significant reward, this hiding was not simply abstaining from complaints to those who knew about the disease. Instead, it was precisely an act of *satr* or "covering" of the calamity inflicted by God that was rewarded immediately by God's *satr* or "covering" of one's vices and bad deeds.

In these accounts, speech acts were seen as uttered in the presence of God. Even if these words were directed to people, the possibility that God might be insulted or blamed or that any form of annoyance and impatience might be directed at him was behind these pietistic restrictions on speech. The presence of God in this disease-scape was further emphasized by showing that complaining about diseases could indeed be a complaint levied against God as the ultimate cause of these conditions. Ibn Abī al-Dunyā's selections went further to emphasize this presence:

> The prophet said, "if a servant is afflicted [with illness], God sends him two angels telling them, 'Go to my servant. If he speaks good and does not complain to his visitors, I will replace his flesh with a better flesh, and his blood with better blood. If I bring him to me [meaning if he dies], I guarantee him paradise. If I release him [from illness], he will be [free from sin] and would recommence his [good] deeds.'"[87]

God was physically present, not only through his omniscience, but also through physical emissaries that sat with the patient and reported his or her deeds.

In all these cases, the goal was not simply to govern actual words or enunciations, but also to develop a unique and conscious disposition that governed speech. Although certain words were mentioned explicitly in the traditions, such as 'Ā'isha's saying "O my head!" and were therefore deemed permissible in themselves, the disposition behind these words was central to the role they played in this pietistic environment. For instance, saying "O my head!" in a manner that intended to complain or that was indeed as a sign of impatience would invalidate the original permissibility of these words and render them offensive to God. As such, the words and the different situations reported in these various traditions aimed to create a web of references that allowed pious Muslims to develop a conscious disposition infused with fear and gratitude to God and that governed and regulated their speech beyond specific examples.[88]

'Urwa ibn al-Zubayr: pain and gratitude

Ibn Abī al-Dunyā traced an anecdote about the companion 'Urwah ibn al-Zubayr that seemed to embody the discussion surrounding affliction and patience and show a model for proper behavior. Focusing on different aspects of the story at different times, Ibn Abī al-Dunyā repeated the story about ten times with varying details and from varying sources, using it to start some of the discussions and questions delineated earlier. In this account, 'Urwah's leg was afflicted with maggots or gangrene on his way back to Damascus from Medina. When the Umayyad caliph, al-Walīd ibn 'Abd al-Malik (r. 705–715), heard about this, he insisted that 'Urwah see a physician (in other versions also reported by Ibn Abī al-Dunyā, it was 'Urwah's friends who suggested that he see a physician). After resisting and consistently belittling his suffering, 'Urwah either agreed or was forced to see a physician. The physician decided the leg would need to be amputated and offered to give 'Urwah a medication that would cloud his mind during the amputation. 'Urwah refused to take the medication. In one account, he explained his decision by saying, "One is not to take a drink that clouds his mind so that he does not know his Lord."[89] In another, he added, "I would not take a drink that would prevent me from praying to my Lord."[90] More indicative of the notion of patience, Ibn Abī al-Dunyā reported another version where 'Urwah explained his rejection of medication by saying, "God has afflicted me with this to see my patience, should I then object to his will by removing [the suffering]?"[91]

In the various accounts of the amputation, Ibn Abī al-Dunya demonstrated how the process was exceptionally painful. In one account, the physician chose to cut part of the living flesh to make sure no gangrene was left. In another, they used three different saws, one after the other, to cut through the flesh and bone or used a sword to cut through the flesh and (one or more) saws to cut the bone. In all these cases and despite the clearly agonizing pain, the people around 'Urwah reported, "[W]e have not heard him utter a sound" that would show his pain, even though some reported that the pain caused him to faint by the time the amputation was completed.[92] Instead, he kept saying, "[Lord!] If you have taken, you have also left; and if you have afflicted, you have also healed."[93] Soon after the amputation was completed, ʻUrwah was told that he lost his favorite (or eldest) son, Muḥammad, who died after being kicked and stepped on by camels or horses. To that ʻUrwah responded by thanking God and saying:

> Lord! You have endowed me with four limbs. Then you took one and left me three, for that I thank you. And you have endowed me with five sons. Then you took one and left four. For that I thank you. You have taken but you have left. And You have afflicted but You have healed.[94]

Despite his pain, ʻUrwah was able to place his calamity within the context of divine blessing, understanding that God's gifts have exceeded the calamities – not to mention that these calamities were a blessing in themselves as they helped him reach heaven.

The centrality of the ʻUrwah account and its attractiveness to Ibn Abī al-Dunyā was likely because this anecdote touched on a variety of questions at the heart of his narrative. First, ʻUrwah was injured while returning from either a pilgrimage or a visit to the Holy Cities, therefore establishing that, to reap reward, one must maintain piety and religious commitment before illness. Second, ʻUrwah's initial rejection then reluctant acceptance of treatment in the form of amputation reflected the ambivalence between seeking cure and withstanding the calamity with the hope of a better reward. Here, ʻUrwah belittled the suffering, keeping his focus on the more central question: God's reward. Third, and building from the previous point, ʻUrwah rejected medications that were to cloud his mind. This was not framed as a legal discussion on the use of alcohol or other drugs in treatment.[95] Instead, ʻUrwah's interest was in maintaining his ability to worship God and pray at all times. Also, in focusing on the rewards attached to suffering, ʻUrwah would not give away the blessing of pain that came with forgiveness and reward.

ʻUrwah's behavior and response to first losing his leg and then losing his son demonstrated his gratitude to God by remembering what God has endowed him and not focusing solely on what God has deprived him or has taken away. In this context, Ibn Abī al-Dunyā recalled al-Ḥasan al-Baṣrī's interpretation of the verse, "Man is an ingrate unto his Lord" [Q100:6]. Al-Ḥasan al-Baṣrī, a well-respected authority, explained that the verse did not only refer to humanity's lack of gratitude at moments of plenty. Instead, it also reflected how humans, when afflicted with trial, often forget the blessings that had been given to them and only "remember the calamities."[96] Faced with calamity, ʻUrwah immediately recalled the various blessings that far outmatched these calamities.[97] In Ibn Abī al-Dunya's narrative, the polar opposite of ʻUrwa's attitude was presented by a Bedouin, who fell sick and was visited by the prophet. When the prophet told him, "A cleansing God willing" (meaning that the disease would cleanse the man of his sins), he replied, "Cleansing?! No! Rather a burning for an old man that would drive him to his grave." The prophet replied, "It is so then!"[98]

At the end of two different versions of ʻUrwah's anecdote, he asked for his leg after it was cut, held it in his hand, and spoke to it, "God knows that I have never stepped with you in the direction of sin."[99] ʻUrwah's discourse with his leg was reminiscent of various contemporary accounts on how God would call on body parts to stand witness to the deeds committed by their owners. For instance, in the exegesis of the verse, "This day We seal up their mouths, and their hands speak out to Us and their feet bear witness as to what they used to earn" [Q36:65], al-Ṭabarī (d. 923) reported a tradition from al-Aʿmash and al-Shuʿabiyy who said:

> On the Day of Judgement, a man is told, "you did this and this," so he says "I did not." Then his mouth is sealed and his limbs testify [to his sins]. He then says to them, "May God curse you! I have not sinned except for you."[100]

Similar to Abū Hurayra's description of fever as a cleansing of each joint, ʿUrwah's discourse with the amputated leg underscores the physical infrastructure of this pietistic narrative. Piety, as well as sin, manifested physically in the organs and body parts that undertook them. At the same time, the individual, or the human being subject to divine reward and punishment, was separated from their own bodies and rendered guardians of these tools granted to them by God.

As mentioned before, diseases discussed in these writings were undoubtedly physical and their manifestations deeply embodied. Moreover, the narratives of ʿUrwah, Abū Hurayrah, and others further emphasized the corporeal nature of the pietistic narrative. Not only were these texts concerned with physical pain and embodied suffering, they were also interested in explicating how this physicality governed reward and regulated the divinely inhabited disease-scape. Reward was regulated and adjudicated based on the degree of physical and embodied suffering. Speech, as a corporeal performance, was regulated en route to regulating one's thoughts and dispositions. God was not only following one's deeds due to his omniscience, He also sent angels to physically surround the diseased and report on his deeds. Angels inspected the places that a diseased person used to frequent and was prevented because of illness. In all these examples, among many others, this pietistic narrative underscored the deeply embodied nature of illness and the equally corporeal and physical nature of the piety that it required.[101]

Diseases and social piety

The pietistic cosmology diseases existed in was a social one that involved not only the sick person and God, but also caretakers, friends, relatives, and others who knew the sick person. Although caretaking and the obligations related to such activities were organized in a variety of contexts that related to gender, the identity, and the relationship between caretakers and the cared for (such as discussions of caring for children, spouses, parents, etc.), the pietistic social cosmology of diseases was organized around visiting patients. The act acquired its own term *ʿiyādah*, rarely used to describe any other form of visits. Developing as a unique term, *ʿiyādah* became a locus of pietistic epistemology, where scholars like Ibn al-Mubārak, Hannād, Ibn Abī al-Dunyā, al-Bukhārī, and others contributed to the knowledge of this practice, what it meant, and how it should be conducted. Hannād dedicated a chapter to visiting patients, which he entitled *ʿIyādat al-Marīḍ*. He started the chapter with a tradition that highlighted the obligation to visit the sick, "The prophet said, 'Respond to the caller [in the call for prayers], and visit (*ʿūdū*) the sick."[102] Ibn Abī al-Dunyā cited Ibn ʿAbbās to define the legal status of visiting patients and whether it was an obligation. Ibn ʿAbbās explained that "visiting a sick person once is a sunna. More visits are additional good deeds (*nāfila*)."[103]

Whereas Ibn ʿAbbās, cited by Ibn Abī al-Dunyā, did not seem to believe that visiting patients was a religious obligation, al-Bukhārī, followed by Ibn Baṭṭāl, disagreed. The first chapter dedicated to visiting patients in al-Bukhārī's ṣaḥīḥ was entitled, "On the obligation to visit the sick (*wujub ʿiyādat al-marīḍ*)." This chapter contained one tradition where the prophet ordered his companions to participate in funerals and to visit the sick.[104] Ibn Baṭṭāl explained that the obligation to visit the sick is a communal obligation (*farḍ kifāyah*), which means that it would be fulfilled for all when even one person fulfills it and does not require every person to visit every sick person they know.[105] In either case, visiting a patient was not seen as a personal duty that drew from a person's relationship to the sick. Instead, it was either a communal obligation that ensured that the sick would be visited, a sunna, or a recommended act that individuals were encouraged to engage in.

Authors emphasized that proper intentions and true desire to seek God's favor were necessary to perform this pietistic act of visitation. In one tradition, the prophet was reported to have said, "Whoever visits a sick person, hoping for God's reward and the accomplishment of God's promise, God assigns him seventy-thousand angels to pray for him until he returns to his home [from the visit]."[106] In another tradition that also recalled the theme of angels praying for one who visits the sick, a caller from heaven calls on the visitor, "May you and your steps be blessed, and may you find your place in heaven."[107] In both cases, the reward is not precisely defined; however, the angels' prayers and the heavenly caller indicated the significant, though unspecified, rewards promised to the visitor. Other traditions reported by Hannād and Ibn Abī al-Dunya, among others, utilized different metaphors to express the type of reward that is given to the visitor. In one tradition, the prophet explained that, "A visitor walks under a shade from heaven" as he walks to the house of the sick person.[108] In another, the prophet explained that, "A visitor wades in mercy up to his knees, and when he sits, mercy covers him all."[109]

In all these traditions, emphasis was placed on the process of visiting – leaving the house, walking to the sick, and sitting there – creating a ritualized framework for the visit as part of this emerging pietistic cosmology. This ritualized space was regularized and organized in many details from the time of the visit, the duration one should spend in a sick person's house, to what to say and what not to say and whether or not to touch the patient or eat at their house. For instance, and as an example of the details that conditioned such ritualized practice, Hannād, followed by Ibn Abī al-Dunyā, explained that this ritualized pietistic visit should occur only after three days of a person's falling sick.[110] In a couple of traditions, Ibn Abī al-Dunyā addressed the proper duration and frequency of these visits. Visits should not be daily but rather every other day or every fourth day, if repeated at all.

If the patient or their family are overwhelmed by disease, poverty, or both, then they should not be visited to reduce the burdens on them. If the person dies, a single visit for consolation should be made.[111] In different places, Ibn Abī al-Dunyā selected traditions that explained that the best visit is a light one that lasts for a short time and does not require much effort on the part of the sick person and their families.[112] In one instance, the prophet was reported as saying that visitation should last for the duration it takes a she-camel to recover from a milking session before being ready for a second.[113]

During a visit, visitors should pray for the sick person to be cured and to receive God's mercy. Ibn Abī al-Dunya reported two prayers that a visitor could say to help the patient.[114] Hannād reported a detailed tradition, where the prophet instructed on what one should do during a visit,

> The prophet said, "It is of the completion of visiting the sick (*ʿiyādat al-marīḍ*) that you extend your hand to him, ask him how he is, put your hand on him. And it is of the completion of your greeting him that you shake his hand."[115]

Similarly, al-Bukhāri dedicated two chapters to the type of behavior required of or expected from those who visit the sick. In the first, he addressed the recommendation to put a hand on the sick person's body and to touch the area of pain while praying for the sick.[116] In the second chapter entitled, "What should be said to the patient and how he should reply (*mā yuqāl lil-marīḍ wa mā yujīb*)," al-Bukhārī reported traditions that mentioned specific prayers recited by the prophet and particular responses given by the patient that aimed to show patience and acceptance of God's will.[117] For Ibn Baṭṭāl, placing a hand on the patient was a sign of care and a way of understanding how much the patient was hurting. The prayers, and more importantly for Ibn Baṭṭāl, the responses given by the patient, were important in providing evidence for accepting God's will and showing patience.[118]

At another level, this ritualized practice also reflected the social and gendered organization of the society. Al-Bukhārī was, for example, interested in the organization of the space of visitation with the jurisprudential implication that such organization entailed. One of his chapters dealt with visiting the Bedouins and mentioned a tradition where the prophet visited a Bedouin when sick.[119] For Ibn Baṭṭāl, the tradition fell within the general obligation to visit the sick but it was useful in indicating that

> [I]t is not blameworthy if a ruler visits a sick person of his flock or a person in the rural [areas of his domain], or if a scholar visits an ignorant person. This is because Bedouins are known for their ignorance as mentioned by God in the Quran.[120]

In the same vein, al-Bukhārī's chapter on visiting sick children indicated, in Ibn Baṭṭāl's view, that people of power and privilege could visit even sick children. Chapters discussing visiting women served a similar purpose and proved the permissibility of men visiting women when sick.

When it came to visiting sick nonbelievers, al-Bukhārī's choice was a tradition where the prophet visited a servant of a Jewish neighbor, who was likely also Jewish. The prophet invited the servant to convert and he converted. Al-Bukhārī also referenced a tradition by Saʿīd ibn al-Musayyab who mentioned that the prophet visited his uncle Abū Ṭālib, who died a polytheist, when the latter was on his deathbed.[121] The two traditions showed that visiting the non-Muslim sick was at least permissible. However, Ibn Baṭṭāl argued that the traditions implied an obligation to invite these non-Muslims to Islam:

> [Such visits are meant] to invite them [the non-Muslim sick] to Islam, if their conversion was deemed possible. Don't you see that the Jew converted when the prophet invited him? And that the prophet invited his uncle to Islam but God did not will [the uncle] to convert? However, if the conversion of the unbeliever was not sought or seen as possible, he should not be visited when sick.[122]

In this view, visiting the sick was placed within the context of establishing the connections among Muslims and maintaining solid relations in the community or, at least, attempting to expand the community by converting or seeking to convert non-Muslims. However, it was less desirable, if not entirely prohibited, when it was directed to those outside the community.

For al-Bukhārī and others, visitations were important social acts that symbolized and reinforced the cohesion of the community as a whole. As such, it was important to discuss visiting nonbelievers or those who did not belong in the community. In the same manner, the jurisprudential regulations of these visitations contended with the socio-cultural organization of the society in manners that both underscored socio-gendered hierarchies and provided for the unique occasion of crossing boundaries. In all these cases, al-Bukhārī, followed by Ibn Baṭṭāl, looked to define the socio-legal parameter for visitation and to embed it within a socio-religious ordering of the society that addressed differences in status, age, and gender. This attention to status was also reflective of al-Bukhārī's interest in the social function of this particular pietistic ritual, which he considered to be a communal obligation.

The ritualized space created through visitation was one inhabited by God himself. In a state of sickness and patient enduring, the sick person was close to God and the visitor was walking under the shades of heaven. In a tradition reported in Muslim ibn al-Ḥajjāj's (d. 875) *Ṣaḥīḥ* and in various writings by Aḥmad ibn Ḥanbal (d. 855) and others, the prophet is reported to have said:

> On the Day of Judgement, God says, "O son of Adam, I have fallen sick and you did not visit me." [The servant] would say, "O Lord! How could I visit you when you are the Lord of all the living?" God says, "Did you not know that my servant so and so has fallen sick and you did not visit him? Had you visited him, you would have found me there."[123]

Here, the presence of God within the confines of this disease-scape becomes the heart of how a Muslim needed to perceive the obligation to visit the sick. Although the visitation was seen as a communal obligation that did not fall on each Muslim to fulfill, the visit referred to consistently as *ʿiyāda* was framed as a visit to God who resided in the houses of the sick waiting and lamenting the absence of his servants who failed to visit him. The formulaic call and response, presented in the various prayers reported from the prophet and his companions and the responses to them, the ritualistic regulations that indicated how visits should be conducted, and the physical ritualization of touching further typify the visit within a narrative of ritual wherein God has given words and indicated specific acts that must be fulfilled as part of worship to him. In this context of divine presence, Ibn al-Mubārak and Hannād reported a tradition that advised visitors to ask patients to pray for them.[124] Here, the roles seemed to be reversed. Although the patient was allowed to ask his visitors to pray for him, they, too, were advised to ask him to pray for them as he resided in the confines of divine presence. Here again, and as explained before, the disease-scape was deeply corporeal and the connection between the sick, the visitors, and God was embodied and deeply physicalized.

Disease-scape as a space of piety

As mentioned before, in pietistic literature and beyond, the term *ʿiyādah* became a specific term for visiting a patient to fulfill the religious obligation or follow the sunna of the prophet. The specificity of the term helped create particular pietistic categories that governed the social life of illness. First, illnesses needed to be understood as caused by, and only by, God. Yet this view had little to do with discussions about causality in a theoretical sense and did not seem to affect the role of humors or other natural factors in making diseases. Attributing the ultimate agency and causality to God was a sign of belief and acceptance of the specific pietistic cosmology that diseases and diseased people inhabited.[125] Second, illnesses were seen as gifts from God that produced forgiveness and mercy for the sick person and also for those who took care of them or visited them.[126] Third, in all these cases, sickness in this pietistic landscape was transformed into a ritual to build and emphasize this relationship. At the same time, this pietistic discourse around illness was rooted in the overarching emphasis on intentions and sincerity, which governed much of Islamic pietistic discourse. In accepting illness, exhibiting patience, or visiting the sick, the pious subject needed to have the proper intentions and to keep God's rewards in mind.[127] Here, the physical introduction of God into the disease-scape served to heighten the immediacy of the recommended acts and the necessity of sincerity and proper intentions. One's behavior during sickness became a behavior toward God with no intermediary that required remembering God's blessings and gifts – or what He left and had not taken. It also required a specific language and demanded avoiding any sign of impatience that would be essentially directed at God.

The relationality in this construction of piety was not restricted to diseases but was rather part and parcel of a more extended discourse about one's relationship with God. This relation relied on layers of embodiment and anthropomorphisms to emphasize the connections between a person and God. Sickness, both as a personal and social condition, played an important role in the production of this relational space. Not only were diseases and cures the domain of God and his will, but they also affected people differently and occasioned layers of ambivalence that served to distinguish the believer from the nonbeliever. The first layer of ambivalence is caused by the fact that diseases should be seen as a sign of mercy while being a source of suffering. At a second level, God was to be perceived as the only cause of illness but should never be blamed. Finally, the pious subject needed to comprehend and reflect on how the severity of their illness delivered them more reward but to also consistently belittle such illness, whether publicly or in contemplating and reflecting on other blessings endowed by God, including the illness itself. More significantly, it was the ability to perceive and inhabit this ambivalence that authorized the reward. Perceiving and inhabiting such an ambivalent sphere of pietistic lexicology differentiated the believer, or those who would emerge benefitting from illness, from nonbelievers, or those who would emerge with no reward, possibly even with damnation. Ambivalence demanded constant and consistent contact, whereby the sick established a deeper connection with God and continued to communicate with Him in accepting pain and suffering and also demanding, if subtly, reward and mercy.

At another level, visibility and enunciation played a rather important role in this dynamic. Hiding one's illness was presented in the language of *satr*, a word used to denote covering one's faults or shameful behavior. In this case, hiding one's illness becomes a covering of God's affliction, which is then rewarded with God's covering and then forgiving sins. Visibility, in this case, became a sign of impatience or a form of implicit blame directed at God. The valued position of invisibility gave space to belittling the suffering as a sign of patience. For instance, ʿUrwah kept belittling the pain and injury that he suffered in his leg until it was necessary to amputate it. Such belittling was deployed as a sign not only of reliance on God to cure ailments, but more commonly as the embodiment of an ambivalent position toward healing itself, even if it was granted miraculously by God. Physical suffering should be belittled as it paled in comparison to the potential rewards of patience and to the blessings already given by God. It was also negligible in comparison to the punishment in the afterlife that diseases might protect one from. Yet it was the degree of this physical suffering and the enormity of the trial or affliction that conditioned the reward. This degree was to be reckoned with by the pious sick as they contemplate God's reward. In this context, words and even sounds made to express pain or exasperation or attempts to alleviate pain were causes for concern. God was to be thanked for afflicting one with illness. Moreover, one needed to always be reminded and to remind others of God's blessings and not to be an ingrate by remembering only his afflictions. The emphasis on enunciations and on the dynamics of visibility of suffering underscored the closeness as well as the anthropomorphic and performative nature of this relational behavior toward God. Although God knew of one's thoughts and ideas, He was to be respected and honored through the explicit deeds and enunciations that should rise from inner feelings, but could also stand to modify inner feelings in a continuous self-reflexive dialogue that was rooted in a consistent and constant reckoning of one's behavior toward God.

This is particularly evident in the single tradition that Ibn Abī al-Dunya reported in relation to what one should do when healed or recovered:

> Khawāt ibn Jubayr [a companion] said, "I fell sick so I visited the prophet. He said to me, 'May your body be healthy.' I replied, 'and your body, prophet of God.' [Later, my body] was healed. [When I saw the prophet,] he said, 'Give God what you pledged to Him.' I said, 'O prophet of God, I have not pledged anything to God.' He said, 'Yes you did! Not a person who falls sick but he speaks to himself of doing good [when cured]. So repay God what you pledged.'"[128]

In such intensified divine presence, thoughts, even if not articulated, became part of a conversation with the divine that created obligations and provided privilege.

Conclusion

On his deathbed, the prophet spoke to God, asking him for mercy, forgiveness, and relief in death and in His encounter. Although several traditions indicated that the prophet, like other prophets, engaged in some conversations with God, this particular conversation with God was not unique and did not constitute a special privilege of prophecy. Sick companions, followers, and others engaged consistently in these conversations with God and were to think of His presence in their company as they suffered. After all, God was reported to have said that he resides with the sick, awaiting visitors with them. Ibn Abī al-Dunyā reported a tradition from the famous ḥadīth reporter, Sufyān ibn ʿUyaynah, where he recounted, "We went to visit [Ibn al-Ḥarith] Zubayd al-Yāmī [when he was sick] and told him, 'ask God for healing.' He said, 'Lord! Choose for me! Lord! Choose for me!'"[129] Within this relationship between the pious patient and God, it was God who chose what was better for His servant in the now and the hereafter. These conversations with God were not one-sided either. The wealth of prophetic traditions that discussed experiences of illness contained descriptions of God's wishes, demands, and even literal responses to his servants as they suffer in their sickbeds and to those who visit and pray for them. Precisely because the responses were affirmed in advance, the conversation with God became a scripted ritual that a pious Muslim was expected to enter and to perform in hopes of divine reward. Specific things were to be said and repeated, and specific responses were expected. Certain prayers were more effective to request healing and were also important in ensuring reward and affirming piety. Illness, in this context, was a ritual space where the communication with God was reenacted.

In the various works of zuhd by Wakīʿ, Ibn al-Mubārak, and more prominently in the work of Hannād and Ibn Abī al-Dunyā, as well as in the ḥadīth compilations of al-Bukhārī and others, the question of proper thought and correct understanding was key to the construction of this pietistic ritual space. Thoughts and intentions, even more than words or acts, were the main differences between Muslims and non-Muslims – or believers and nonbelievers. First, a believer needed to perceive a divine causality in which God is the only source of illness and the only source of cure. No one should be blamed for sickness and suffering but God, and no one but him should be asked for help. This firm belief in the origin of illness further underscores the fact that annoyance, impatience, or simple boredom of illness were seen as directed at God. Indeed, such annoyance and impatience would be misplaced precisely because illness was a conduit of forgiveness, a sign of reward, and a bearer of good news of divine favor. Yet such forgiveness and reward hinged precisely on harboring the correct thoughts and the proper intentions, a process that entailed constant reflection and demanded deep considerations of one's own views and behaviors.

In this context, illness created an ambivalent space. Illness invited the construction of a social pietistic space and conditioned the making of a series of public performances, but it was ultimately an occasion for individual pietistic reflection and for "correcting" one's intentions. Illness, as a space that entailed the presence of God along with caretakers, was a space for visitations that were constructed around communal lines: the sick Muslims should be visited, but not the unbelievers, unless their conversion was possible. This public side of the disease-scape was heavily ritualized through specific discussions of the length and frequency of visitations and through specific prayers and sayings that the visitor was supposed to utter. This ritualized space was organized along lines of gender and was disciplined across lines of wealth, power, and knowledge as scholars attempted to answer questions about who should visit whom and why. In providing a vivid imagery of the visitor wading through mercy, which resembled high waters, and sitting to be fully immersed in this water of mercy, authors constructed a parallel divine space that changed the imagery of visitation and provided the ritualized visit with its mythical equivalent, which it recreated and recalled at the same time.

The logic of these ritualistic structures posed important questions related to the legality or the piety implied in seeking cure, whether from a physician or even by asking God for deliverance from disease through cure or death. To be sure, neither al-Bukhārī nor Ibn Abī al-Dunyā showed any hesitation in pronouncing cure and seeking help to be legally permissible. However, for both of them, as was the case for Ibn Abī Shaybah and others, withstanding was always better, and patience was the surest conduit to divine reward. Seeking cure within the parameters of this ritualistic space, including admission of God's responsibility for health and disease and gratitude for His blessings, can function positively for believers and provide them with reward. Ultimately, it was what resided in their hearts and what they truly believed that would affect how God looked at them. In this case, and many others, the pietistic space extended beyond the space of legality, creating layers of ambivalence and allowing for a better understanding of one's place in relation to God.

Notes

1 In her 1985 piece on zuhd, Leah Kinberg observed that most Western scholarship dealt with zuhd (renunciation) within the context of Sufism and that, even there, zuhd was still ill-defined (Kinberg, "What Is Meant by Zuhd"). Since then, a number of scholars provided important contributions to the definition of zuhd and its role in society. For instance, Maneula Marin presented an overview of the development of zuhd as a concept in al-Andalus (Marín, " Early Development of Zuhd in al-Andalus"). Christopher Melchert's work on piety, mysticism, and asceticism engaged with the meaning of zuhd and its connection to piety at various levels (Melchert, "Transition from Asceticism to Mysticism;" "Piety of the Hadith Folk"). Michael Bonner analyzed how zuhd related to commerce and financial gains (Bonner, "Kitāb al-Kasb," 411–15). More recently, Hannah-Lena Hagemann's dissertation explored the concept of zuhd in Kharijite writings and how it related to similar concepts in Sunni thought (Hagemann, "History and Memory," 73–84). Denise Aigle explored the role of zuhd in establishing religious authority (Aigle, "Les Autorités Religieuses dans l'Islam Médiéval," 3–4). The study of zuhd within mysticism and Sufism continued as well but paid more attention to the concept and its deployment. See for instance, Schimmel, *Mystical Dimensions of Islam*. See also, Anjum, "Sufism in History," 255. Similarly, zuhd played a central role in the hagiographies of various figures and in how these figures established authority. For instance, on Ibn al-Lyth, see Tor, "Historical Representations of Yaʿqūb b. al-Layth." See also Sizgorich, "Narrative and Community." Other scholars followed up on the connections between zuhd/asceticism and mysticism by looking at authors known for their animosity toward Sufis. See, for instance, Assef, "Le Soufisme et les Soufis Selon Ibn Taymiyya" and Anjum, "Sufism Without Mysticism?" Most recently, on zuhd books, some of which are discussed in this chapter, see Yaldiz's dissertation, "The Afterlife in Mind."

2 In the same vein, and on modeling selves through pietistic discourses, see Munim Sirry, "Pious Muslims in the Making." On imitating the prophet as a central practice of piety in Islam, see, among many others, Annemarie Schimmel, *And Muhammad Is His Messenger*; and Gordon D. Newby, "Imitating Muhammad in Two Genres."

3 On Ibn Abī al-Dunyā, see Bellamy, "Makārim al-Akhlāq;" Librande, "Ibn Abī al-Dunyā."

4 The word *raqāʾiq* comes from the verb *raqqa*, meaning to become softer and finer. It is used in this context to refer to the softness or brittleness of the hearts through purification. The term was used to describe a genre of pietistic writings that included exhortations and stories about the prophet and his companions aimed to soften and purify the hearts.

5 Studies have shown that scholars of ḥadīth dealt with prophetic traditions on piety, renunciation, or other *raqāʾiq* differently from how they dealt with legal traditions. While they emphasized increasingly stricter rules for authenticity in the case of legal traditions, they were more accepting of various reports that intended to provide moral guidance. See Brown, "Even If It Is Not True It Is True"; Daaïf, "Dévots et Renonçants."

6 In her new book, Feryal Salem looks at the life and career of ʿAbd Allāh ibn al-Mubarak and the role that his works played in structuring discourses around piety and scholasticism. See Salem, *The Emergence of Early Sufi Piety and Sunnī Scholasticism*. On Ibn al-Mubarak's piety, see Salem's fourth chapter.

7 On the different versions of Aḥmad ibn Ḥanbal's *zuhd* and the different sources, in which the text survives, see Melchert, "Aḥmad ibn Ḥanbal's Book of Renunciation."

8 "Follower" or *tābiʿ* referred to important scholars and pious figures of the second generation of Muslims, following the companions, who encountered the prophet themselves.

9 By sensorium, I refer to a culturally produced shared feeling and vocabulary that define these feelings and give them social and cultural meanings. Here, I rely on Charles Hirschkind's work on the secular body, where he defines a pious sensorium as, "the embodied aptitudes and affects necessary for the achievement of a virtuous life as defined by those traditions" (Hirschkind, "Is There a Secular Body?," 635). At another level, Javier Moscoso provided a longue durée cultural history of pain that showed how pain was felt in various contexts (Moscoso, *Pain: A Cultural History*). In the Islamicate context, Henry Corbin explored how the concept of a common sensorium (*ḥiss mushtarak*) developed in Islamic philosophy (Corbin, "Theory of Visionary Knowledge," 231). The concept and the importance of common sensoria were developed in a number of ethnographic writings. See, for instance, Griffin, "Moroccan Sensorium;" Eisenlohr, "Technologies of the Spirit;" Jouili and Moors, "Islamic Sounds."

10 On this style of writing and the utilization of ḥadīth as "little narratives" to be deployed in various situations and for different purposes, see Sperl, "Man's 'Hollow Core'" and Khalidi, "Premodern Arabic/Islamic Historical Writing."

11 Al-Baghdādī, *Tārīkh Madinat al-Salām*.

12 Jacqueline Chabbi and Christopher Melchert argued that Ibn Abī al-Dunyā's work was not embraced by scholars of ḥadīth because of his deep interest in adab and his seemingly relaxed standards in selecting ḥadīths for his *raqāʾiq* writings. See Chabbi, "Remarques sur le développement historique des mouvements ascétiques et mystiques au Khurasan" and Melchert, "Piety of the Hadith Folk." A deeper look at Ibn Abī al-Dunyā's works and the evidence of their reception during his time supports, but modulates, some of Chabbi's and Melchert's conclusions. Indeed, Ibn Abī al-Dunyā was one of the more prolific authors, but he was not considered a significant authority in ḥadīth. Yet his works continued to be cited, and many scholars of ḥadīth reported traditions on his authority. Contrary to Melchert's argument, Ibn Abī al-Dunyā presented an image of piety and asceticism that was consistent with his teacher Hannād ibn al-Sarī, who was respected by Ibn Ḥanbal and other ḥadīth scholars, and also similar to the works of Ibn Ḥanbal in his pietistic writings.

13 On zuhd writings, see Yaldiz, "The Afterlife in Mind."

14 As Christopher Melchert has shown, the surviving manuscripts of Ibn Ḥanbal's zuhd appear to be much shorter than the original version that seemed to have been available as late as Ibn Ḥajar al-ʿAsqalānī's (d. 1449) time, if not later. The chapters and traditions on pre-Islamic prophets in the surviving manuscripts appear to exceed the size of similar materials in other writings about zuhd. Melchert argues that this may be because of the loss of other materials. See Melchert, "Aḥmad ibn Ḥanbal's Book of Renunciation."

15 Al-Bukhārī, among other contributors to the *ṣaḥīḥ movement*, was also interested in collecting ḥadīth that covered the major questions in law and ritual. Qasim Zaman argued that even the treatise on the prophet's battles (*maghāzī*) in al-Bukhārī was compiled with an eye toward the law and legal questions compared to earlier works by ʿAbd al-Razzāq al-Ṣanʿānī, for instance (see Qasim Zaman, "Maghāzī and the Muhaddithūn"). Brown cites Abū Dāwūd (d. 889), himself a student of Ibn Ḥanbal and a contemporary of al-Bukhārī and Muslim, as claiming he knew nothing, after the Quran, more essential for people to know than his book (Brown, *The Canonization of al-Bukhārī and Muslim*, 57). Of course, Abū Dāwūd explained in the same *Risāla* (or treatise to the people of Mecca) that he only discussed issues of law and did not include traditions on piety. Although Abū Dāwūd's collection was reviewed and recommended by Ibn Ḥanbal himself, his first commentator was al-Khaṭṭābī (d. 996), almost a century after the composition of his collection. Al-Khaṭṭābī was also the first to write a commentary on al-Bukhārī's *Ṣaḥīḥ*.

16 Burge argued that al-Bukhārī's selections and his ordering of different traditions should be read as part of his authorial voice and that he utilized these techniques to provide coherent narratives (Burge, "Reading between the Lines"). See also, Burge, "Myth, Meaning and the Order of Words."

17 Al-Ṭabarī, *Tafsīr al-Ṭabarī*.
18 Al-Dunyā, *Al-maraḍ wa al-Kaffārāt*, 94, 108.
19 Ibid., 94, 110.
20 Ibid., 179.
21 Al-Kūfī, *Kitāb al-Zuhd*, 235.
22 Abū Bakr was Muḥammad's closest friend and companion. He was also the first caliph and is an important authority in matters of piety and law for Sunnis.
23 Ibid., 248.
24 Al-Rāzī, *Tafsīr Ibn Abī Ḥātim*, 4: 1072.
25 Ibid., 4: 1071.
26 Ibid., 4: 1071–2. For this verse, Ibn Abī Ḥātim relied on traditions reported in the "book of exegesis" in Al-Tirmidhī's *Jāmi'*.
27 Al-Bukhārī, *Ṣaḥīḥ al-Bukhārī*, 7: 114–15.
28 The earliest commentary on al-Bukhārī's *Ṣaḥīḥ* was a brief one authored by Abū Sulaymān al-Khaṭṭābī (d. 988), who also wrote a commentary on Abū Dāwūd's compendium. See Tokatly, "A'lām al-Hadīth of al-Khaṭṭābī." Ibn Baṭṭāl (d. 1057) authored a rather longer commentary, which was likely the second commentary on *Ṣaḥīḥ al-Bukhārī* and was one of the more cited commentaries for centuries to come up until Ibn Ḥajar's (d. 1449) detailed and celebrated *Fatḥ al-Bārī*. By the eleventh century, al-Bukhārī's ḥadīth collection *al-Ṣaḥīḥ* had become the most celebrated and authoritative Sunni ḥadīth collection.
29 Ibn Baṭṭāl, Sharḥ Ṣaḥīḥ al-Bukhārī, 9: 372.
30 Ibid., 9: 372–3.
31 Ibid., 9: 373.
32 Ibid., 9: 373.
33 Ibid., 9: 373.
34 Al-Dunyā, *Al-Maraḍ wa al-Kaffārāt*, 14–15.
35 Al-Kūfī, *Kitāb al-Zuhd*, 241–2.
36 Ibid., 239.
37 Al-Bukhārī, *Ṣaḥīḥ al-Bukhārī*, 7: 115.
38 Ibn Baṭṭāl, Sharḥ Ṣaḥīḥ al-Bukhārī, 9: 372.
39 Al-Dunyā, *Al-Maraḍ wa al-Kaffārāt*, 160. Ibn Baṭṭāl also reported this tradition citing Ibn Abī al-Dunyā (Ibn Baṭṭāl, Sharḥ Ṣaḥīḥ al-Bukhārī, 9: 377). The tradition was reported in a number of ḥadīth compilations in chapters related to piety. For instance, al-Tirmidhī (d. 892) reported the tradition in the treatise dedicated to zuhd, where he explained that it was a rare tradition that occurred only through this line of transmission (Al-Tirmidhī, *Al-Jāmi' al-Kabīr*, 4: 276). Similarly, Al-Ḥāfiẓ al-Ṭabarānī also reported the tradition in his *Al-Mu'jam al-Kabīr*. In the late twelfth century, Ibn al-Jawzī (d. 1201), on the other hand, rejected this tradition and considered it to be fabricated commenting in his *Al-Mawḍu'āt* (the book of fabricated traditions) that this tradition had no merit especially that the prophet ordered believers to pray for health. Regardless, the tradition survived, occurring, for instance, in the *Al-Targhīb wa al-Tarhīb* (recommendation and admonitions) composed by al-Ḥāfiẓ Zakiyy al-Dīn 'Abd al-'Aẓīm al-Mundhirī (d. 1258), which also focused on various pietistic questions (Al-Mundhirī, *Al-Targhīb wa al-Tarhīb*, 4: 142). Jonathan Brown has explained that scholars of ḥadīth normally accepted "weaker" traditions in relation to issues concerning piety, and when told by preachers (*qaṣṣāṣīn*) highlighting the pietistic impact that these traditions had on commoners. He explained that Ibn al-Jawzī was one of the few who rejected the use of these traditions even for the purposes of preaching. See Brown, "Did the Prophet Say It or Not?," 283.
40 Al-Dunyā, *Al-Maraḍ wa al-Kaffārāt*. The same tradition was cited by Ibn Baṭṭāl in his commentary: Ibn Baṭṭāl, Sharḥ Ṣaḥīḥ al-Bukhārī, 9: 391. Here, as in other traditions, the character of the Bedouin is invoked to show ignorance and, even, dim fate. However, the character was sometimes deployed to refer to some form of nativist morality, goodness, and propriety. See Sadan, "An Admirable and Ridiculous Hero."

41 Al-Dunyā, *Al-Maraḍ wa al-Kaffārāt*, 160. This anecdote occurred in the biography of Khālid ibn al-Walīd in different places, such as Ibn ʾAsākir's history (Ibn ʿAsākir, *Tārīkh Madinat Damashq*, 106). In both Ibn Abī al-Dunyā and Ibn ʾAsākir, the story was a sign of Khālid ibn al-Walīd's own piety and commitment as he rejected his wife because he was concerned about her potential impiety.

42 Ibn Abī Al-Dunyā, *Al-Maraḍ wa al-Kaffārāt*, 155. The tradition appears in Abī Dāwūd's (d. 889) collection under the treatise dedicated to death and funerals (Abū Dāwūd, *Sunan Abī Dāwūd*, 3: 182–3. In both Abī Dāwūd and Ibn Abī al-Dunyā, a Bedouin asks the prophet, "What is sickness?" The prophet responded, "And haven't you been sick before?" When the man affirmed that he was never sick before, the prophet told him "Then leave us! You are not one of our nation." Here again, the narrative of sickness as a sign of faith and of God's favor was articulated and posed in relation to the value of sickness for the believers. The tradition was also reported by al-Bayhaqī (d. 1066) in his *Shuʿab al-Imān* (The Branches of Faith) in relation to patience and acceptance of God's will.

43 Al-Dunyā, *Al-Maraḍ wa al-Kaffārāt*, 155.

44 As explained in the introduction, I draw in my discussion of reflexivity in pietistic narratives on Ebrahim Moosa's analysis of al-Ghazālī's work and the production of the self in his narratives (Ebrahim Moosa, *Ghazali and the Poetics of Imagination.* From a comparative perspective, this discussion is also informed by the work of Jonathan Schofer. See Schofer, "Ethical Formation and Subjection"; *Confronting Vulnerability*; "Embodiment and Virtue in a Comparative Perspective" and *The Making of a Sage*.

45 Al-Jarrāḥ, *Ṣaḥīḥ Kitāb al-Zuhd*, 94.

46 Al-Marūzī, *Kitāb al-Zuhd*, 69–70.

47 Al-Dunyā, *Al-Maraḍ wa al-Kaffārāt*, 193.

48 Traditions linking fever and hellfire were rather common in writings of prophetic medicine. In many texts, the discussion was related to a tradition recommending the use of water to treat fever, which some physicians disagreed with. Authors of prophetic medicine attempted to clarify how the tradition referred to specific fevers caused by sun heat and that these were to be cured by water (see Al-Kaḥḥāl, *Al-Aḥkām al-Nabawīyah fī al-ṣināʿah al-ṭibbīyah*). See also Al-Jawzīyah, *Al-ṭibb al-Nabawī*. The interest in this aspect of the ḥadīth can be traced back to the work of Ibn al-Sunnī and Abū Nuʾaym al-Isfahānī as explained in Chapter 2 (Al-Aṣbahānī, *Al-ṭibb al-Nabawiyy*). Ibn Abī al-Dunyā, however, was not interested in this aspect of the ḥadīth, further demonstrating the treatise's overall dedication to pietistic rather than medical questions.

49 Although there is little concrete information on the prevalence of particular diseases during this period, fevers continued to be a central condition that animated much medical writings and occupied important chapters in various medical textbooks. For instance, Cristina Alvarez Millan's work on medical cases shows that fevers constituted a stable aspect of medical thinking at the time (Álvarez-Millán, "Practice Versus Theory" and "The Case History in Medieval Islamic Medical Literature"). Similarly, Efraim Lev's and others' works on pharmacopeia in the Geniza documents, which show as close a look at actual practice as possible, showed the consistent presence of fever as well (Lev and Amar, " 'Fossils' of Practical Medical Knowledge from Medieval Cairo"; Lev and Chipman, *Medical Prescriptions in the Cambridge Genizah Collections*; and Lev, "An Early Fragment of Ibn Jazlah's Tabulated Manual") Popularized medical texts showed similar interest in fever as well (Al-Jazzar, *Ibn al-Jazzar On Fevers*).

50 Al-Dunyā, *Al-Maraḍ wa al-Kaffārāt*.

51 Ibid.

52 Al-Kūfī, *Kitāb al-Zuhd*, 232.

53 Ibid., 233.

54 Al-Bukhārī, *Ṣaḥīḥ al-Bukhārī*, 7: 116.

55 Ibid., 7: 116–17. This tradition was the first that Hannād listed in his chapter on "Patience in the Face of Calamity" (Al-Kūfī, *Kitāb al-Zuhd*, 229). Al-Tirmidhī cited the same tradition in his *muṣannaf* – the treatise on zuhd. On blindness and other similar deformities in medical, religious, and literary writings, see Richardson, *Difference and Disability in the Medieval Islamic World*.
56 Ibn Baṭṭāl, Sharḥ Ṣaḥīḥ al-Bukhārī, 9: 376.
57 Ibid., 9: 377.
58 On patience and the needed awareness of such act being performed for God's sake, see Avner Gil'adi, " 'Ṣabr' " (steadfastness) of bereaved parents. Also Moosa, *Ghazali and the Poetics of Imagination*, 91–2. This knowledge of the reason and the reward behind a practice was part of the construction of intention or *niyya*, as will be seen in Chapter 5. See Powers, "Interiors, Intentions, and the "Spirituality" of Islamic Ritual Practice."
59 As will be seen later, praying for cure and the attendant practice of *du'ā'* entailed more than leaving the matter in the hands of God. Instead, it animated a specific spiritual economy where *du'ā'* was part of a continuous communication with God. See Khalil, "Is God Obliged to Answer Prayers of Petition (du'a)?"
60 Al-Dunyā, *Al-Maraḍ wa al-Kaffārāt*.
61 Ibid.
62 Al-Kūfī, *Kitāb al-Zuhd*, 232. The tradition was also reported by Ibn Ḥanbal and Ibn Ḥibbān, among others.
63 As mentioned in the first and second chapters, these questions were addressed extensively in the medicine chapters of ḥadīth collections and in later volumes of prophetic medicine. See Perho, *The Prophet's Medicine*.
64 Although this ambivalence was not as clearly visible in the canonical ḥadīth collections of the late ninth century and beyond, one can find such contradictory reports in the longer and more comprehensive collection of Ibn Abī Shaybah, among others. Scholars have demonstrated that collections like al-Bukhārī's and Muslim's were developed with an eye toward legal and jurisprudential questions, which may explain their reluctance to show such ambivalence (see Brown, *The Canonization of al-Bukhārī and Muslim*; Melchert, "Bukhārī and Early Ḥadith Criticism"; and Brown, "The Canonization of Ibn Mājah").
65 Al-Kūfī, *Kitāb al-Zuhd*, 230; Ibn Ḥanbal, *Kitāb al-Zuhd*. The tradition was also reported in Ibn Abī Shaybah's *Muṣannaf*.
66 Al-Kūfī, *Kitāb al-Zuhd*, 230–1; Al-Marūzī, *Kitāb al-Zuhd*, 25; Ibn Marthad and al-Rāzī, *Zuhd al-Thamāniyah min al-Tābi'īn*, 4.
67 Ibn Ḥanbal, *Kitāb al-Zuhd*, 111.
68 Ibn Baṭṭāl, Sharḥ Ṣaḥīḥ al-Bukhārī, 9: 390.
69 Ibid.
70 Al-Jarrāḥ, *Ṣaḥīḥ Kitāb al-Zuhd*; Al-Kūfī, *Kitāb al-Zuhd*, 254; Ibn Ḥanbal, *Kitāb al-Zuhd*, 240–41. As seen in Chapter 3, this saying was reported from a number of companions, including Abū Hurayrah. Some of the companions said this statement to the prophet, who accepted it.
71 Ibn Baṭṭāl, Sharḥ Ṣaḥīḥ al-Bukhārī, 9: 391–2.
72 Ibid., 9: 391.
73 Al-Dunyā, *Al-Maraḍ wa al-Kaffārāt*.
74 Al-Bukhārī, *Ṣaḥīḥ al-Bukhārī*.
75 Ibn Baṭṭāl, Sharḥ Ṣaḥīḥ al-Bukhārī, 9: 387–8.
76 Al-Dunyā, *Al-Maraḍ wa al-Kaffārāt*, 74–5.
77 Al-Kūfī, *Kitāb al-Zuhd*, 251.
78 Al-Dunyā, *Al-Maraḍ wa al-Kaffārāt*, 52, 161. In his *Al-Targhīb wa al-Tarhīb*, al-Mundhirī reported this tradition citing Ibn Abī al-Dunyā (Al-Mundhirī, *Al-Targhīb wa al-Tarhīb*, 4: 280).

79 This view on causality did not necessarily contradict the belief in natural causes for health and disease, which many of the scholars cited here and beyond ascribed to, as explained in Chapter 3. On debates around causality and God's omnipotence, see Morrison, *Islam and Science*, 95–105. In relation to medicine, albeit in a later period, see Stearns, *Infectious Ideas*, 6–9, 106–39. See also, Livingston, "Science and the Occult." Irmeli Perho addressed the question of causality in her work on prophetic medicine and explained that most authors of prophetic medicine believed in the natural causes of diseases that operated within divine will. See Perho, *The Prophet's Medicine*, 67–70.
80 Al-Dunyā, *Al-Maraḍ wa al-Kaffārāt*, 172.
81 Ibid., 195.
82 Ibn Ḥanbal., *Kitāb al-Zuhd*, 109–10.
83 Al-Bukhārī, *Ṣaḥīḥ al-Bukhārī*.
84 Ibid., 7: 120.
85 Ibn Baṭṭāl, Sharḥ Ṣaḥīḥ al-Bukhārī, 384.
86 Ibid., 9: 384.
87 Al-Dunyā, *Al-Maraḍ wa al-Kaffārāt*, 78. Ibn al-Jawzī considered this tradition to be fabricated and included it in his book on fabricated traditions *Kitāb al-Mawḍūʿāt*, perhaps, based on *matn* (content) criticism explaining that such a tradition could not come from the prophet.
88 Christopher Melchert has explored the theme of intense fear of God in early pietistic literature, including materials by authors discussed here as well as figures like Abū Nuʿaym al-Isfahānī and others. In his analysis, Melchert explains that this form of piety was built on asceticism and cultivating anxiety, fear, and reverence toward the divine (see Melchert, "Exaggerated Fear in the Early Islamic Renunciant Tradition"). In the accounts discussed earlier, fear, reverence, and anxiety toward God were on full display and were further heightened by the physical, albeit mediated, presence of the divine in the disease-scape. Most recently, Karen Bauer's discussion of emotions in the Quran highlighted the importance of fearing God and the interplay of fear, reverence, mercy, and forgiveness in the relationship between God and pious Muslims (see Bauer, "Emotion in the Qur'an").
89 Ibid., 113.
90 Ibid., 134.
91 Ibid., 140.
92 Ibid., 113.
93 Ibid., 113, 119.
94 Ibid., 138. The story of ʿUrwah was also mentioned in Abū Nuʿaym al-Isfahānī's *Ḥulyat al-Awliyāʾ* and in Ibn al-Jawzī's *Ṣafwat al-Ṣafwah*.
95 The legality of using alcohol and other similar materials in treatment was discussed in various texts on prophetic medicine (see Al-Jawzīyah, *Al-ṭibb al-Nabawī*; Perho, *The Prophet's Medicine*).
96 Al-Dunyā, *Al-Maraḍ wa al-Kaffārāt*, 175.
97 Remembering God's blessings and the rewards for patience was a common theme in literature around piety and steadfastness. See, for instance, Gilʿadi; Gobillot, "Patience (ṣabr) et rétribution des mérites."
98 Ibid., 120–1.
99 Ibid., 114.
100 Al-Ṭabarī, *Tafsīr Al-Ṭabarī*, 545.
101 The corporeal manifestations in pietistic discourses was not limited to this discourse on illness but extended to various other issues. On paradise, for instance, see Al-Azmeh, "Rhetoric for the Senses," 215–31; and Rustomji, "Early Views of Paradise." On pietistic corporeal discourses surrounding Jihad and martyrdom, see Denaro, "The Most Beautiful Body."

102 Al-Kūfī, *Kitāb al-Zuhd*, 224.
103 Al-Dunyā, *Al-Maraḍ wa al-Kaffārāt*, 167.
104 Al-Bukhārī, *Ṣaḥīḥ al-Bukhārī*. The tradition, which ḥadīth scholars saw as a variant report of Hannād's tradition noted earlier, was reported by Ibn al-Mubārak and Ibn Ḥibbān in the form that links visiting patients to attending funerals. The connection between visiting patients and following or participating in funerals was not unique to al-Bukhārī. In fact, in many other works, the entire discussion of illness and piety was located within chapters dedicated to funerals and death (see, for instance, Al-Mundhirī, *Al-Targhīb wa al-Tarhīb*.). This connection may be related to the fact that death may follow illnesses, or that loss was a calamity similar to illnesses. They may also be connected as manners in which certain social obligations are created and propagated.
105 Ibn Baṭṭāl, Sharḥ Ṣaḥīḥ al-Bukhārī.
106 Al-Dunyā, *Al-Maraḍ wa al-Kaffārāt*, 124. The tradition, in slightly different wording, was also reported by Hannād, Al-Kūfī, *Kitāb al-Zuhd*, 224–5.
107 Al-Dunyā, *Al-Maraḍ wa al-Kaffārāt*, 146.
108 Al-Kūfī, *Kitāb al-Zuhd*, 224–5.
109 Al-Dunyā, *Al-Maraḍ wa al-Kaffārāt*, 171.
110 Al-Kūfī, *Kitāb al-Zuhd*, 228.
111 Al-Dunyā, *Al-Maraḍ wa al-Kaffārāt*, 168.
112 Ibid., 131.
113 Ibid., 142.
114 Ibid., 132, 140.
115 Al-Kūfī, *Kitāb al-Zuhd*, 226. Al-Tirmidhī placed this tradition in his treatise on shaking hands.
116 Al-Bukhārī, *Ṣaḥīḥ al-Bukhārī*.
117 Ibid.
118 Ibn Baṭṭāl, Sharḥ Ṣaḥīḥ al-Bukhārī.
119 Al-Bukhārī, *Ṣaḥīḥ al-Bukhārī*.
120 Ibn Baṭṭāl, Sharḥ Ṣaḥīḥ al-Bukhārī. 9: 379.
121 Al-Bukhārī, *Ṣaḥīḥ al-Bukhārī*.
122 Ibn Baṭṭāl, Sharḥ Ṣaḥīḥ al-Bukhārīk, 9: 380.
123 Muslim ibn Al-Ḥajjāj, *Ṣaḥīḥ Muslim*; Ibn Ḥanbal, *Al-Musnad*.
124 Al-Kūfī, *Kitāb al-Zuhd*, 226.
125 Perho, 67–70.
126 On this question, but in relation to plague as an example of severe calamity, see Conrad, "Tāʿūn and Wabāʾ."
127 For more detailed discussion on intentions, see Chapter 5. See also, Powers, "Interiors, Intentions, and the 'Spirituality' of Islamic Ritual Practice" and Katz, *Prayer in Islamic Thought and Practice*. Recently, ethnographic studies have explored the question of intentionality and sincerity in Muslims pieties, see Haeri, "Unbundling Sincerity" and "The Sincere Subject." See also, Mahmood, "Ethics and Piety."
128 Al-Dunyā, *Al-Maraḍ wa al-Kaffārāt*, 134.
129 Ibid., 168.

4 Spiritual medicine

In the introduction to his book *Al-Ṭibb al-Rūḥānī* (Spiritual Medicine), Abū Bakr al-Rāzī (d. 925) explained how he came to write the book.[1] He related how, after completing his more famous medical textbook *Al-Manṣūrī*, his patron, the Samanid emir Abū Ṣāliḥ al-Manṣūr (d. 915), approached him to write another book that addressed questions of spiritual medicine. For al-Rāzī and his patron, the two books were therefore parts of the same endeavor: seeking the health of both the body and the spirit. This particular connection between spiritual medicine and physical medicine was not unique nor novel. In fact, al-Rāzī drew on Galen's *On the Affections of the Soul* and *On Character Traits* – both were translated into Arabic in the ninth century and addressed the same topic. Moreover, al-Rāzī followed Galen in relying on Plato's work in the *Republic* and *Timeaus* – with al-Rāzī likely depending on Galen's commentary on the medical aspects of *Timaeus*.[2] Al-Rāzī's contemporary Abū Zayd al-Balkhī (d. 935) also included a treatise on the spirit in his book *Maṣāliḥ al-Abdān wa al-Anfus* (Benefits for Bodies and Spirits). Including a section on the health of the spirit after one on the body may have inspired al-Rāzī, who attempted to produce the same result in coupling his two volumes *Al-Manṣūrī* and *Al-Ṭibb al-Rūḥānī*.[3] In this same context, al-Kindī (d. 873) also referenced the ills of the spirit in his *Dispelling Sadness* (al-Ḥīlah li Dafʿ Al-aḥzān).[4] In the following century, the works of Yaḥya ibn ʿAdī (d. 974) and Miskawayh (d. 1030), both entitled *Tahdhīb al-Nafs* (Refinement of the Spirit), also referenced medical narratives in constructing ethical claims. Many of these ethical claims paralleled what al-Balkhī and al-Rāzī explained and mirrored the Hellenistic Islamicate archive of the period distinguished by the works of Plato, Aristotle, and Galen, among others.[5]

Along with these writings, authors and scholars of adab and ḥadīth engaged frequently and consistently in writings about manners and ethics, which discussed similar topics but utilized sources that were different from those used by the earlier mentioned authors who possessed more Hellenistic learning. For instance, the writings of adab and *raqāʾiq*, especially books on zuhd or the renunciation of earthly pleasures, played a significant role in creating pietistic narratives about refinement and modeling of the spirit around pietistic and religious ethics. As seen before, the writings of Ibn al-Mubārak (d. 798), Wakīʿ ibn al-Jarrāḥ (d. 813), Aḥmad ibn Ḥanbal (d. 813), and Hannād ibn al-Sarī (d. 858) as well as authors like Ibn Abī al-Dunyā (d. 894), among many others, were deeply concerned with arranging and organizing prophetic materials in treatises that addressed the main ethical questions of the period from modesty to moderation and to controlling passions and desires, among others. Similarly, the works of al-Ḥakīm al-Tirmidhī (d. 869) and others often labeled as early Sufis or mystics were also concerned with these ethical conversations.[6] Although many of these writings engaged with similar questions to those posed by al-Rāzī, al-Balkhī, or Miskawayh, they relied more heavily on materials from Quran, ḥadīth, and other materials that fit more neatly within the adab archive.[7]

Living close to three centuries after al-Rāzī, Ibn al-Jawzī (d. 1200) used a framing similar to al-Rāzī's and explained that his book on spiritual medicine, which carried the same title as al-Rāzī's – *Al-Ṭibb al-Rūḥānī* (Spiritual Medicine) – was the second part of his other book on physical medicine, *Luqaṭ al-Manāfiʿ*[8]:

> After I had compiled a book on physical medicine (*ṭibb al-abdān*) and called it "The Beneficial Gleanings" (*luqaṭ al-manafiʿ*), I decided to follow it with a book in the medicine of the spirits (*ṭibb al-nufūs*) and call it "Spiritual Medicine." That is because physical medicine [aims] to fix the images, and the medicine of the spirit aims to fix the meanings [entailed in them], which is more honorable and dignified.[9]

Ibn al-Jawzī, a respected scholar and preacher, composed a number of books that addressed the good deeds that Muslims were supposed to follow and outlined the parameters of good pious life.[10] As such, the content of his *Spiritual Medicine* was not, by any means, new to him or to his readers and followers. In fact, and as will be seen later, most of the chapters and topics covered in Ibn al-Jawzī's *Spiritual Medicine* were covered in his other books, especially the more famous and more voluminous *Kitāb Dhamm al-Hawā* (Disparaging Passion).[11] Although Ibn al-Jawzī never cited or referenced al-Rāzī by name in his *Spiritual Medicine*, there is little doubt that he was deeply influenced by him. In addition to the framing of the book and the invocation of a book on physical medicine, Ibn al-Jawzī followed the same arrangement and the same chapters that al-Rāzī had chosen for his book with minor modifications, as will be seen later.

Although similar to al-Rāzī's and al-Balkhī's works in framing and overall content (more to al-Rāzī than al-Balkhī actually), Ibn al-Jawzī's book was also part of a larger textual and literary tradition that was dominated by scholars of ḥadīth, mystics, preachers, and other religious scholars. These writings were concerned with the refinement of morals and with instilling piety in their readers. Writings of this sort, which ranged from ḥadīth collections to books on zuhd to even hagiographies of saints and pious people,[12] utilized narratives from ḥadīth and anecdotes about the companions and followers to deliver their message of piety and self-refinement. Although they addressed many of the same topics that were discussed in the writings of al-Balkhī, al-Rāzī, Miskawayh, and others, these writings were also interested in other topics. For instance, in his book, Ibn al-Jawzī added chapters that corresponded to other issues directly concerned with piety and worship, such as pride and hypocrisy, as well as topics like "hiding good tidings from people," which was frequently addressed by other scholars of ḥadīth.[13] Beyond Ibn al-Jawzī, scholars like Ibn Taymiyah (d. 1328) and his student and associate Ibn Qayyim al-Jawziyyah (d. 1350) followed with similar works that addressed asceticism and the training of the spirit. Although Ibn Taymiyah's and Ibn al-Qayyim's books fall outside the scope of this chapter, it is instructive to see that similar concerns continued to be discussed and expressed over these centuries.

This chapter looks at the pietistic narratives embedded in and deployed through spiritual medicine. Although this mini-genre (to use Peter Adamson's description)[14] was located within the writings of Galen and others, the work of Ibn al-Jawzī, as well as that of the Isma'īlī scholar Ḥamīd al-Dīn al-Kirmānī (fl. 996–1021) and others, presented a particular interest in providing a pietistic discourse that redeploys these medicalized pietistic and ethical narratives within the long-established traditions of adab, raqā'iq, and shamā'il. Here, I focus primarily on three texts that ostensibly placed themselves within this particular discursive space: Abū Bakr al-Rāzī's *Spiritual Medicine*, Ḥamīd al-Dīn al-Kirmānī's *Golden Statements*, and Ibn al-Jawzī's *Spiritual Medicine*. First, I look at the meaning and the subject of spiritual medicine conveyed in these volumes and how such meaning related to other topics in medical and pietistic literature. I then examine the spiritual nosology: the diseases, their etiologies, and their symptoms. From there, I turn to the various treatments proposed and the sources from which they were derived. Finally, I attend to a number of social issues (such as dealing with children, wives, and slaves) that were addressed in al-Kirmānī's and Ibn al-Jawzī's works. In conclusion, I will offer an image of the ideal pious self and will reflect on how these authors envisioned their contemporary audiences witnessing and living their pious good lives.

The subject of *Spiritual Medicine*

In his work on al-Rāzī's *Spiritual Medicine*, Peter Adamson explained that the medical framing of these ethical writings should not be taken as a metaphor. Instead, such medical framing should be viewed as key in a conception of the spirit as similar to the body, requiring treatment and care, and consequently, also requiring medicine and physicians to help it. This particular view conditioned a specific understanding of health and sickness in relation to ethics and manners, with virtues being signs of the health of the spirit.[15] As explained before, this connection between ethics and medicine can be traced back to Galen, whose writings were at the heart of the works of al-Balkhī and Abū Bakr al-Rāzī as well as Miskawayh and others.[16] The medical framing poses more questions in relation to Ibn al-Jawzī, who addressed these ethical, moral, and pietistic topics in a variety of other contexts, the most prominent of which was his *Dhamm al-Hawā* (Disparaging Passion), from which he borrowed extensively in *Spiritual Medicine*. A perusal through Ibn al-Jawzī's works show an undeniable interest in medicine and a deftness in handling medical topics and questions. Although most of his biographies did not mention any formal medical training, his writings, especially in the previously discussed *Luqat al-Manāfi'*, demonstrated that he was deeply familiar with medical writings and interested in medical narratives. Similar to other scholars of his time and beyond, Ibn al-Jawzī seemed to be particularly interested in utilizing medical language in many of his writings – a tendency that continued with later Ḥanbalī scholars such as Ibn Taymiyah and Ibn Qayyim al-Jawziyah, who respected Ibn al-Jawzī and were familiar with his writings.[17] In this work and others, framing these pietistic questions in medical language and couching them in a medical framework produced a number of significant rhetorical and discursive consequences that influenced how piety and pietistic behaviors were conceived and understood. Although these writings could not be firmly placed within a trajectory of Galenic ethics, despite clear influences and exchanges, and although their commitment to the nonmetaphorical use of medicine was not as firm as it was for al-Balkhī and al-Rāzī, this medical framing created a "supplementary play of meaning," in the Derridean sense, that influenced the production of pietistic narratives.

The Isma'īlī scholar Hamīd al-Dīn Abū al-Ḥasan al-Kirmānī (fl. 996–1021) was perhaps most forceful in his deployment of this medical framework in the discussion of spiritual medicine. Al-Kirmānī, a student and admirer of the Isma'īlī missionary and scholar, Abū Ḥātim Aḥmad ibn Ḥamdān al-Rāzī (d. 935), and a protégé and favorite scholar of the Fatimid Caliph al-Ḥākim bi-Amr Allāh (r. 996–1021), encountered the writings of Abū Bakr al-Rāzī (the physician) perhaps during his stay in Iraq or Iran.[18] He was particularly interested in the debates between the two Rāzīs: Abū Ḥātim, a prominent Ismā'īlī missionary and thinker, and Abū Bakr, the celebrated physician and (less celebrated) philosopher.[19] This is not surprising because al-Kirmānī had devoted his energy to completing and augmenting the arguments of Abū Ḥātim al-Rāzī in the latter's debates with al-Firghānī – a debate that was evidently consequential to both Abū Ḥātim and al-Kirmānī. In *Al-Aqwāl al-Dhahabiyyah* (The Golden Statements), al-Kirmānī suggested that his patron, the caliph and Imam al-Ḥākim, had asked him to comment on Abū Bakr al-Rāzī's *Spiritual Medicine*. Al-Kirmānī obliged and wrote both a critique of Abū Bakr al-Rāzī's book and a version of his own that addressed the central problems that he saw in Abū Bakr al-Rāzī's work.[20] For al-Kirmānī, a key underlying problem that manifested itself throughout Abū Bakr al-Rāzī's *Spiritual Medicine* lay with al-Rāzī's views on prophecy and on the legitimacy of prophets and imams – a question at the heart of the debates between the two Rāzīs and documented in Abū Ḥātim's account of such debates in his *A'lām al-Nubuwwah* (Signs of Prophecy).[21] Al-Kirmānī acknowledged this debate and explained how it related to Abū Bakr al-Rāzī's handling of *Spiritual Medicine*. As such, in the first part of al-Kirmānī's *Al-Aqwāl al-Dhahabiyyah*, he decided to augment Abū Ḥātim's arguments in relation to the question of prophecy. He rehearsed some of Abū Bakr al-Rāzī's claims, then cited Abū Ḥātim's attacks, before expanding on Abū Ḥātim's arguments to bolster them against potential criticism. Al-Kirmānī did not intend to expand on the entire discussion of prophecy, which Abū Ḥātim explored in *A'lām al-Nubuwwah*. Instead, he highlighted specific points, which he believed were central to his discussion of Abū Bakr al-Rāzī's *Spiritual Medicine*. In the second part of *Al-Aqwāl*, al-Kirmānī then proceeded to discuss Abū Bakr al-Rāzī's *Spiritual Medicine*. First he culled long quotations from almost each chapter of al-Rāzī's book and commented on them in detail, showing the problems that he found in them. Then, he proceeded to discuss his own views on *Spiritual Medicine* so as to provide what he thought was a sounder approach to this topic.

Al-Kirmānī was respectful of Abū Bakr's celebrated medical knowledge. In fact, he summarily acknowledged that Abū Bakr al-Rāzī's *Al-Manṣūrī* was an excellent example of medical books and that it deserved the reputation that it had received.[22] However, in his view, *Spiritual Medicine* was a different affair. On one hand, Abū Bakr al-Rāzī's problematic views on prophecy negatively affected the book and led it astray – weakening its arguments and rendering most of it useless to readers. On the other hand, al-Kirmānī argued that the book was misleading because it was not truly spiritual medicine. In al-Kirmānī's view, a discussion of spiritual medicine needed to stay true to its analogy to physical medicine:

> I have found what he [Abū Bakr al-Rāzī] wrote what he claimed to be spiritual medicine, unlike what he has established in physical medicine (*al-ṭibb al-jismānī*). [. . .] He fell short in his composition from what he was required to discuss and what is needed in spiritual medicine, [such as:] the patient, what is he? The disease and its treatment, what are they? And following the route of treatment and cure, how is it?"[23]

Here and in other places, al-Kirmānī accepted al-Rāzi's medical authority: "[in physical medicine,] he is like a knight of great might pacing up and down in the field of battle."[24] He lamented that Abū Bakr al-Rāzī's *Spiritual Medicine* failed to follow the rigorous and systematized structures of his physical medicine books.

Al-Kirmānī's contention that a serious and proper discussion of spiritual medicine required a clearer definition of what diseases were, who the patients were, and how to craft a treatment showed that, at least to al-Kirmānī, the medical framing carried important epistemic significance and allowed for a specific organization that benefited the overall meaning and goal of the book. In his own work, al-Kirmānī was also clear that his book on spiritual medicine was indebted in terms of content to some of his other books that addressed questions of piety more directly. He linked the composition of his book to three other treatises that he had composed, *Iklīl al-Nafs* (The Crown of the Spirit), where he addressed the meaning of the spirit and the differences between humans and animals in God's view, and *al-Maqāyyīs* (The Measures) and *al-Risālah al-Wāḥidah* (The Singular Treatise), both of which were concerned with various pietistic questions. As he completed these books, and after seeing Abū Bakr al-Rāzī's text, and presumably also upon the request of the caliph, he decided to write the book at hand, which he entitled *Al-Aqwāl al-Dhahabiyyah* (The Golden Statements).

Similar to Ibn al-Jawzī's explicit mention of his other books on piety and on manners, al-Kirmānī's references served to locate his spiritual medicine within larger narratives of pietistic writings, which he believed offered a more detailed discussion of the topics summarily discussed in *Al-Aqwāl al-Dhahabiyyah*. For both al-Kirmānī and Ibn al-Jawzī, along with other authors who deployed terms of medicine within the discussion of piety, spiritual medicine was epistemologically and discursively medical but not necessarily ontologically so. Whereas al-Balkhī and al-Rāzī relied on a Galenic ontology that understood the spirit as equivalent to the body in its being subject to ills and imbalances, al-Kirmānī and Ibn al-Jawzī perceived these vices and ills of the spirit not as ontological equivalents to bodily ills but as epistemological analogs. The medical framing invited an epistemological inquiry into meanings of health and illness, how to maintain and achieve health, and the role of recommendations and expertise. Although all these topics were also important for al-Balkhī and al-Rāzī, they, and others, were also invested in the ontology of spiritual diseases and how these diseases were sometimes linked to or caused humoral imbalances in the body.

In the Galenic perspective, psychology was deeply linked to physiology. The body was composed of four humors that should exist in a form of balance or equilibrium in the case of health, but the functions of the body – from eating, drinking, and moving to thinking – were carried out by certain powers or faculties of the spirit (or three different parts of the spirit), each residing in one of the central organs of the body:

> The concupiscible or appetitive power of the soul was located in the liver and was responsible for conception, growth, and nourishment; the irascible power in the heart generated the emotions, such as courage, anger, and joy; and the rational power in the brain was unique to human beings and was corporeal. This last power was responsible for three functions: the senses, voluntary movement, and autonomous intellectual activity.[25]

Islamic Galenic authors debated whether these powers/spirits/pneumata were faculties of a single soul, if they were parts of a tripartite soul, or if they were three different entities.[26] Nahyan Fancy has shown that many Muslim scholars agreed on considering these as either parts of a single but tripartite soul or faculties of the single soul of the human. This formulation corresponded better with the Islamic view on the soul, which insisted on every human having one soul endowed by God.[27] This psychology had implications on Galenic pathologies and diagnostics. Afflictions of the humors or of the central organs of the body reflected itself on the functioning of the pneumata and affected other parts of the body because of their ability to spread throughout the entire body. At another level, mental illness and other similar conditions were understood and explained from a humoral perspective relying heavily on the increase and corruption of black bile, which led to various mental and psychological problems. Conditions like madness, passion, epilepsy, and others were possible to explain from a humoral perspective but were understood to manifest in specific behavioral patterns and specific actions distinct from the manifestations of other purely physical conditions. As such, and although these conditions were rooted in a humoral context, they existed on a different level from fever or diarrhea.[28]

Although al-Balkhī and al-Rāzī, who were both well-known physicians, were aware of these questions, their books featured rather limited, if any, direct references to humors or any detailed discussions of the possible influences that humors might have on spiritual health.[29] With the exception of brief references in al-Balkhī's discussion of obsessions and of sadness and in al-Rāzī's discussion of passion, most such references could be found in books of physical medicine concerning diseases of the head.[30] In the same manner, al-Kirmānī seemed also uninterested in the effect of humors on behaviors or how complexions affected dispositions. Even in criticizing al-Rāzī for not being sufficiently committed to his claim of writing a book of medicine, al-Kirmānī did not find the lack of discussions of humors to be problematic. Ibn al-Jawzī, who was keenly aware of these issues and discussed some of these (humoral-spiritual) conditions in his *Luqat al-Manāfi*ʿ also did not have any direct reference or discussion of humoral influences on spiritual health. Ibn al-Jawzī presented his spiritual medicine as concerned with "the affairs of the hidden" (*al-bāṭin*), referring to the matters of the spirit rather than issues affecting the body. In this context, all authors paid attention to a number of vices and virtues, discussing questions like pride, greed, sadness, happiness, and excessive thought. The main purpose of these books was the refinement of the spirit through learning and training into proper social practices.[31] In this sense, writings on spiritual medicine shared similar purposes with writings on adab,[32] as well as other writings of shamāʾil and raqāʾiq, not to mention pietistic hagiographies and biographies of learned and pious individuals.[33]

In this way, spiritual medicine, in its focus on self-refinement, reflected specific values and social virtues that were seen as central to living a pious and socially respectable life. Values like honesty, courage, and thoughtfulness were to be cultivated both through religious writings and recommendations, as in Ibn al-Jawzī's writings, or through intellectual discussion and arguments, which one could find in both al-Rāzī and Ibn al-Jawzī. At the heart of this discussion was the belief that the soul, self, or spirit was inherently interested in the consummation of its earthly and most basic desires and was controlled by passion. Such passions were created by God for the purpose of protecting the body, but they were also the root for the various evils that might afflict the soul:

> Know that all that was created in the human was created for his wellbeing; either to bring about a benefit such as the passion for eating, or to fend off a harm such as anger. If the passion for eating increases, it becomes gluttony; and if anger increases, it leads to depravity. This book was composed to [guide oneself] to using the rules of righteousness within oneself, and to prevent passion from leading to harm, and to treat behaviors that resulted from passion exceeding proper rules.[34]

Ultimately, the goal of writings on spiritual medicine was to provide a tool for the readers to manage their passions and desires and behave in a way worthy of the pious and/or educated.

Al-Kirmānī did not fully agree with this characterization of the role of spiritual medicine as seen by both al-Rāzī and Ibn al-Jawzī. In his view, this characterization contained a logical fallacy: If the problems befalling the individual and causing these diseases of the spirit were indeed inherent in the spirit, how could one be trusted to correct such problems himself?

> It is not useful to a sick man, suffering from excess yellow bile that gave him fever, headache and back pain, to be told by the physician: "You have to suppress your yellow bile and reduce it because [its increase] is increasing your pain, insomnia and constipation." A saying like this by the physician is not a treatment that will cure the fever. And would not a statement like this demonstrate lack of knowledge about what is at hand?![35]

In his view, a physician sometimes is required to force his patient to follow specific rules and could not always trust the patient to adhere to the right behavior. Al-Balkhī agreed partially with this assessment, explaining that exhortations from the outside are often more effective than self-convictions. He explained that "it was the habit of resolute kings to have in their company wise men who would treat their spiritual symptoms, such as anger or fear [. . .] through advice."[36] Yet al-Balkhī, similar to al-Kindī and al-Rāzī, also accepted that the spirit can correct its own diseases with proper education and training.[37] For al-Kirmānī, there was no way that the spirit, being admittedly the seat of passion and the culprit of these faults, could be trusted to right its own course. Instead, al-Kirmānī argued, divine revelation was the only true path that would allow for correcting the behaviors of the spirit. In other words, divine revelation presented the external factor that was needed for the spirit to evaluate its actions and to understand what was required of it. divine revelation and law was the sole way through which a person could correct their behaviors and avoid spiritual ills.

The centrality of divine revelation in al-Kirmānī's view of spiritual medicine explains why he thought al-Rāzī's view on prophecy was relevant to this discussion. If al-Rāzī was correct that prophets were not necessary – that they were but talented and highly educated individuals, that God has supplied evidence for his existence and his laws in nature and endowed humans with intellectual powers so that any human could reach these laws through the intellect – then indeed the spirit or the intellect was capable of correcting one's behaviors and was able to treat its various spiritual complaints. Al-Kirmānī cited Abū Ḥātim's various arguments against this view and explained that divine existence and divine laws were not discoverable without the aid of the prophets and imams. The intellect was required to follow the dictates of the prophets and imams in order to reach salvation in this life and the next. It followed then that spiritual medicine could not be conducted without strict adherence to God's laws and without understanding the tools that God has provided to guide humans.

This interest in religious law and in the instructions that it provides could also be found in the writings of Miskawayh. For instance, in discussing the instructions given to children, Miskawayh explained that the first step in educating children will be to teach them the commandments of religious law (*sharīʿa*) as the basic form of learning that they require.[38] This, however, was only the beginning, which should be followed by additional refinement through reading books on ethics, presumably like his own, and learning from educators. Unlike al-Kirmānī, who believed that divine guidance was necessary for all humans to attain the refinement of the spirit, Miskawayh's interest in the role of religious law was probably related to his view on the needs of the commoners, who required clearer recommendations and orders similar to how children needed these basic instructions.

The ethical agent

In all these works and other similar texts, the reader is certainly not the spirit. Although the main subject of spiritual medicine is the spirit and how it can be bettered at various levels, the reader was consistently addressed as the person controlling the spirit, training it, or complaining about its various diseases. The reader could be controlled by the spirit and its various passions; however, this was a state of being of which neither the reader nor the authors were supportive. In other words, the reader was seen as the one reigning over (or supposed to be reigning over) the spirit and controlling its behaviors.[39] For instance, all previously mentioned authors addressed the question of training the spirit in order for it to be used to behaving properly. Ibn al-Jawzī dedicated a separate chapter to training the spirit, which he placed close to the end of the book and close to chapters about training and educating children, spouses, and slaves, presenting it as a culmination of the fixes and treatments he had described throughout the book. He explained:

> Know that training [the spirit] is to be done nicely and by moving slowly from one state to another, and should not be done by force in the beginning. It also involves mixing desires with fear [. . .]. [For example,] when some of the pious ancestors would feel a desire for sweets, he would promise his spirit that he would eat after praying through the night. When [Sufyān] al-Thawrī ate a thing that he desired, he would say [God's] servant has fed his child. Some of Mālik ibn Dīnār's neighbors reported "I heard him saying one night 'Like this, behave!' The next morning I asked him who he had at home, and he said no one. I asked then who he was talking to. He said, 'My spirit asked me for bread and persisted so I prohibited it from food for three days. Last night, after the end of these three days, I found a piece of dry bread so I told it wait and I will get you soft bread. It said, 'that is enough for me,' so I said, 'like this, behave!' "[40]

After giving instructions similar to the ones that he provided for raising children, Ibn al-Jawzī reported Ibn Dīnār's anecdote to illustrate how one can train their spirits. In the anecdote, the spirit acquired an independent persona on which Ibn Dīnār acted – recognizing demands, imposing punishment, and even accepting and recommending behaviors. In all cases, Ibn Dīnār, the reporter of the anecdote, and Ibn al-Jawzī were clear on the fact that the spirit inhabited and affected the same body that Ibn Dīnār was controlling. After all, Ibn Dīnār used his first person pronoun to describe his own attempt to eat the old bread before offering better bread to his spirit. In the same way, the long and arduous punishment of starvation for three days was directed at the spirit through its immediate connection to the body, which it used to manifest its various desires. Ibn al-Jawzī followed with a saying by another pious follower, where he explained, "I continued to drive my spirit to God while it cried, until I was able to drive it while it was laughing."[41] Training the spirit and forcing it to follow the demands and commands of God eventually allowed it to recognize the joy in worship and to seek such nearness to the divine.[42] The duality between the actor and his or her spirit was further underscored. Ibn al-Jawzī's view on this duality was even clearer in his instructions to preserve and protect the spirit's divinely ordained rights:

> After this, one should not forget its [the spirit's] rights. It is within its right to be given its share [of its desires], that could not be denied even for the intention of training. If this share was withheld in total, the heart would go blind [to the light of God], the resolve will be in disarray and worship will be burdensome. Know that, for God, the value of the spirit is higher than that of the rituals (*al-ʿibādāt*) and this is why He permitted breaking the fast for the traveler.[43]

Self-care, in this context, is a demand and obligation from God that prevented people from abusing their spirits through starvation or excessive unneeded worship. Rituals are important to train the spirit and to reach higher and more prominent spaces, but the spirit was, in itself, valued by God and protected by His orders and the licenses that He gave to people.

The three spirits

Ibn al-Jawzī's understanding of the spirit was based on his acceptance of a singular spirit with three faculties, as explained in the works of Galenic physicians, among others. He explained that these three faculties were the enunciative or rational faculty (*al-quwwah al-nāṭiqah*), the passionate or appetitive faculty (*al-quwwah al-shahwāniyyah*), and the irascible faculty (*al-quwwah al-ghaḍabiyyah*). These faculties were mentioned by al-Rāzī as well, who cited Plato when calling them three spirits, "The first is the enunciative or the divine, the second [is] the irascible or the animalistic, and the third is the vegetative, the growing or the passionate."[44] He then explained that, for Plato, the animalistic and vegetative spirits did not have a particular essence that survived after death, unlike the enunciative, which survives after death.[45] Al-Kirmānī, in responding to al-Rāzī, rejected the idea of three spirits, explaining that it was only one spirit that had various functions and faculties and that "philosophers" tended to describe it as three spirits because they mistook its actions for its essence. He referenced his various writings on the topic in his *Rāḥat al-ʿAql* (The Comfort of the Intellect), *Tāj al-ʿUqūl* (The Crown of Intellects), *al-Iklīl* (The Crown), and *al-Ḥadāʾiq* (The Gardens):

> The spirit is one in essence and it earned these three names due to its various acts. If it sought what replenishes what is lost from its body, it is called growing *nāmiyah*. If it sought refuge [from danger] to preserve itself, and traced knowledge by the senses from outside itself, it is called sensual *ḥissiyyah*. If it sought divine knowledge and understood the forms of intellectual being and what is needed for the perfection of its essence, it is called enunciative.[46]

Al-Kirmānī was keen on rejecting the existence of a tripartite spirit or three spirits and was adamant in identifying the philosophers' error in equating actions with essence.

Although Ibn al-Jawzī expressly used these qualities as faculties of a singular spirit, he soon reverted to calling each of them a spirit in order to explain his overall point:

> Man, who is honored by God with the love of knowledge, should care to perfect his enunciative *spirit*, with which God had privileged him over all animals and which he shares with angels, and make it the controller over the other two *faculties*; meaning the passionate and the irascible. So that [the enunciative spirit/faculty]'s place in the body is like the rider to the horse. As such, this enunciative faculty should be higher than other faculties, use them as it likes and withholds them when it likes. Whoever does this can indeed be called a human.[47] [Emphasis added]

He further explained that a man controlled by appetitive faculty was like a dumb beast and one controlled by his irascible faculty was similar to a predatory animal. Al-Kirmānī agreed on the desire to train the spirit. Whereas Ibn al-Jawzī utilized examples that likened the spirit to a child (and he followed the chapter on training the spirit with one on training children), al-Kirmānī preferred an example that further underscored his view on spiritual medicine as a discipline deeply connected to physical medicine. To him, training the spirit was akin to dieting imposed by physicians on the sick, preventing them from eating things that they desire and forcing them to eat undesirable foods and foul-tasting medicines.[48]

To be sure, the spirit was largely embodied and connected to the body and its various desires. Food, drink, sex, and many other physical needs and desires were understood as implicit in the desire of the spirit, which was seen as often driven by desires and needs – or at least, by the faculties of the spirit that were more connected to the body, such as the appetitive and irascible faculties. Al-Rāzī explained that these two spirits would perish with the body.[49] And, although al-Kirmanī, and possibly Ibn al-Jawzī, rejected the multiplicity of spirits and accepted a framework where these were powers or faculties of the singular spirit, they also accepted that these faculties/spirits perished with the body and that only the enunciative spirit or faculty survived in the afterlife. Yet one other actor within the body of the reader was to be addressed at length: the intellect.

The intellect

The intellect (*al-ʿaql*) played an important role in the pietistic cosmology of Ibn al-Jawzī and al-Kirmānī along with many others. For al-Kirmānī, the notion of the intellect was connected to a deeper understanding of the order of creation that had significant theological implications.[50] The divine First Intellect was in many ways separate from the world and shielded by the Spirit from which creation manifested and emanated. The First Intellect was the source and site of all knowledge. In this context, the human intellect, a faculty that al-Kirmānī placed in the human heart based on various traditions and verses, was the reflection of the divine intellect. However, this reflection required its own acculturation and should not be thought of as containing knowledge in itself. Instead, al-Kirmānī continued to stress the importance of divine guidance delivered by the prophets and imams in acculturating the human intellect and creating proper behavior. Al-Kirmānī understood the intellect to be the source of good nature and behavior and the spirit to be the source of various issues and problems.

For both al-Rāzī and Ibn al-Jawzī, the intellect was also at the center of some of the vices that they sought to correct in their work. For instance, al-Rāzī, followed by Ibn al-Jawzī, explained that the root of stinginess could be found in the intellect. After all, stinginess was a quality that intended to preserve oneself through the hoarding of food and other substances necessary for life.[51] In the same way, anger also had value in that it provided oneself with the impulse to protect their own bodies and their properties.[52] In these examples and many others, the intellect was responsible for these useful and seemingly rational behaviors that intended to protect the animal (or the human in this case). It was the spirit that would exaggerate these laudable or necessary behaviors, such as the protection of the body, and allow them to exceed their needed limits. The "rationality" of these acts attributed to the intellect was rooted in the goal-oriented act of self-preservation – a rational and legally sanctioned goal in itself.[53] As such, these behaviors, such as protecting the body, were attributed to the intellect, which was trusted to conduct itself with moderation. Al-Kirmānī seemed to accept that this was a form of rationality; however, at the same time, he refused to accept that some of these vices could contain a core of reasonableness.

Al-Kirmānī engaged with al-Rāzī's discussion of stinginess as an example of the role of the intellect in creating vices or condemnable behavior. At issue was the question of whether the hoarding of goods was, even in part, an act of the intellect directed at the protection of oneself against harm. First, al-Kirmānī explained that hoarding goods only benefitted the mortal body and protected against physical dangers. It did not protect against psychological or spiritual dangers. If it was indeed the intellect that provided for such hoarding, one would assume that it would try to "hoard" spiritual goods to protect the entirety of oneself and not only the body. As such, "the stinginess of the spirit is only part of its passion for increase in its body and flesh in the same way that a mouse, an ant, or a bat [aim to] grow [their bodies]."[54] In fact, if it were the intellect behind such an act, it would have realized that the proper way to protect and preserve oneself was to give rather than to hoard:

> A person of good faith and good belief does not fear poverty or death, and does not care for what afflicts his body, in the example of Socrates or Pythagoras and those like them of the ancients, who rejected [the earthly goods]. [This is also the example] of ʿAlī ibn Abī Ṭālib, the heir to the prophet: Once when he was fasting, he had only four biscuits that he needed to break his fast. When a pauper and an orphan came to his door asking [for food], he gave [his biscuits] to them not caring about his own hunger or the hunger of whoever was in his household, seeking only the perfection of his spirit by giving in good and charity. [Similarly,] Abū Dharr al-Ghaffārī never kept excess food in his house because he did not care about poverty or death. How could there be praiseworthy stinginess when no prophet, messenger, heir [to the prophet], Imam or scholar was known for meanness.[55]

Ultimately, al-Kirmānī accepted that the intellect provided for reasonable and defensible behaviors. However, he rejected what al-Rāzī proposed in evaluating such reasonableness based on material self-preservation – a position that Ibn al-Jawzī later adopted as well. Instead, al-Kirmānī considered the reasonable behavior to be the one that matched the dictates of the religious law. In this view, he marshalled the examples of ʿAlī and Abū Dharr, along with Socrates and Pythagoras, as examples of perfect intellects with perfect control over their bodies and spirits.[56]

For Ibn al-Jawzī, the intellect, its nature, and its role were central questions to be addressed in the first chapter of his book. The rather brief chapter was complemented by a reference to a longer and more detailed discussion in Ibn al-Jawzī's book *Dhamm al-Hawā* (Disparaging Passion), where the first chapter was dedicated to the intellect and its nature, place, and importance.[57] In *Spiritual Medicine*, Ibn al-Jawzī chose to only mention what he considered the intellectual proofs for the importance of the intellect, "[The value of] a thing is known by its fruits, and the fruit of the intellect is the knowledge of God."[58]

In *Dhamm al-Hawā*, Ibn al-Jawzī started by explaining the nature and the place of the intellect. He explained that some scholars believed that the intellect was a kind of knowledge, an instinct or a faculty that enabled the acquisition of knowledge. Others opted for a more material explanation, arguing that it was a simple or transparent body. Citing scholars of religion and ḥadīth, such as al-Ḥārith al-Muḥāsibī, a known ascetic and scholar in Baghdad, and Abū al-Ḥasan al-Tamīmī, jurisconsult of the ḥanbalī school like Ibn al-Jawzī, Ibn al-Jawzī explained that the intellect was a light (*nūr*), which emanated into the heart and allowed for the acquisition and discovery of knowledge.[59] Ibn al-Jawzī also cited the celebrated Ibrāhīm al-Ḥarbī, a known student of Aḥmad ibn Ḥanbal, who explained that the intellect was an instinct (*gharīzah*). Giving clear preference to the opinions of these three scholars, who were the only ones he mentioned by name, Ibn al-Jawzī concluded:

> The intellect is an instinct, which is similar to a light that is thrown in the heart so that [the heart] becomes ready to perceive things, and [is able to] know the possibility of the possible, the impossibility of the impossible and understand the consequences of various matters. This light can increase or decrease. If it increases, it suppresses the urgency of passion (*ʿājil al-hawā*) by virtue of observing the consequences.[60]

As such, the intellect was not a stable body that existed in all beings, but was rather a quality – or light – that was different from one person to the next and that influenced a person's ability to control their passion and, therefore, behave properly. The notion that the intellect's role manifested primarily in controlling passion was rather common in various pietistic writings. For instance, in a book entitled *al-ʿAql wa Faḍluhu* (The Intellect and Its Privilege), Ibn Abī al-Dunyā (d. 894) cited ʿAlī ibn Abī Ṭālib as saying that the Arabic word for the intellect (*al-ʿaql*) was indeed derived from the word for a camel's leash (*ʿiqāl*) because the former was to control passions in the same way that the leash drove and controlled a camel.[61] In the same vein, al-Māwardī (d. 1058) reported in his book *Adab al-Dunyā wa al-Dīn* (The Refinement of the Earthly Life and of Religion) a saying by the celebrated ascetic ʿĀmir ibn ʿAbd Qays: "If your intellect controlled you from [engaging in] what is not proper, then you are a reasonable person."[62] This saying was structured around the similar roots of intellect (*ʿaql*), control (*yaʿqil*), which is derived from the word for a leash, and the subjective form (*ʿāqil*) – further emphasizing the intriguing morphological similarity between the words for intellect, control, and leash.

Ibn al-Jawzī, similar to al-Kirmānī, used a number of verses in the Quran to explain that the heart is the site of the intellect. Although Ibn al-Jawzī explained that the hanafīs believed the intellect to be located in the head – a view that al-Rāzī agreed with – locating the intellect in the heart was not unique to Ibn al-Jawzī. For instance, the famous Sufi scholar al-Ḥakīm al-Tirmidhī (d. 869) explained in his *Adab al-Nafs* (The Refinement of the Spirit):

> Knowledge and the intellect are placed in the heart. Passion is outside of the heart and stands between the heart and its God. It sheds darkness over the hearing and the vision of the heart, imprisons what is inside of it and overcomes the heart. The heart is then like a lamp, in a house, but is placed inside a clay vassal and is covered so the house is dark.[63]

Although al-Ḥakīm al-Tirmidhī did not explicitly engage with the question of the nature of the intellect and its being a light, as Ibn al-Jawzī explained, he employed a metaphor used to portray the intellect as the light burning inside the heart – the lamp – and intending to illuminate the house – the person. In his metaphor, passion, located in the spirit, was the cover that obscured and obstructed the light of

God. al-Kirmānī was rather explicit in linking the intellect to the divine and in deploying a narrative of illumination that placed piety and belief both inside and outside the heart by virtue of such emanation of the intellect from the divine origin; however, Ibn al-Jawzī, as well as Ibn Abī al-Dunyā and al-Ḥakīm al-Tirmidhī, utilized a similar narrative without engaging directly in the theological implications.

Ibn al-Jawzī followed his discussion of the nature and place of the intellect with a discussion of prophetic traditions and anecdotes that praised the intellect and explained its importance. He was, however, aware of the fact that most prophetic traditions concerning the intellect were seen by scholars of ḥadīth as doubtful at best because of their problematic chains of transmission. He cited the famous scholar and compiler of ḥadīth Abū Ḥātim ibn Ḥibbān (d. 965) as saying, "I do not deem any tradition from the prophet about the intellect as authentic."[64] Ibn Ḥibbān enumerated a number of reporters to whom most of the traditions about the intellect were attributed and explained that he did not trust their reports. As Jonathan Brown explains, weak and even rejected or fabricated traditions were used by preachers and deployed in many books related to piety and asceticism.[65] Ibn al-Jawzī, Brown argues, belonged to a small but ultimately growing group of preachers and scholars who had some reservations on the use of these traditions, even in the context of preaching and pietistic narratives, preferring to always use more trustworthy traditions.[66] This explains Ibn al-Jawzī's decision to limit his use of traditions about the intellect to only a few: "The traditions transmitted from the prophet about the intellect are numerous. However, they are unreliable. So we will limit ourselves to these few."[67] This, of course, is different from Ibn Abī al-Dunyā, who belonged to a different generation but also a different school in relation to utilizing weaker traditions in pietistic narratives.[68]

In either case, the rather small selection that Ibn al-Jawzī deployed focused on one issue: that the intellect was essential to proper worship and that the true believer is one who enjoyed a sound intellect. In one tradition, ʿĀʾisha was asked which of two people – one of them prayed all night and the other slept all night – was better in the eyes of God? She explained:

> I have asked the prophet the same question and he said, "Whoever has a better intellect." I said, "O prophet of God, but I asked about their worship!" he said, "They will not be questioned [by God] about their worship but about their intellects. Whoever of them has a better intellect would be better off in this world and in the hereafter."[69]

Ibn Abī al-Dunyā reported this tradition along with a few other similar traditions. In one, the companions explained that whenever the prophet was told about the worship of one of his companions, he would ask, "How is his intellect?"[70] In another, the prophet advised his companions, "Do not admire one's belief before you know about his intellect."[71] Similarly, both Ibn Abī al-Dunyā and Ibn al-Jawzī reported a tradition about Adam when he was first sent to earth:

> Gabriel came to Adam with religion, the intellect and good manners and told him, "God is asking you to choose one of these three." Adam exclaimed, "O

> Gabriel, I have not seen anything better than these three since I left paradise." Adam then grabbed the intellect and took it and told the other two [religion and good manners], "you two ascend [back to God]." They said, "No! we will not!" Adam said, "Do you disobey me?!" They said, "No. But God has commanded us to be always with the intellect wherever it is" So the three became Adam's.[72]

In Ibn Abī al-Dunyā's and Ibn al-Jawzī's narratives, the value of the intellect in pietistic discourse went beyond its role in controlling passion and regulating one's behavior. Ibn Abī al-Dunyā reported a tradition where the prophet was reported to have said that people are rewarded in the hereafter based on their intellects. In another tradition, reported by both Ibn Abī al-Dunyā and Ibn al-Jawzī, the famous scholar Wahab ibn Munabbah said, "God is never worshipped with something that is better than the intellect."[73] In this context, and when thinking and reflecting on the divine represented the most exalted form of worship, the intellect became the main tool for performing such worship. This was the reason God was reported to have said that He has never created something that was dearer to Him than the intellect.[74]

Yet the intellect had various meanings, including ones related to the earthly affairs that people engaged in. Ibn Abī al-Dunyā cited Wakīʿ ibn al-Jarrāḥ as saying, "The intellectual (*al-ʿāqil*) is the one who intellects his affairs based on the commands of God and not the one who intellects the management of his daily affairs."[75] "Intellecting" one's affairs in accordance to divine law was also a guarantee of surviving inevitable sins and errors. Ibn al-Jawzī reported a known tradition from Muʿādh ibn Jabal, who explained:

> A man with an intellect and with sins that are as numerous as the sand is closer to survival [in the afterlife] than an ignorant man with good deeds as numerous as the sand. This is because the man with the intellect understand [his situation] and resorts to repentance by virtue of the intellect that he possesses, while the ignorant is like a man who builds and then destroys so he may be inflicted with the destruction of his good deeds because of his ignorance.[76]

As mentioned before, in his *Spiritual Medicine*, Ibn al-Jawzī focused on what he considered to be the intellectual arguments for the value of the intellect. He followed al-Rāzi in explaining that the intellect was the difference between humans and beasts: "It is the thing that separated us from beasts, children or the mad."[77] The intellect was to be valued for its main fruits:

> Through the intellect, we learned what elevates us, improves our lives and takes us to our goals. Through the intellect, we learned the making of ships and used it to cross the various seas.[78] And through the intellect, we came to know about the Creator, which is the most significant knowledge and benefit that we acquired.[79]

Even among animals, the intellect was the sine qua non of excellence as it allowed for mastering passion and controlling the spirit's basic desires. Ibn al-Jawzī brought an example that explained how mastering passions was the definitive feature of higher beings:

> The privilege of the human over the beastly animal is by the intellect, which was ordered [by God] to control the passion. If the person does not accept the judgement of the intellect and [allowed] passions to rule [over him], the beastly animal would be [better than the human]. As evidence for the benefit of disobeying passion, [one can observe] the privilege awarded to hunting dogs over other dogs. That is because [a hunting dog] disobeys its passion and holds on what it hunts for its owner whether out of fear or gratitude.[80]

The sign of a functioning intellect was the control it was able to exercise on the body and on the basic desires of the spirit. It is notable here that the intellect was also a reason for honor and distinction precisely because of this controlling role.

In all these cases, the intellect played two important roles in these pietistic and spiritual-medical narratives. On one hand, it served as the site of knowledge, blessing, and light emanating from the divine and the means by which a person was able to control his passions.[81] On the other, the intellect was God's best creation and the tool with which God should be worshipped. In this pietistic cosmology, the intellect stood as the sight of knowing God and as an adversary to the spirit, which was more concerned with basic needs and often consumed by its passion. The intellect's desires and interests were seen as intellectable ones, meaning that their reasons and their goals could be understood and deduced through organized thought. Some of these desires were seen as aimed at protecting the body and preserving oneself, whereas others were more concerned with the refinement of the spirit and the acquisition of higher status in this world and in the hereafter. The desires of the spirit, on the other hand, were connected to the basic instincts and desires. And although some of these desires could be understood, in al-Rāzī's and Ibn al-Jawzī's views, as originating in forms of self-protection and preservation, they were still basic in their being unintellectable and rooted in simple animalistic desires and passions. The passions of the spirit were therefore the significant danger affecting the intellect and posing a threat to its ability to control one's behavior and guide it.

The duality of reason and passion

Regardless of their differing views on the nature, place, or exact acts of the spirit and the intellect or whether the intellect was the function of the rational spirit, the pietistic and spiritual medical narratives discussed before agreed on a form of duality whereby a person's acts are governed through the balance of the intellect and the spirit. Such duality was evident in the exchanges that people had with their spirits, ordering them or demanding them to undertake specific acts. It was also evident in the recommendations offered by authors of spiritual medicine and others to train the spirit and provide for its edification. Moreover, and on top of this duality, the person, or the ethical agent these books addressed, presided over both the intellect and the spirit, exercising choice in which they would listen to. Both the spirit, here equated with the appetitive and irascible faculties, and the intellect, sometimes equated with the rational faculty, provided resources for actions and thoughts, but the ethical agent (or person) was to choose either the path of the intellect, organized around proper and deductive thinking and following the dictates of religious law, or the spirit, controlled and consumed by its passions. For Ibn al-Jawzī, this ethical agent existed separately from both the intellect and the spirit. It desired pleasure but could also be persuaded that immediate pleasures were fleeting, whereas eternal pleasures required waiting and oftentimes suffering. As such, certain authors considered the proper course of action for treating spiritual ills was to uncover some of the intelligible arguments for disobeying the passions of the spirit and convincing the person to see the intellect's point of view. Al-Balkhī was most forthcoming about the need to remind the ethical agent of what they originally knew of the importance of following the dictates of the intellect and to reject or tame passions and desires.[82]

Similarly, in his discussion of the need to disobey passion, Ibn al-Jawzī, following al-Rāzī, explained that those who followed their passions ended up losing even the pleasures they so diligently sought:

> The intellectual should know that whatever hardship he suffers in disobeying passion is easier than what he would endure by obeying it. For the least that obeyers of passion endure is becoming in a state where they neither enjoy their passion nor are able to survive its absence because [their passion] becomes an addicted habit, as in the case of sex addicts and alcoholics.[83]

This complete separation between the intellect/rational spirit, the (appetitive and irascible) spirit(s), and the overruling ethical agent was at the heart of the medical narrative advanced by al-Balkhī, al-Rāzī, and Ibn al-Jawzī and rejected by al-Kirmānī. This separation meant that the diseases of passion did not affect all of the person – or ethical agent – but rather her or his spirit, whereas the intellect remained capable of functioning and understanding the consequences of such acts. Moreover, the person was ultimately able to remedy all of these problems by better understanding and obeying the commands of the intellect and bringing the spirit and its passions under control. Ibn Ḥibbān agreed:

> The intellect and the passion are enemies. It is incumbent upon a person to be swift in affirming his [intellect][84] and slow to accepting his passion. If the difference between the two was unclear, he should avoid the thing that is closer to his passion because avoiding the passion is conducive to mending the interior.[85]

In this context, al-Rāzī, followed by Ibn al-Jawzī, proceeded in providing intellectual and, in the case of Ibn al-Jawzī, transmitted proofs for what one should do and for what one should reject, arguing in essence that knowledge of these proofs would strengthen the person and allow him or her to reject passion and control the spirit.

Al-Hakīm al-Tirmidhī presented a similar cosmology, though organized physically in a manner different from al-Rāzī and more clearly than Ibn al-Jawzī. For him, the heart became the site of this reigning personhood that governed and ruled over the body. The heart, in al-Ḥakīm al-Tirmidhī's view, was made of two layers: the heart (*al-qalb*) and the bosom (*al-fuʾād*). The heart, which is the innermost part, was the site of God's light "because it is driven from Him" and is capable of recognizing God. The bosom, which is the engulfing layer made of flesh and membranes could, however, obscure this light and prevent it from shining over the body and affecting one's deeds.[86] As explained before, al-Tirmidhī explained that the heart was the site of the intellect as well as knowledge and experience. Passion, however, existed outside the heart (possibly affecting the bosom) and obscuring the light of God from reaching the heart and shining from it. While the heart always contained the knowledge of and belief in God, it could be overcome with passion, which would prevent the required manifestations of belief in sayings and in deeds,

> [God] has made the heart the sovereign over all the body. [But] passion moves the still body and bothers the heart; and the devil gives it false hope and false promises; and passion sways and drives it. [Although] the believer has his heart set on belief and monotheism is clear on his tongue, desires act on [the heart] when it is time to perform the rituals, passions sway it until [the believer] does what makes him look like he has not believed yet. While he is indeed a believer by heart and by tongue, passions and desires overcome his heart but do not change what is inside his heart. For the heart has its knowledge [of God] but has become imprisoned and oppressed [by passions].[87]

Al-Ḥakīm al-Tirmidhī's view on the heart and its connection to the divine light was similar in a number of ways to al-Kirmānī, who argued that the intellect was a divine gift that emanated from the First Intellect. This core belief existed within every person because it was part of the divine. However, passions were able to overcome and overwhelm such belief leading to improper behaviors and the appearance of unbelief. Similar to al-Kirmānī, who rejected al-Rāzī's perspective, al-Ḥakīm al-Tirmidhī seemed suspicious that the intellect or the trained spirit can overcome its own passions through argument and conviction. For both al-Kirmānī and al-Ḥakīm al-Tirmidhī, the effective way to lead a pious and upright life was to follow God's commandments, which would enable the heart (or the intellect) to overcome the powers of passion.

Ibn Ḥibbān (d. 965) also agreed on the existence of basic and innate knowledge along with acquired knowledge that was to be derived from divine instructions. Citing the ḥadīth scholar Abū Ḥātim Muḥammad ibn Idrīs al-Rāzī (d. 890),[88] he explained that the intellect is of two types: the innate (*maṭbūʿ*) and the auditory (*masmūʿ*) (or the learned). The innate was similar to fertile land, which had the basic qualities needed to grow crops, but the auditory (or learned) was akin to seeds, "There is no way for the innate intellect (*al-ʿaql al-maṭbūʿ*) to grow crops without the auditory intellect (*al-ʿaql al-masmūʿ*) visiting it, awakening it from its slumber, and releasing its potentials."[89] Using the term *auditory* to refer to the learned intellect and to externally acquired learning, in part, indicated that such learning required *listening* to God's word and obeying His orders. In this same context, al-Ḥakīm al-Tirmidhī viewed remembrance, or *dhikr*, as the central worship that allowed the believer to achieve nearness to God and control over the passions of the self. Dhikr was a simple form of worship that could be performed in all places and at all times. Al-Ḥakīm al-Tirmidhī argued that dhikr was preferred by God to all other forms of worship precisely because of how it connects the servant to the God and allows for purification of the spirit.[90]

Al-Rāzī, al-Kirmānī, and Ibn al-Jawzī agreed on another role for the intellect, that is to understand and to know God. For all three, such knowledge was the utmost goal and the most sublime intellectual activity. Al-Kirmānī and Ibn al-Jawzī were even more emphatic in explaining that the real reason behind creation was to know God and, therefore, render Him the worship that He is due. Al-Ḥakīm al-Tirmidhī proposed a similar point but went further in explaining how worship was affected by the intellect and by the true knowledge of God. First, he explained that God has ordered His servants to declare God to be one (*waḥḥada*) by their hearts, tongues, and deeds. Such unity of belief, which mirrored the belief in the unity of God, could only be achieved through true knowledge of God established in the intellect. Only in this way could a person be a true servant of God:

> That is because you do not become a servant to Him, until he becomes a Lord to you, with no partners. Whoever takes a partner to God has departed the institute of monotheism. Although that person remains a servant to Him by virtue of ownership, the servant himself has not rendered himself a servant because he has not declared [God] as one and worshiped him. Nor did he obey God because he was ordered to obey. Since he who obeys God is obedient to God.[91]

Al-Tirmidhī's seeming tautology intended to clarify the difference between the true and established relationship between a person and God, on one hand, and the confessed and professed relationship between a believer and God. Whereas the first is built on the 'fact' of God's ownership of the human body and His ability to force obedience and achieve His will, the second is built on the knowledge and recognition of these facts. Therefore, the believer submits to the divine and declares himself an obedient servant by virtue of knowing his true relationship to God. Knowledge, which al-Tirmidhī explained was a light that resided in the heart,[92] was a tool to achieve piety, "If you know [about] your Lord, how would your heart be towards Him, [and how would it receive] His promises and His power?!"[93] True knowledge of God and His powers was to allow the servant to submit to God and to tame his spirit with ease. Al-Tirmidhī explained that this was the reason why God has ordered people to truly know Him.[94] The intellect, whether placed in the heart or in the head, was responsible not only for choosing reasonable behaviors, but also for achieving true knowledge of God, making piety and worship easier and more available to the servant.

In this pietistic context, such duality of the intellect and the spirit enforced discursively the pietistic habit of self-reckoning whereby believers were asked to consider their own deeds and to carefully reflect on their acts. The ostensible duality permitted pious actors to assume distance from their own passions, to claim superiority over their own basic desires – which were affixed to the spirit – and to enact self-reckoning and self-discipline. In fact, if the pious actor was unable to see the faults of his own ways, Ibn al-Jawzī instructed that he "imagine these [deeds] done by another person and reflect on their results with his intellect. He would then see what he should have known from the beginning."[95] Pious actors presided over the constant animosity between the intellect and the passions that inhabit the spirit, to use Ibn Ḥibbān's imagery. They were to listen keenly to their intellect and to disobey their passions. However, they were also responsible for the wellbeing of their intellects and their spirits. Their intellects required training through learning and through listening to the wisdom of divine revelation.[96] The spirit required rearing and restraint, but some of its legally acceptable needs should be provided for, as Ibn al-Jawzī explained and as discussed before.[97] The spirit itself was not the enemy. The spirit was the house of the main spiritual disease: passion (*al-hawā*).

To be sure, questions related to the meaning and place of the intellect, the nature of the soul and its parts or faculties, and the relation between the spirit and the intellect carried significant theological and philosophical implications. Adamson has shown how al-Rāzī's *al-Ṭibb al-Rūḥānī* (*Spiritual Medicine*) was connected to his larger body of philosophical works. Al-Kirmānī was also open about the connections between a critique of al-Rāzī's advice and larger and more crucial theological questions he addressed elsewhere.[98] However, similar to what Adamson observed in al-Rāzī's *Spiritual Medicine*, all of these authors, such as al-Kirmānī and Ibn al-Jawzī, steered clear of any of these questions and focused entirely on rather simplistic and action-oriented narratives that aimed to benefit their readers. Al-Rāzī refrained from discussing the nature of the soul, explaining that this was a discussion that exceeded this book and was not needed there.[99] Al-Kirmānī's critique of al-Rāzī's *Spiritual Medicine* was loaded with significant theological and philosophical arguments – some of which were made explicit. However, al-Kirmānī was clear that the point of the second part of his book, which included his own spiritual medicine, was meant to show diseases of the spirit, diagnose them, and prescribe treatments that are available to all. Even in his discussion of rather sophisticated philosophical questions, he was ostensibly brief and employed references to some of his other works to focus on a more accessible illustration of al-Rāzī's errors and his own advice to his readers. Even less interest in philosophical questions can be detected in the works of Ibn Abī al-Dunyā or Ibn al-Jawzī, who relied heavily on prophetic traditions and deployed a pietistic narrative that was accessible to large swaths of believers either directly or through preachers. Ibn Abī al-Dunyā's book, which was largely a curated collection of ḥadīths, served in a manner similar to his other writings as a source for ḥadīths on the discussed questions that other authors and preachers used. Ibn al-Jawzī's book can be securely placed within a large corpus of books, which he composed and directed to preachers aiming at helping them speak to their congregants.[100] Similarly, Ibn Ḥibbān explained that he wrote "a light book" to help people understand what proper behaviors were.[101] As such, the discussion of the spirit, its passions, and the intellect was not intended to necessarily clarify philosophical or theological questions but rather to provide a background for pietistic or ethical elaborations that aimed to instruct the believers in ways of piety. This is not claiming that these authors were uninterested in these questions, unable to engage in these discussions, or unwilling to do so. Rather, they presented these texts with the clear intention of public edification.

Etiology and diseases

In writings about spiritual medicine as well as in other pietistic and moralistic literature, passion (*al-hawā*) was always portrayed as a problem affecting the spirit and compromising the thoughts and deeds of the educated or the pious.[102] Al-Rāzī was emphatic on the importance of disparaging and controlling passion in his *al-Ṭibb al-Rūḥānī* (*Spiritual Medicine*). He explained that he commenced the book with a discussion of the intellect (in the first chapter) and passion (in the second) because, "They act as the principles for this [discussion] of spiritual medicine."[103] Although he explained that philosophers, theologians, and other scholars had varying views on the spirit and the intellect and their roles, he insisted that any worthy endeavor required a measure of controlling passions and that any sensible or reasonable person agreed on this rule, "Disparaging passion (al-hawā) and controlling it is necessary in all opinions, in the view of any reasonable person (ʿāqil) and in all religions (dīn)."[104] In al-Kirmānī's insistence on following a strictly medical narrative in his discussion, he categorized passion as one of the three main diseases that affect the spirit and that were at the heart of spiritual medicine's task. As such, many of the acts that would guarantee spiritual health are related to the control of passion. Following al-Rāzī, Ibn al-Jawzī also placed his chapter on passion as the second chapter and used the title "Disparaging Passion," which was reminiscent of his more celebrated and larger text under the same title. As mentioned before, Ibn al-Jawzī referenced his *Dhamm al-Hawā* (Disparaging Passion) text few times in his *Spiritual Medicine*. More significantly, *Disparaging Passion* contained chapters and advice similar to *Spiritual Medicine* but was not organized or justified by a medical paradigm. This similarity was perhaps natural, seeing that passion was the main cause of the ailments of the spirit. In both texts, Ibn al-Jawzī defined passion as "nature's inclination to what suits it."[105]

The universality of this view on passion and on moderation, which al-Rāzī claimed, underscored the fact that much of the recommendations of spiritual medicine, whether in the writings of al-Rāzī, al-Kirmānī, or Ibn al-Jawzī, represented general principles of comportment that applied to the educated and learned elites in society. Self-control; disregard for earthly passions and desires; and the consistent striving for knowledge, learning, and refinement were hallmarks of how educated elites understood themselves and thought about their position in society.[106] Of course, the works of al-Kirmānī, Ibn Abī al-Dunyā, Ibn Ḥibbān, and

Ibn al-Jawzī relied on prophetic traditions and transmitted religious materials in explaining the importance of their recommendations, which imbued their work with layers of religious piety that were not in the works of al-Rāzī, al-Balkhī, or Miskawayh. However, in all of these cases, both the pietistic and the Galenic-ethical writings shared central dictates and behaviors and exhibited similar principles and views. In all of these writings, a learned or pious person needed to control (almost always) their passions and to behave according to the dictates of their intellect.[107]

Ibn al-Jawzī was emphatic in his rejection of passion and his insistence on the need to disparage and disobey it. In his book *Disparaging Passion*, he reported a tradition where King Solomon said, "The one who defeats his passion is more powerful than one who conquers an entire city on his own."[108] In the same vein, al-Ḥasan al-Baṣrī was asked what the best form of Jihād was, and he responded, "Fighting *jihāduk* your passion."[109] The narrative linking Jihad to fighting passion was rather common and relied on a number of prophetic traditions that circulated widely during this period and beyond. Passion was akin to another god that controlled a person and prevented them from worshipping the one true God. Ibn al-Jawzī chose a tradition where the prophet said, "There is no god under the sky that is worshipped and that God [detests] more than a passion that is being followed."[110] In the same vein, al-Kirmānī placed passion and following it at a similar level to denying God or disbelieving in the prophets, imams, and angels.[111] Following Ibn Ḥibbān, Ibn al-Jawzī admonished his readers to disobey passion in all possible ways. If one was in doubt about a particular matter, one should do the thing that was further away from his passion,

> Al-Aṣma'ī said, I heard a Bedouin say, "If you are confused by two matters and you do not know which of the two is more proper, disregard the one that is closer to your passion because most error results from following passion."[112]

Different authors encouraged their readers to reject acts that were incited by passion, regardless of the matters at hand and even if some of these acts were mandated by religious law or seemed to be pietistic in nature. In fact, piety and pietistic acts can be contaminated by passion, resulting in a hypocrisy where one performed acts of devotion only because they made him or her feel better or made people speak highly of him or her.[113] Even if passions had no adverse effects and represented no harms in this life or the next:

> Know that if a man agrees with his passion even if it did not harm him, he will find himself to be despicable because he was defeated. If he conquers his passion, he will find majesty in himself since he was a victor. You see that when people find an ascetic, they marvel at him and kiss his hand. This is only because he is strong enough to disregard the passions that they could not.[114]

For al-Rāzī, followed by Ibn al-Jawzī, disparaging and disobeying passion distinguished humans from animals. Rephrasing al-Rāzī, Ibn al-Jawzī explained that animals obtain more passion-related pleasures than humans: "A camel eats more [than a man] and a bird copulates more. And beasts are free to pursue their passions without a limit and without thought or worry."[115] As such, humans were not created to follow their passions. If they were, God would have endowed them with the capacity to attain more of these desires than any inferior animal could. As explained before, Ibn al-Jawzī cited the example of hunting dogs, which are more prized than other dogs because of their ability to defeat their passions and bring their hunt to their owners.[116] In the same way, al-Ḥakīm al-Tirmidhī explained that trained falcons change their habits and their natural desire to live in high mountains and escape humans, controlling their passions when they hunt for their owners rather than themselves.[117] Thus, training and refinement – be it in comparing humans to animals or trained and well-bred animals to untrained ones – involved the controlling of passions, which became a sign of such refinement and of superior intellects. Throughout these cases, and as will be further explained later, passion emerges as a force that drives humans and animals to immediate gratification throughout the fulfillment of immediate needs, whereas the intellect, whether in humans or that which is cultivated in trained animals, allows them to consider larger consequences and to take actions that enable them to garner more benefits.

The values of passion

For al-Rāzī, al-Kirmāni, and Ibn al-Jawzī, among others, passions were necessary to maintain the survival of the individual and the species. Passion for eating and drinking drove beings, whether human or animal, to fulfill their needs and maintain their health. As such, passion itself, and in the abstract, was not to be disparaged, only excess passion:

> Know that passion is the inclination of nature to what suits it. This inclination was created in humans to ensure their survival. For if it were not for a human's inclination to food, he would not eat; or to drink, he would not drink; or to copulate, he would not copulate; etc. Passion is, therefore, a harbinger of what is useful and anger is to spell out what is harmful. As such, it is not proper to disparage passion in general. Instead, we disparage excess passion, that is passion that exceeds bringing benefits or expelling harm. However, since most of those who obey passion do not stop at the limits of what is useful, disparaging passion was generalized because of the commonality of harm. This is because it is difficult to understand the purpose of placing passion in the spirit. And if this was understood, it was seldom applied.[118]

Al-Ḥakīm al-Tirmdhī explained that passion was "the core of the spirit."[119] In his view, passion was a product of the earthly elements from which Adam was created. Because God created Adam of clay, composed of dust, and a spirit, the spirit relied on the clay as another key component of the human. Passion was the expression of this dusty core that made humans. For humans who were created from flesh and blood after Adam, the dust/clay element was replaced by the food the mother ingested. Passion was the product of her breathing. In this context, al-Tirmidhī used the morphological similarities between hawā (passion) and hawā' (air) to emphasize his point on the origins of passion and its centrality to the making of humans. Al-Tirmidhī explained that passion always drove the spirit toward earthly pleasures, as it inclined to what it was made of: earthly dust and clay. Al-Rāzī, al-Kirmānī, Ibn al-Jawzī, and others agreed that moderation was the key and that it was not possible, let alone desirable, to extinguish passion altogether. For al-Rāzī and Ibn al-Jawzī, this entailed detailed arguments for the benefits of controlling passion.[120] Although al-Kirmānī agreed on the purposes of passion, he did not seem to believe that it could exist in moderation. Instead he criticized al-Rāzī, explaining that because passion was inherent in the spirit, the spirit was unable to control it on its own. In other words, passion, although necessary for survival, was not possible to moderate. Instead, it was to be brought under the control of God's commands and the rule of divine law.[121]

In all these accounts, passion was presented as a character of the spirit, if not one of the central ways that the spirit manifested its desires and needs. Passions for food and sex were part of the functions of the appetitive spirit. Passions that lead to anger and fear were part of the irascible spirit or the animalistic functions and faculties of the spirit. As such, the dual nature of passion, a necessary quality for the preservation of life and a dangerous fault in excess, was reflective of the dual nature of the spirit itself. The spirit was naturalistic and animalistic, often connected to nature (*al-ṭab'*) and to the basic needs of the body and also likened to animals and children in its inability to perceive dangers or to contemplate the consequences of its actions. The spirit, controlled and driven by its passion, required training, harnessing, and control through the intellect (or the rational part of the spirit itself). Spiritual medicine was then based on this dual nature. Similar to how bodies contained the causes of their illnesses as part of their compositions, namely the humors, the spirit also contained the causes for its illnesses, namely its passions. Al-Kirmānī explained:

> Similar to how the body is composed of four humors: blood, yellow bile, phlegm and black bile, the spirit [. . .] has four qualities: thought [of God's orders], deeds according to God's orders, knowledge of the obligations of God's religion, and knowledge of the intellectual [issues] related to monotheism [. . .]. Similar to how the body has diseases that affect it through increase or decrease in its humors, the spirit has ills that corrupt it. These are either corrupt belief in the unity of God, in his angels, in his friends, in the law of his religion, bad habits or manners, and [following] passion.[122]

As such, the dual nature of passion and of the spirit provided for the medical narrative to acquire more depth. Moreover, it allowed for the production of narratives related to training and harnessing the spirit as a tool for the betterment of one's fate in this life and beyond.

At another level, the disparaging of passion left a space that accepted its importance and that allowed for the seemingly naturalistic or animalistic qualities and needs to exist and be recognized. Yet such a space served to highlight a more central virtue, namely, moderation. Al-Kirmānī and Ibn al-Jawzī, among others, were less enthusiastic about al-Rāzī's interest in the full rejection of all earthly goods. Whereas al-Rāzī explained how some philosophers and mystics were able to reject passions entirely and to disparage the passions of the spirit with no exceptions, both al-Kirmānī and Ibn al-Jawzī were keen on highlighting the importance of some of these passions and the need to maintain moderation rather than reject all passion. Al-Kirmānī explained all acts emanating from the spirit were originally intended to benefit the spirit and the body. As such, any such act performed in moderation was therefore virtuous.[123] Ibn al-Jawzī warned that the spirit had rights mandated by God and that one should not violate its rights, as this will result in rebellion and would ultimately prevent one from taming their spirits fully.[124]

Passion and sensual pleasures

The question of sensual pleasures, whether in this world or in the afterlife, was a recurrent issue in the writings of many scholars. Ultimately, passion forced people to seek sensual pleasures which would lead them to error. For instance, al-Rāzī, argued on several occasions that one should abstain from immediate pleasures in order to attain longer and more sustainable pleasures.[125] This was not only related to the pleasures of the afterlife that one earns through reining passion in this world and committing to good deeds, but also to the immediate pleasures of this life. He explained that those addicted to sex, wine, or music tend to slowly lose the pleasure of these particular desires: "They do not enjoy it to the same degree that those not addicted to them do because [these passions] become a habit that they cannot stop and they become necessary to living not a privilege or a pleasure."[126] Although al-Rāzī's argument may seem to indicate hedonistic or Epicurean narratives, as L. E. Goodman suggested,[127] Adamson has convincingly argued that this characterization might be misleading. As Adamson explained, al-Rāzī's writings show instead that he adhered to Plato's view in Timaeus that pleasure has no value but was rather the absence of pain or harm.[128] In fact, this particular view on pleasure did not escape al-Rāzī's main critic, Ḥamīd al-Dīn al-Kirmānī, who rejected this view on pleasure and its connection to pain:

> [Al-Rāzī argued] that it is known that a person who was not exposed to the heat of the sun or encountered harm [from this heat], would not yearn to shade or enjoy cold water like that who was hurt by heat. If this was indeed the case, [. . .] pleasure thus could not exist except following harm, and that it is transient. [However,] this is not true for all pleasures. Some pleasures are eternal and do not end, and exist without harm before it. This is like the pleasures of the afterlife that was promised in paradise, which do not end and do not involve harm.[129]

Miskawayh agreed with al-Rāzī's views on pleasure. He admitted that arguments emanating from the hedonistic logic that justified abstaining from fleeting pleasures as means to acquiring lasting ones were useful. However, these arguments were fit only for commoners and children.

Miskawayh's rejection of bodily pleasures and his view that these pleasures only appealed to the feeble in mind and soul extended to his view of the pleasures of the afterlife. He explained in a few occasions how the commoners clang to the materially portrayed pleasures of heaven:

> If they [the commoners *al-ʿāmah wa al-riʿāʿ wa juhhāl al-nās wa al-siqāṭ*] follow the rituals and abstain from the earthly [pleasures] and renounce it, it is by way of commerce or bargaining on their part – as if they left the few [pleasures] to attain the many, and rejected the finite to reach the eternal. However, despite [their] beliefs and acts, when angels or higher beings are mentioned, you find [the commoners] agreeing that [angels and these beings] are closer to God and of higher status than humans and that they do not require any of the needs of humans.[130]

Although Ibn al-Jawzī followed al-Rāzī and explained that one of the harms that afflict those who follow their passions was precisely the loss of the pleasure they so diligently sought,[131] he did not seem to have accepted the rest of the argument about pleasures being perceptible only after harm. For Ibn al-Jawzī, the rhetorical pseudo-Epicurean argument of choosing eternal and lasting pleasures over transient ones was rather convincing and corresponded to the promise of heaven in the afterlife. Contrary to Miskwayh, neither al-Kirmānī nor Ibn al-Jawzī saw this "bargain" to be blameworthy.

Although al-Kirmānī did not reject bodily pleasures in the same manner that Miskawayh did or that al-Rāzī hinted at, angels and higher beings, who included the prophets and imams in the afterlife, occupied the pride of place in his narrative, as he was keen on the similarities between a well-trained spirit and angels. In fact, he followed this specific goal throughout his book explaining, for instance, that the point of washing and ablution was to be as clean as angels and as the honorable deceased prophets and imams.[132] The same applied to praying[133] and to performing the pilgrimage,[134] each of which engaged the believers in physical acts that resembled those that angels and deceased prophets and imams engaged in. Fasting was similarly an act that likened the believer to angels but it also imposed strict regulations on the body and bodily desires that made other forms of worship and piety even easier.[135] Although resembling angels was a goal, al-Kirmānī did not consider the promised seemingly sensual pleasures of the afterlife to be an impediment. Instead, he argued that these were different from earthly pleasures and were lasting and free of pain.

The dangers of passion

As explained before, both al-Rāzī and Ibn al-Jawzī explained that passion drove people to seek immediate and short-term gratification. From a pietistic point of view, following one's passion could lead to disobeying God or, at least, neglecting religious obligations. Because obeying religious obligations led to heaven, obeying one's passions led to immediate gratification but loss of eternal happiness. Ibn al-Jawzī reported a number of traditions that indicated how passion was a conduit to hellfire. In one tradition, the prophet told a story about God creating heaven and hell:

> When God created paradise and hell, he called Jibril [and showed him] paradise [. . .]. Jibril said, "By your honor, anyone who would hear of [paradise] and what you prepared in it, would want to go there." God ordered that paradise be covered under difficult obligations. Then he asked Jibril to go back and look at it. Jibril said, "I am afraid that no one will ever get to it." God told him to look at hellfire. Jibril said "By your honor, anyone who would hear of hellfire and what you prepared in it would never go to it." So God ordered it to be covered with desires and passions and told Jibril to go back and look at it. Jibril said, "By your honor, I am afraid that no one will ever survive it."[136]

Passion was a conduit to hellfire, which was covered in desires, whereas heaven was concealed behind onerous tasks and difficult obligations.

Al-Ḥakīm al-Tirmidhī agreed with the dangers of passion explicated by these authors and others. In a chapter entitled "The Fruit of Passion (*thamarat al-hawā*)," he aimed to provide an account of the finality of passion and its ultimate result, "If one asks, 'what is the fruit of this passion?' [I] say, 'Its fruit is for one to claim divinity.'"[137] Because the ultimate submission to passion would result in one following all of his or her desires and refusing to submit to any rule or regulation, such full sovereignty over oneself amounted to or resulted in a claim of divinity or a desire to combat the divine, which obviously amounted to the gravest of sins that could ever be committed. Al-Ḥakīm al-Tirmidhī recalled the example of Moses's pharaoh, whom the Quran explained had claimed divinity. Al-Ḥakīm al-Tirmidhī explained that the pharaoh was one who followed his passion blindly and could not accept that he needed to submit to a higher authority. The result was that he claimed divinity, telling his people that he knew of no God but himself. Similarly, the biblical and Quranic disbeliever, Nimrod, attempted to fight God

> because he could not tolerate the burden caused by the strength of his passion and his desire to follow it. He was unable to accept that someone else was capable of more than him. As such, he showed the people of his kingdom that he fought [God] and killed him.[138]

For believers, the knowledge of God's unity and power forced their spirits, under the influence of their passion, to despair from claiming divinity. Such despair, which was inspired by God and by the dictates of religion, saved believers from the gravest error of claiming divinity. However, it did not prevent passion from influencing them, and they remained exposed to lesser evils and excesses that their passions drove them to.[139]

Conclusion: gender, sovereignty and taming the spirit

In a rather well-known anecdote, a man traveling through the desert came across a woman crying by the carcass of a she-goat with a growing wolf cub by her side. The man stopped to ask her what happened. She explained, in verse, that the wolf cub had killed the goat:

> You have devoured my goat and saddened my people . . .
> yet you have been raised by this goat!
> You were nourished by her milk and grew up with her . . .
> Who then advised you that your father was a wolf?!
> If the nature is evil . . .
> no upbringing or instructor can help

The famous anonymous anecdote, which continued to be known as the story of "Who advised you that your father was a wolf," was often mentioned as a sign of how nature often overcomes nurture and that there was little recourse to changing one's nature. Ibn al-Jawzī used this shorthand in the beginning of his chapter on "Training the Spirit (*riyāḍat al-nafs*)," explaining that

> training would have no effect except in the highbred [. . .] much like a predator, even if brought up [among people] when young, would not let preying when grown. And you must know this anecdote *who advised you that your father was a wolf.*[140]

Unlike al-Rāzī, Ibn al-Jawzī wrote three chapters on training children, spouses, and slaves in his *Spiritual Medicine.* He placed these chapters immediately following his chapter on training the spirit, which resembled similar chapters in al-Rāzī and others. The three chapters displayed similar titles (all included the word training [*riyāḍah*]) and symmetry in their contents. Close to the end of the book and followed only with a chapter on dealing with relatives and on cultivating a "praiseworthy mention," the chapters provided the final advice for readers on how to deal with those that they were responsible for.

Pietistic writings discussed in this chapter, throughout the book, and beyond displayed clear gendered hierarchies. Free men were the authors and main audience of these books. This meant that the books were written for their benefit as the main subjects of the pietistic discourse and the main ethical agents responsible for applying such discourse to other people they were responsible for, including their children, spouses, and slaves, among others. To be sure, many of these texts included important examples of pious women. As explained in previous chapters, an anecdote about a woman suffering from epilepsy who sought the prophet's help and ended up accepting her illness in hope of divine reward, was consistently used to symbolize the value of patience and of accepting God's will and calamities. In the same way, stories of Job's wife and her commitment to her husband and ʿĀʾisha's nursing of the prophet when sick were also marshaled in pietistic writings about illness. These examples of 'ideal pious women' helped complete a narrative about pietistic behavior that included people of different genders and involved various people in the household. Such anecdotes, including even stories about Muḥammad's wives and daughters, remained in the minority and continued to emphasize the relative difference and gendered hierarchies embedded in much of these writings. However, at the same time, they represented anchoring points that allowed for such pietistic discourses to also apply to women and people of other genders.[141]

Unlike pietistic writings on physical medicine, writings on spiritual medicine were devoid even of these brief or symbolic mentions. In fact, al-Rāzī, al-Kirmānī, Miskawayh, Ibn al-Jawzī, and others were explicit in their condemnation of women and people of other genders, using them as examples of decadence and an inability to control passion.[142] Al-Rāzī, followed by al-Kirmānī in a rare occasion of agreement, mentioned feminized men and hermaphrodites as examples of people who were unable to control their sexual passions. In their view, women, hermaphrodites, and children were examples of those who would follow their passion as opposed to their intellect precisely because they had defective or incomplete intellects.[143] Ibn al-Jawzī reiterated these points and, as mentioned before, added special chapters that detailed how the reader, here explicitly identified as a free man, could deal with his children, spouses, and slaves. In relation to passion and lovesickness, women, young boys, and hermaphrodites were dangerous conduits to moral corruption.[144] Compared to other pietistic writings, and particularly compared to pietistic writings about medicine and illness, writings on spiritual medicine were exceptionally masculine and presented themselves as such with little ambiguity.

In the previous chapters, we have traced how piety in relation to illness was tethered to patience and tolerance. The two cardinal pietistic rules that patients needed to adhere to were to accept that God was, indeed, the cause of illness and of cure alike and that illness was an opportunity for reward that should be embraced with patience and acceptance. Many questions arose from these two cardinal rules pertaining to the legality of treatment, the types of treatments used, what patients should think or say, and what visitors should think or say. Yet the central tenet remained patience and acceptance. In spiritual medicine, patience was not a fundamental rule but rather another virtue to be installed in the well-trained and healthy spirit. Instead, the narrative of spiritual medicine was one about sovereignty and control. The reader was to understand "his" place as sovereign over his spirit, intellect, and body, and he was to undertake the duties of such sovereignty. These duties involved the maintenance of religious obligations as well as the preservation of the spirit and the body and caring for them. Obeying passion gave rise to a false sense of sovereignty that could lead as far as claiming divinity, in al-Tirmidhī's view. Conquering passion, Ibn al-Jawzī promised, would bring about even more pride and feelings of greatness as one emerged victorious from such battles with the spirit.[145] Similes and metaphors related to conquest and battle were not accidental but were part of a larger narrative about sovereignty and control.[146]

Rooted in sovereignty, the main audience for these writings were those who enjoyed such position in society – namely free men. As sovereigns over their own bodies and their own destiny, they were demanded to also control their passions and to show the moderation and restraint worthy of their gendered sovereignty.[147] Such display of control and power was not only linked to their gender but also to their position as Muslims. For instance,

> ʿUqbah al-Rāsibī said, "I once visited al-Ḥasan [al-Baṣrī] while he was eating. He said, 'Come [and join the meal]' I said, 'I had eaten so much that I cannot eat anymore.' He said, 'Praise be to God! And does a Muslim eat so much that he could not eat anymore?!!'"[148]

For al-Ḥasan al-Baṣrī, control over oneself was a character of Muslims who were able to exercise their power over their bodies and their passions. In this context, children, spouses, and slaves were natural additions to Ibn al-Jawzī's discussion of one's control over oneself. As much as a Muslim man was responsible for controlling his body and his passions as well as for caring for his body and his spirit and ensuring their survival and flourishing under divine law, he was also responsible for training, upbringing, and managing his children, spouses, and slaves to ensure that they flourish in this world under his sovereignty and perform their duties under religious law.

In this view, the similarities between advice on training the self and on training children and spouses are no longer surprising. The medical discourse in which these pietistic writings were placed served to queer the spirit, coloring it similar to the objects of women, children, and slaves – in need of protection but also stubborn and requiring cunning management in order to properly bring it under control. The reader's sovereign masculinity emerged not only in relation to his children, spouses, slaves, or people of other genders, who fell under his direct or indirect sovereignty (including people of other religions), but also in relation to his own queered spirit, which represented the animalistic desires that must be conquered and trained as part of the sacred and pietistic duties of the masculine ethical agent. In this context, masculine piety was formulated as a form of agency and sovereignty over oneself in contradistinction to the practices of submission and acceptance that were equally a part of the larger pietistic discourse. The masculine pious actor stood, in this framework, as an intermediary between the sovereign divine, who demanded and was owed submission, and the spirit, which demanded training and control and which resembled the children, spouses, and slaves the masculine pious actor was responsible for.

In this context, and as shown before, the spirit (or *al-nafs*: a morphologically feminine word in Arabic) was spoken to and trained by pious companions and followers, "Some of the followers would desire sweets so he would promise it to himself (his spirit) [if he prays at night]. If he prays, he would feed her."[149] Similar to children, training the self needs to be, "with ease and by moving from one condition to the next. It should not be done with force or violence."[150] Al-Ḥakīm al-Tirmidhī explained that some people had enough willpower to practice "dieting, to reject all passions and to disrupt all the [earthly] pleasures of the spirit until [the spirit] submitted to him." Others did not have such power. These would seek God's help and learn about him more every day, bringing their spirits closer to God and "becoming more certain in their faith until the light of knowledge conquers the darkness of passion."[151] In the same vein, the spirit, being vulnerable to various corrupting influences, benefitted from accompanying good and pious people and avoiding evil people.[152] A steady diet of the prophet's sīra (biography), the stories of pious people, of remembering God, and of various forms of worship were necessary for its training. In the same way, children and wives were to be trained smartly and without resorting to excessive force and violence to avoid possible rebellions. Both were to be protected from corrupting influences. Children were to be kept away from evil people, from singers, poets, and others who might inspire rebellion. Women were to be kept away from other women, especially older women, who may have a corrupting influence over them.

Although the queered spirit remained in a fixed gendered state that required control, children, spouses, and slaves were in danger of transgressing gendered boundaries. Ibn al-Jawzī explained that boys should not be allowed to wear colored clothes, "[a boy] should be dressed in white. If he asks for colored clothes, his father should tell him that these are the clothes of women and hermaphrodites."[153] A boy should not be fed much or allowed to sleep a lot. Instead, he should be taught to withstand hardship and to be instructed to walk a lot or do other physical exercises.

Similar gender boundaries were to be enforced in relation to spouses. Ibn al-Jawzī advised that an old man should not marry a young girl because she would hate and despise him. An ideal wife for an old man was a woman who is older than girlhood but not yet old. She would be easier to live with and more respectful. As for young men, they are free to choose whom they want. However, Ibn al-Jawzī suggested that they might start with young slave girls who knew no one other than them, as they would be easier to train and educate, "[They would also appreciate] his power to sell and exchange them."[154] In all cases, women should be kept at home as much as possible and always prevented from "talking to those of her gender." A man would do well if he had an older woman that would train his spouse and teach her how to respect her husband.[155] Slaves' sexuality was to be equally monitored. Young male slaves should not be allowed to mingle with women because their passion might overcome them and they may violate the rules of ownership and privacy. However, Ibn al-Jawzī advised care in dealing with slaves, "They are in fact the owners of their owners since they are entrusted with food and drinks. One ought to be kind to them so as they do not conspire to kill [their owners]."[156]

As mentioned before, although writings on spiritual medicine and the attendant ethical and pietistic discussions emerged from a variety of places and were composed by many authors of diverse backgrounds and with different priorities, these narratives shared general outlooks on the good and pious life that was advised to their readers. To be sure, authors differed in their views on who was ready to receive or act on such advice, with religious and pietistic narratives ostensibly directed toward a more general public and attempting to address more general concerns for Muslims. It is evident that the selections in the works of Ibn al-Mubārak, Ibn Ḥanbal, Ibn al-Jawzī, and Ibn Abī al-Dunyā, among many others, informed the choices that preachers made and affected the production of popular pietistic narratives in ways that writings by al-Kindī, al-Balkhī, al-Rāzī, or Miskawayh may not. Yet throughout, these narratives shared a general view about the necessity of moderation and self-control and propagated social virtues that were imbued with views of sovereignty in gendered and sociocultural manners. The good person, whether as described by the philosophers and physicians or by the ʿulamā and preachers, was one who practiced this sovereignty over "himself" and who imbued his acts with this pietistic ethical sovereignty.

Notes

1 Al-Rāzī is known most of all for his medical works, which have received a fair amount of attention in recent scholarship. See, for instance, Tibi, "Al-Razi and Islamic Medicine"; Pormann, "Qualifying and Quantifying Medical Uncertainty"; Richter-Bernburg, "Al-Rāzī and Al-Fārābī on Medicine and Authority"; and Adamson, "Al-Rāzī (d. 925), the Spiritual Medicine." Cristina Alvarez-Millan has shed light on some of al-Rāzī's work, particularly in relation to medical practice. See Álvarez-Millán, "Practice Versus Theory" and "The Case History in Medieval Islamic Medical Literature." On al-Rāzī's work in relation to sex differences, see Ragab, "One, Two, or Many Sexes."

2 Adamson, "Abū Bakr al-Rāzī (d. 925), the Spiritual Medicine," 66, 68. See also Bar-Asher, "Quelques Aspects de l'Éthique d'Abū-Bakr al-Rāzī."

3 Al-Balkhī, *Maṣāliḥ al-Abdān wa-al-Anfus*.

4 Adamson, "Abū Bakr al-Rāzī (d. 925), the Spiritual Medicine," 67.

5 Ibn Adī's work may have carried the title *Siyāsat al-Nafs* (management of the soul). See Griffith, "Yaḥyā b. ʿAdī 's (d. 974) Kitāb Tahdhīb Alakhlāq," ibid., 130. Although there is some doubt on the authorship of the treatise, which was attributed to a number of later authors, it is generally accepted that Yaḥyā ibn ʿAdī is the author of this work. See Endress, "The Works of Yahyā Ibn 'Adī", and, Wisnovsky, "New Philosophical Texts of Yaḥyā ibn ʿAdī." On Miskawayh, see Arkoun, *Contribution à l'Étude de l'Humanisme Arabe au IV/XE Siècle*; *Humanisme Arabe au IV/XE Siècle*.

6 On al-Hakīm al-Tirmidhī, see Gobillot, "Patience (ṣabr) et Rétribution des Mérites"; O'Kane and Radtke, *The Concept of Sainthood in Early Islamic Mysticism*; and Radtke, "Al-Hakim al-Tirmidhi on Miracles." On the pietistic implications and attitudes among scholars of ḥadīth to the writings of Ibn Abī al-Dunyā and al-Hakīm al-Tirmidhī, see Chabbi, "Mouvements Ascétiques et Mystiques au Khurasan" and Melchert, "Piety of the Hadith Folk" and "Transition from Asceticism to Mysticism."

7 This is not to say that the writings of al-Rāzī, al-Balkhī, or Ibn ʿAdī were disconnected from these adab materials. As will be seen later, they were equally invested in similar frames of reference and often addressed similar audiences. On these influences, in the work of Ibn ʿAdī for instance, see Hossein Nasr and Leaman, *History of Islamic Philosophy*; Griffith, "Yaḥyā b. ʿAdī 's (d. 974) Kitāb Tahdhīb Alakhlāq."

8 Ibn al-Jawzī, *Al-Ṭibb al-Rūḥānī*; See Mohaghegh, " 'Spiritual Physic' of al-Razi," 7.

9 Ibn al-Jawzī, *Luqat al-Manāfiʿ fī ʿIlm al- Ṭibb*, 5.

10 Ibn al-Jawzī's main claim to fame was based on his illustrious preaching career, where he came to be recognized as one of the more influential and charismatic preachers in Baghdad. His various writings on *raqāʾiq*, piety, and other refinements, as well as his work on ḥadīth, were directly connected to his interest in preaching and his belief that

preachers reached the majority of Muslims and should therefore be well educated and trained. See Fathi, "Islamic Pulpit," 166–70.

11 Ibn al-Jawzī, *Dhamm al-Hawā.*

12 On biographies and hagiographies and their role in providing narratives of piety, see Cooperson, "Ibn Ḥanbal and Bishr al-Ḥāfī." Brockopp, "Contradictory Evidence and the Exemplary Scholar."

13 See, for instance, Al-Dunyā, *Mudārāt al-Nās.*

14 Adamson, "Abū Bakr al-Rāzī (d. 925), the Spiritual Medicine."

15 Adamson, "Abū Bakr al-Rāzī (d. 925), the Spiritual Medicine" and "Health in Arabic Ethical Works."

16 See Bar-Asher, "Quelques Aspects de l'Éthique d'Abū-Bakr al-Rāzi." On further connections between Galen's philosophical views and those of al-Rāzī's, see Koetschet, "Galien, al-Rāzī, et l'Éternité du Monde."

17 See, for instance, Ibn Al-Jawzī, *Al-Shifā' fī Mawā'iẓ al-Mulūk wa al-Khulafā'*. Terms like *shifā'* (healing), *amrāḍ* (diseases), etc., were common in pietistic writings and were consistently invoked in ḥadīth and in the Quran.

18 On al-Kirmānī and his work and contributions, see Walker, *Hamid al-Din al-Kirmani.* See also Walker, "Chief Qāḍī and Chief Dā'ī." Walker also edited al-Kirmānī's *Al-Maṣābīḥ fī Ithbāt al-'Imāmah* in *Master of the Age*. For additional details on al-Kirmānī's work on the imamate and how it related to the writings of his contemporaries during the reign of al-Ḥākim, see Lalani, *Degrees of Excellence*, 22–3.

19 Mohaghegh, "Spiritual Physic," 6; Adamson, "Abū Bakr al-Rāzī (d. 925), the Spiritual Medicine," 79.

20 Al-Kirmānī, *Al-Aqwāl al-Dhahabiyyah.*

21 See Rashed, "Abū Bakr al-Rāzī;" Kraus, "Raziana II." On the reception of Abū Bakr al-Rāzī's philosophical and theological ideas by Mu'tazilites and Asharites, see Vallat, "Between Hellenism, Islam, and Christianity." See also Stroumsa, *Freethinkers of Medieval Islam*. Al-Rāzī's *A'lām al-Nubuwwah* included long quotatons attributed to Abū Bakr al-Rāzī, where the latter criticized and denied the legitimacy of prophecy. Abū Ḥātim then proceeded to dissect these quotes and refute them (Al-Rāzī, *A'lām al-Nubuwwa fī al-Radd 'alā al-Mulḥid Abū Bakr al-Rāzī*).

22 Al-Kirmānī, *Al-Aqwāl al-Dhahabiyyah.*

23 Ibid., 2.

24 Ibid., 2.

25 Dols, *Majnūn*, 24.

26 Adamson discussed briefly the potential differences between al-Rāzī and al-Balkhī, where the former elaborates more extensively on the existence of three or tripartite souls and the latter seems more ambivalent about this precise division. See Adamson, "Health in Arabic Ethical Works."

27 Fancy, *Science and Religion in Mamluk Egypt.*

28 Al-Balkhī paid special attention to the mutual effects and influences between physical and spiritual ills in a manner that was more pronounced than in al-Rāzī, for instance. See, for instance, his discussion of obsessions, Al-Balkhī, *Maṣāliḥ al-Abdān wa-al-Anfus*, 544. On this point, see Adamson, "Health in Arabic Ethical Works."

29 Al-Rāzī, *Al-Ṭibb al-Rūḥānī.* Al-Balkhī, *Maṣāliḥ al-Abdān wa-al-Anfus*, 543–5; Adamson, "Health in Arabic Ethical Works."

30 See, for instance, Al-Rāzī, *Al- Ḥāwī fī al-Ṭibb*. See Dols, *Majnūn.*

31 Adamson explains that the writings of the Galenic ethicists like al-Balkhī and al-Rāzī focused on the attainment of correct belief as a tool to maintain the health of the soul, Adamson, "Health in Arabic Ethical Works." The question of belief was equally central to the works of Ibn al-Jawzī and al-Kirmānī. This point will be discussed in further detail.

32 On the moral dimensions of adab and its connection to ḥadīth sciences, see Sperl, "Man's 'Hollow Core.'" Khalidi, "Premodern Arabic/Islamic Historical Writing" and *Images of Muhammad.*

33 In fact, al-Balkhī, Miskawayh, al-Rāzī, and Ibn al-Jawzī discussed the importance of surrounding oneself with pious and well-mannered people and listening to the stories and anecdotes of pious and learned individuals as tools to train oneself into good manner.
34 Al-Jawzī, *Al-Ṭibb al-Rūḥānī*, 5.
35 Al-Kirmānī, *Al-Aqwāl al-Dhahabiyyah*, 50.
36 Al-Balkhī, *Maṣāliḥ al-Abdān wa-al-Anfus*, 517.
37 Ibid., 518.
38 Miskawayh, *Tahdhīb al-Akhlāq*, 282–3.
39 Adamson rightly explained that the proper life in the view of these Galenic ethical writings was one where the rational soul controlled or reigned over the other two parts of the soul (the vegetative and irascible), Adamson, "Health in Arabic Ethical Works" and "Abū Bakr al-Rāzī (d. 925), the Spiritual Medicine." See also, Griffith, "Yaḥyā b. ʿAdī 's (d. 974) Kitāb Tahdhīb Alakhlāq." This, however, does not change the fact that the reader/patient was not reducible to the rational soul, but rather reigned over all of these souls and was exhorted by the authors to enable or empower the rational soul.
40 Ibn al-Jawzī, *Al-Ṭibb al-Rūḥānī*, 58.
41 Ibid., 59.
42 A similar view on the benefits of training the soul was also expressed by Miskwayh in the first lines of his treatise. He explained that the goal of the book was "to achieve for ourselves a character (*khuluq*) from which [we] produce deeds that are all good, and yet they are easy on us without pretense or hardship. This is achieved through industry and through education" Miskawayh, *Tahdhīb al-Akhlāq*, 233.
43 Ibn Al-Jawzī, *Al-Ṭibb al-Rūḥānī*, 59.
44 Al-Rāzī, *Al-Ṭibb al-Rūḥānī*, 45.
45 See Adamson, "Abū Bakr al-Rāzī (d. 925), the Spiritual Medicine."
46 Al-Kirmānī, *Al-Aqwāl al-Dhahabiyyah*, 97.
47 Ibn Al-Jawzī, *Al-Ṭibb al-Rūḥānī*, 57, emphasis added. For a general discussion on angels in Islamic thought, see Burge, "Angels, Ritual and Sacred Space." See also Burge's recently published analysis of al-Suyūṭī's "Akhbār al-Malāʾik," Burge, *Angels in Islam*.
48 Al-Kirmānī, *Al-Aqwāl al-Dhahabiyyah*, 92.
49 The appetitive and irascible souls were indeed composed of the mixtures of the heart and the liver, and therefore perished with them. The rational soul, on the other hand, was not composed of the mixture of the brain but acted on it, and as such was to survive after the body perished. See Adamson, "Abū Bakr al-Rāzī (d. 925), the Spiritual Medicine."
50 On the development of the concept of the intellect especially in Shiite thought, see Amir-Moezzi, *Divine Guide in Early Shiʾism*, 6–15. Much work has been done on the question of *ʿaql* (often translated as intellect) in Islamic philosophy, theology, and mysticism. See, for instance, Adamson, "Avicenna;" Umrajī, *Al-Muʿtazilah fī Baghdād wa-Atharuhum fī al-ḥayāh al-Fikrīyah wa-al-Siyāsīyah*; Eichner, "Essence and Existence;" Wisnovsky, "Essence and Existence;" Nasr, "Intellect and Intuition;" and Chittick, "Mysticism Versus Philosophy," 90–3.
51 Al-Rāzī, *Al-Ṭibb al-Rūḥānī*; Ibn al-Jawzī, *Al-Ṭibb al-Rūḥānī*, 18. See also, Druart, "Ethics of al-Razi," 49.
52 Al-Rāzī, *Al-Ṭibb al-Rūḥānī*; Ibn al-Jawzī, *Al-Ṭibb al-Rūḥānī*, 27.
53 Ibn al-Jawzī, *Al-Ṭibb al-Rūḥānī*.
54 Al-Kirmānī, *Al-Aqwāl al-Dhahabiyyah*, 78.
55 Ibid., 78–9.
56 Amir-Moezzi has shown the gradual development of the notion of the 'intellect' and its roles in achieving the knowledge of God. In this context, he argued, the imam's role was manifested both as a representation and a guide to the human intellect. See Amir-Moezzi, *Divine Guide in Early Shiʾism*.

57 Ibn al-Jawzī, *Dhamm al-Hawā*.
58 Ibn al-Jawzī, *Al-Ṭibb al-Rūḥānī*, 7.
59 Ibn al-Jawzī, *Dhamm al-Hawā*, 23–4.
60 Ibid., 24.
61 Al-Dunyā, *Kitāb al-ʿAql wa Faḍlihi*, 49.
62 Al-Māwardī, *Adab al-Dunyā wa al-Dīn*, 1: 19.
63 Al-Tirmidhī, *Adab al-Nafs*, 103. For an overview on al-Ḥakīm al-Tirmidhī, see Al-Geyoushi, "'Qalb' and 'Nafs'" and "Al-Hakim al-Tirmidhi." See also Sviri, "Hakim Tirmidhi and the Malamati Movement" and Radtke, "Al-Hakim al-Tirmidhi on Miracles."
64 Ibn al-Jawzī, *Dhamm al-Hawā*, 27.
65 Brown, "Even If It Is Not True, It Is True."
66 Ibid., 24. As explained before, Ibn al-Jawzī had a similar attitude toward miracle stories, which he explained at length in the introduction to his book on saints where he severely criticized Abū Nuʿaym al-Isfahānī for citing unreliable traditions, among other things. See Brown, "Faithful Dissenters," 153. Ibn al-Jawzī, however, was open to citing multiple weak reports in his biography of Ibn Ḥanbal, which he thought was necessary to establish the privilege of the imam and which were thought of as weak, if not fabricated by al-Dhahabī, among others. See Cooperson, "Ibn Ḥanbal and Bishr al-Ḥāfī," 84.
67 Ibn al-Jawzī, *Dhamm al-Hawā*, 27.
68 Melchert, "Piety of the Hadith Folk," 433.
69 Ibn al-Jawzī, *Dhamm al-Hawā*, 25.
70 Al-Dunyā, *Kitāb al-ʿAql wa Faḍlihi*, 36.
71 Ibid., 34.
72 Al-Dunyā, *Kitāb al-ʿAql wa Faḍlihi*, 44–5; Ibn al-Jawzī, *Dhamm al-Hawā*, 31.
73 Ibid., 43; Ibn al-Jawzī, *Dhamm al-Hawā*, 32.
74 Ibn al-Jawzī, *Dhamm al-Hawā*, 30.
75 Al-Dunyā, *Kitāb al-ʿAql wa Faḍlihi*, 50. I chose the word "intellectual" here to maintain the semantic connection between the noun *ʿaql*, the adjective *ʿāqil*, and the verb *yaʿqil*.
76 Ibn al-Jawzī, *Dhamm al-Hawā*, 32. Ibn al-Jawzī reported two versions of the tradition, one attributed to the companion Muʿādh ibn Jabal and the other *marfūʿ* or elevated to the prophet.
77 Al-Rāzī, *Al-Ṭibb al-Rūḥānī*, 36. Animals played an important role as examples and foils in al-Rāzī's thought. See Adamson, "Abū Bakr al-Rāzī on Animals."
78 In his discussion of the intellectual arguments for the benefits of the intellect in *Spiritual Medicine*, Ibn al-Jawzī also mentioned this same example of shipmaking, citing al-Rāzi word for word without mentioning him by name. In a similar section (also on the intellectual proofs of the value of the intellect) in his *Dhamm al-Hawā*, Ibn al-Jawzī did not mention this example about ships. The rest of the narrative in *Dhamm al-Hawā* is cited in *Spiritual Medicine*. This may indicate that Ibn al-Jawzī encountered, or carefully studied, al-Rāzī's text in the period between his composing *Dhamm al-Hawā* and *Al-Ṭibb al-Rūḥānī*.
79 Al-Rāzī, *Al-Ṭibb al-Rūḥānī*, 35–6.
80 Ibn Al-Jawzī, *Al-Ṭibb al-Rūḥānī*, 8. Al-Ḥakīm al-Tirmidhī, among others, used similar examples that related the differences between types of animals to the role of their intellect and to their ability to control their passions, which was acquired through training. For instance, al-Ḥakīm al-Tirmidhī used the example of trained falcons (Al-Ḥakīm al-Tirmidhī, *Adab al-Nafs*, 37), and Miskawayh also referenced falcons as well as horses (Miskawayh, *Tahdhīb al-Akhlāq*, 281).
81 Adamson has shown that the notion of true knowledge played a central role in the spiritual medicine works of al-Balkhī, al-Rāzī and Miskawayh. See Adamson, "Health in Arabic Ethical Works."

82 Al-Balkhī, *Maṣāliḥ al-Abdān wa-al-Anfus*, 512.
83 Ibn Al-Jawzī, *Al-Ṭibb al-Rūḥānī*. See Mohaghegh, " 'Spiritual Physic' of al-Razi," 10.
84 Ibn Ḥibbān used the word *ra'y* (opinion).
85 Ibn Ḥibbān, *Rawdat al-'Uqalā' wa Nuzhat al-Fuḍalā'*, 19. Ibn al-Jawzī cited this statement in his *Dhamm al-Hawā* (Ibn al-Jawzī, *Dhamm al-Hawā*, 36).
86 Al-Tirmidhī, *Adab al-Nafs*, 52–3.
87 Ibid., 13–14.
88 Al-Rāzī (d. 890) was an important scholar who contributed significantly to the early development of Sunni ḥadīth. He is the father of the famous scholar of ḥadīth Ibn Abī Ḥātim al-Rāzī (d. 938). He is to be differentiated from the Isma'īlī scholar Abū Ḥātim Aḥmad ibn Ḥamdān al-Rāzī (d. 935), who was mentioned earlier in the chapter as the author of *A'lām al-Nubuwwa*, was an important figure of inspiration of Ḥamīd al-Dīn al-Kirmānī, and criticized Abū Bakr al-Rāzī relentlessly. Because of the centrality of the two Abū Ḥātims in their respective domains, they both were referred to as "Abū Ḥātim" without further elaboration by their students, admirers, and followers within the Sunni and Isma'īlī contexts, respectively.
89 Ibn Ḥibbān, *Rawdat al-'Uqalā' wa Nuzhat al-Fuḍalā'*, 17.
90 Al-Ḥakīm al-Tirmidhī, *Adab al-Nafs*, 11–13.
91 Ibid., 13–14.
92 Ibid., 81, 103.
93 Ibid., 81.
94 The connection between real and true knowledge and proper acts was also emphasized in the works of al-Kindī, al-Balkhī, al-Rāzī, and Miskawayh, among others. See Adamson, "Health in Arabic Ethical Works."
95 Ibn al-Jawzī, *Dhamm al-Hawā*, 37.
96 Ibn Ḥibbān, *Rawdat al-'Uqalā' wa Nuzhat al-Fuḍalā'*, 18.
97 Ibn al-Jawzī, *Al-Ṭibb al-Rūḥānī*, 59.
98 Adamson, "Abū Bakr al-Rāzī (d. 925), the Spiritual Medicine," 65.
99 Al-Rāzī, *Al-Ṭibb al-Rūḥānī*, 45.
100 Fathi, "Islamic Pulpit as a Medium of Political Communication," 170.
101 Ibn Ḥibbān, *Rawdat al-'Uqalā' wa Nuzhat al-Fuḍalā'*, 15.
102 Mohaghegh, " 'Spiritual Physic' of al-Razi," 10. In addition to the meanings of *hawā* discussed here, which refers to passions and desires of almost all kinds, the term was used more specifically to refer to love. See Alghani, "Mediaeval Arabic Love."
103 Al-Rāzī, *Al-Ṭibb al-Rūḥānī*, 35.
104 Ibid., 48–9.
105 Ibn al-Jawzī, *Al-Ṭibb al-Rūḥānī*, 8.
106 In this context, adab, being the central literary product of this particular elite, focused on refinement and operated with ostensible moral undertones. See Ashtiany, *Abbasid Belles Lettres*. Among many other works, Pellat has noted the moral dimensions in the adab works of al-Jāḥiẓ, Pellat, *The Life and Works of Jāḥiẓ*. Similarly, Khan's analysis of al-Jāḥiẓ's *Kitmān al-Sirr* has demonstrated the moral and ethical implications in such work and in the notion of secrecy as a theme in adab, Khan, "Chambir of My Thought." Sadan's analysis of the Bedouin as a recurrent hero/antihero in Arabic *belles lettres* also revealed the moralistic undertones embedded in these narratives, Sadan, "Admirable and Ridiculous Hero."
107 Adamson has observed that spiritual health seemed to rely on the rational soul or the intellect controlling the appetitive and irascible souls, as opposed to a general concept of balance akin to humoral physical medicine, Adamson, "Health in Arabic Ethical Works."
108 Ibn Al-Jawzī, *Dhamm al-Hawā*, 46.
109 Ibid., 48.

110 Ibid., 43. This particular tradition was heavily criticized by many scholars during this period, including Ibn Ḥanbal and Ibn Ḥibbān, who considered it to be fabricated.
111 Al-Kirmānī, *Al-Aqwāl al-Ahahabiyyah*, 104.
112 Ibn Al-Jawzī, *Dhamm al-Hawā*, 48. On the use of the Bedouin character in adab writings, see Sadan, "Admirable and Ridiculous Hero."
113 Ibn Al-Jawzī, *Dhamm al-Hawā*, 38.
114 Ibn Al-Jawzī, *Al-Ṭibb al-Rūḥānī*, 10.
115 Ibid., 9. An identical argument was also used by Miskwayh in his *Tahdhīb al-Akhlāq*, 243–4.
116 Ibn al-Jawzī, *Al-Ṭibb al-Rūḥānī*, 8.
117 Al-Tirmidhī, *Adab al-Nafs*, 37.
118 Ibn Al-Jawzī, *Dhamm al-Hawā*, 35.
119 Al-Tirmidhī, *Adab al-Nafs*, 114.
120 Al-Rāzī, *Al-Ṭibb al-Rūḥānī*, 38–9; Ibn Al-Jawzī, *Al-Ṭibb al-Rūḥānī*, 8–10.
121 Al-Kirmānī, *Al-Aqwāl al-Dhahabiyyah*, 81.
122 Ibid., 104. Al-Balkhī, who was not referenced by al-Kirmānī at all, provided similar narrative in relation to the nature of spiritual medicine (Al-Balkhī, *Maṣāliḥ al-Abdān wa-al-Anfus*, 508–9)
123 Al-Kirmānī, *Al-Aqwāl al-Dhahabiyyah*, 107.
124 Ibn Al-Jawzī, *Al-Ṭibb al-Rūḥānī*, 9.
125 Al-Rāzī, *Al-Ṭibb al-Rūḥānī*, 39.
126 Ibid., 40.
127 Goodman, "Epicurean Ethic" and "How Epicurean Was Rāzī?".
128 Adamson, "Platonic Pleasures" and "Abū Bakr al-Rāzī (d. 925), the Spiritual Medicine."
129 Al-Kirmānī, *Al-Aqwāl al-Dhahabiyyah*, 75.
130 Miskawayh, *Tahdhīb al-Akhlāq*, 276.
131 Ibn Al-Jawzī, *Al-Ṭibb al-Rūḥānī*, 8.
132 Al-Kirmānī, *Al-Aqwāl al-Dhahabiyyah*, 146.
133 Ibid., 148.
134 Ibid., 152.
135 Ibid., 151.
136 Ibn al-Jawzī, *Dhamm al-Hawā*, 41.
137 Al-Ḥakīm al-Tirmidhī, *Adab al-Nafs*, 117.
138 Ibid., 118.
139 Ibid., 118–19.
140 Ibn al-Jawzī, *Al-Ṭibb al-Rūḥānī*, 57.
141 On women in pietistic writings, see Ragab, "Epistemic Authority of Women," and Stowasser, *Women in the Qur'an, Traditions, and Interpretation*. See also Schimmel, *My Soul Is a Woman*. On the portrayal of specific women, see Spellberg, *Politics, Gender and the Islamic Past*; Thurlkill, *Chosen Among Women*; and Roded, *Women in Islamic Biographical Collections*.
142 For instance, Miskawayh and Ibn al-Jawzī explained that young boys should not be allowed to wear colorful clothes and should be told that these are more suitable for women, slaves, and hermaphrodites. Miskawayh, *Tahdhīb al-Akhlāq*, 290; Ibn Al-Jawzī, *Al-Ṭibb al-Rūḥānī*, 61.
143 Al-Rāzī, *Al-Ṭibb al-Rūḥānī*; Al-Kirmānī, *Al-Aqwāl al-Dhahabiyyah*.
144 Ibn al-Jawzī, *Al-Ṭibb al-Rūḥānī*, 11–13. Much has been written on the portrayal of women as conduits of lust and corruption. See El-Cheikh, "Describing the Other;" and Merguerian and Najmabadi, "Zulaykha and Yusuf." Similarly, obscenity, another danger to morality, was also seen as connected to sexual indulgence and relation to women and boys. See Lagrange, "Obscenity of the Vizir."
145 Ibn al-Jawzī, *Al-Ṭibb al-Rūḥānī*, 8–10.

146 Ibn al-Jawzī, *Dhamm al-Hawā*, 45–7.
147 Contrary to this ethic of sovereignty, Malamud demonstrates how different gender dynamics based on obedience and submission governed the relationship between sufi masters and disciples, Malamud, "Gender and Spiritual Self-Fashioning." See also Hoffman-Ladd, "Mysticism and Sexuality."
148 Ibn al-Jawzī, *Al-Ṭibb al-Rūḥānī*, 13.
149 Ibid., 58.
150 Ibid., 58.
151 Al-Ḥakīm al-Tirmidhī, *Adab al-Nafs*, 119–20.
152 Ibn al-Jawzī, *Al-Ṭibb al-Rūḥānī*, 58. The same advice was also repeated in Miskawayh and others.
153 Ibid., 61.
154 Ibid., 63.
155 Ibid., 62.
156 Ibid., 64.

5 The pious physician

In addition to being part of a religious discourse that attempted to condition how pious Muslims performed their religious duties and religious thoughts, piety and pietistic behaviors and writings were part of the production of urban elite habitus. As seen in Chapter 4, the ethical traditions that governed the notions of propriety among members of the urban elites emerged both from Galenic and other Hellenistic ethical writings, as well as from pietistic writings that engaged with questions of spiritual medicine and others that existed within the domains of zuhd or renunciation. In this context, concepts and virtues of moderation, control over oneself, and renunciation or disinterest in earthly pleasures combined with ethics of time management, modesty, and honesty, among others, contributed to the pietistic and elite ethics that dominated society at the time. Physicians, of course, were members of this elite. This entailed, as seen before, contributing to the construction of these ethics through their own writings. In Chapter 4, we engaged with the contributions of physicians such as al-Rāzī and al-Balkhī to the writing of Galenic or Hellenistic ethics; however, other physicians, as will be seen later, were more engaged with pietistic writings and contributed to the production of pietistic norms along with other religious scholars.

At another level, as members of learned elites, physicians engaged in various intellectual and learned activities in their societies. For Muslim physicians, in particular, these included engaging with circles of ḥadīth and Quran and encounters with educated religious scholars and jurisconsults, who formed the core of the learned elite in the Muslim urban society from the tenth century on. Similarly, many physicians were themselves educated in Arabic, grammar, ḥadīth, and other related sciences that distinguished the learned communities of that time. Although many of them did not acquire proficiency in these fields, they constituted parts of the learned infrastructure of their contemporaneous societies. As such, these physicians engaged consistently with pietistic writings that discussed questions of health and disease and with the various ethical and pietistic questions that we discussed in the previous chapters. Similarly, and because some of them had careers that spanned medical and religious sciences, they also contributed to the production of these discourses themselves. For instance, Irmeli Perho, in her study of prophetic medicine, looks at the prophetic medicine works of the physicians, Muwaffaq al-Dīn al-Baghdādī (d. 1231) and Ibn Ṭarkhān (d. 1320).

Both physicians were trained in religious sciences and composed their works on prophetic medicine relying on their knowledge of ḥadīth. Perho credits these two authors with starting a new trend in prophetic medicine writings, lending increased focus to the details of medical knowledge. She argued that the experience and knowledge of the two physicians allowed for more sophisticated engagement with medical theory and practice, which was novel in the history of prophetic medicine. Although I agree that these two books were indeed influential, they cannot be fully credited with such a change. In fact, both books relied heavily on the works of Abū Nuʿaym al-Isfahānī, whose book on prophetic medicine remained a central text in the field for centuries. At another level, the work of Ibn al-Jawzī, particularly his *Luqat al-Manāfiʿ* (The Gleanings of Benefits) which was dedicated to medicine, showed deep and solid engagement with medical theory by a renowned religious scholar. Both Abū Nuʿaym and Ibn al-Jawzī were more influential in the writings of prophetic medicine than al-Baghdādī or Ibn Ṭarkhān.

As part of a learned elite, Muslim physicians were interested in locating their practice within larger frameworks of epistemic pieties. Pious physicians, much like many other practitioners of various sciences and professions in the marketplace, were interested in presenting medical learning and medical practice as pious endeavors that merited appreciation. This pietistic investigation into learning and practicing medicine entailed locating medicine within the different hierarchies of knowledge, which in turn entailed structuring a relationship between medicine, a field of knowledge and practice that relied on ancient knowledge, and the more pietistic and religiously esteemed professions such as Quran, ḥadīth, and law. Moreover, physicians' engagement with pietistic questions also involved issues related to the legality and piety of seeking medical care and treatment. As explained before, the proper behaviors of pious Muslims in case of illness included specific ways of accepting illness and of seeking cure or complaining. For physicians, the engagement with these questions was necessary to their endeavor to locate the practice of medicine within the hierarchies of knowledge at the time. At another level, physicians also engaged with more explicit legal questions, which included the legality of using illicit materials, such as alcohol, in treatment. Moreover, and as they engaged more concretely with the prophetic literature, physicians also needed to grapple with possible contradictions between the prophetic corpus and medical recommendations, whether these contradictions touched on theoretical or practical issues.

At the heart of all these questions, the image of the pious physician emerged as a member of the urban learned elite connected to discourses about piety and self-fashioning discussed in the earlier chapters. Although all of the previously discussed issues relating to accepting and following the model of the prophet, understanding the blessing of health, accepting and pietistically comprehending illness, and managing one's spiritual ills applied to physicians as much as they applied to others, this chapter dives deeper into the making of the pious physician as a special figure whose intellectual and professional life entailed the constant encounter with illness, medicine, and patienthood. This chapter will focus on the works of three physicians: Muwaffaq al-Dīn ʿAbd al-Laṭīf al-Baghdādī (d. 1231),

Muwaffaq al-Dīn Aḥmad ibn Abī Uṣaybiʿah (d. 1269), and ʿAlāʾ al-Dīn ʿAlī ibn Ṭarkhān al-Kaḥḥāl (d. 1320) to investigate the production of pietistic medical practice and to uncover the textual and practical resources that conditioned the making of pious physicians.

As mentioned before, the works of the two physicians ʿAbd al-Laṭif al-Baghdādī (d. 1231) and Ibn Ṭarkhān (d. 1320) were seen as significant moments in the history of prophetic medicine. Known for their religious knowledge and their experience in ḥadīth and other religious sciences, the two physicians were able to compose treatises on prophetic medicine. Al-Baghdādī dictated a commentary on the medical chapter in Ibn Mājah's ḥadīth compilation, and Ibn Ṭarkhān compiled his own collection of medical traditions, which became rather popular in the following decades and helped inform later writings in the thirteenth and fourteenth centuries. In addition to these two physicians, Ibn Abī Uṣaybiʿah composed one of the more famous biographical dictionaries of physicians. Although the dictionary remains an important source of the history of medicine in the region, it is expectedly rife with biases and inaccuracies that limit its value as a historical source. However, the central message that Ibn Abī Uṣaybiʿah intended was not only to document the histories of physicians, but also to present important and key examples of how good, pious, and skilled physicians should act. Here, I will focus on his biography of al-Baghdādī, which he claimed to have copied from al-Baghdādī's work, as well as his biography of his own uncle, which he presented as a testimony to his and his own family's thoughts about how physicians should behave.

This chapter explores how these physicians understood their own professions from a pietistic viewpoint. Here, I look at al-Baghdādī, Ibn Abī Uṣaybiʿah, and Ibn Ṭarkhān as examples of self-claimed pious physicians who composed texts that intended to provide a narrative of pietistic medical practice. The chapter investigates how their work provided a template for how Muslim physicians should understand their own practice, how they should practice pietistically, and how they should attend to the pietistic needs of their patients. First, the chapter looks at how these physicians placed medicine within a pietistic epistemic hierarchy and how they viewed the place of medicine in relation to other fields of knowledge. The chapter then analyzes how they understood the pietistic debates around seeking care or abstention from seeking cure and relying on God. Finally, the chapter examines how they understood the process of treatment within this pietistic cosmology, including understanding the materials prescribed or prohibited by the prophet and his companions and the potential conflicts between medical knowledge and the prophetic corpus.

The authors and their narratives

Muwaffaq al-Dīn Al-Baghdādī was reported to have written a few books on ḥadīth. Perhaps the most important among these books was his work on *mukhtalif al-ḥadīth*, or confusing and contradictory traditions. In this book, he relied on the writings of Ibn Qutaybah and al-Khaṭṭābī on the topic, compiling the traditions that they listed into a single volume. Later, he authored a summary of his own *mukhtalif*.[1] Although the book, by the admission of al-Baghdādī himself, did not include new traditions or particularly new ways of explaining them as it relied on the famous books of Ibn Qutaybah and al-Khaṭṭābī, it represented al-Baghdādī's foray into one of the more established genres of ḥadīth. At another level, al-Baghdādī's education put him in a particularly important lineage in relation to *Sunan Ibn Mājah*.[2] As Jonathan Brown has shown, *Sunan Ibn Mājah* was not an uncontroversial addition to the Sunni canon of ḥadīth. However,

> in the first decades of the seventh/thirteenth century we see that Ibn Mājah's *Sunan* was gaining increased acceptance as part of the ḥadīth canon. Part of this acceptance was the construction of a canonical culture around the book that celebrated its reliability as a representation of the Prophet's Sunna.[3]

When al-Baghdādī was a child, his father sent him to learn ḥadīth with a number of scholars, including Abū Zar'ah al-Maqdisī (d. 1171).[4] Abū Zar'ah al-Maqdisī was one of the people who had a short and solid isnād (or chain of transmission) for Ibn Mājah's *Sunan* – he had read it with Abū Manṣūr al-Muqawamī (d. after 1091), who was known as the *rāwī* (or reporter) of Ibn Mājah's *Sunan* through al-Qāsim ibn Abī al-Mundhir al-Khaṭīb. Al-Khaṭīb studied with Ibn Mājah's most prominent student and reporter, Abū al-Ḥasan al-Qaṭṭān al-Qazwīnī. It appears that, later in his life, Abū Manṣūr al-Muqawamī possessed the most authenticated and perhaps shortest line of transmission for Ibn Mājah's *Sunan*, earning him the title of *Rāwī Sunan Ibn Mājah*, or the reporter of Ibn Mājah's *Sunan*. As such, and as the interest in Ibn Mājah's *Sunan* was on the rise in the beginning of the thirteenth century, Muwafaq al-Dīn al-Baghdādī was in a rather important position to report and explain the book in the Levant and Egypt, where very few had an isnād as short or as prominent back to Ibn Mājah.[5]

The appreciation of al-Baghdādī's isnād was evident in the comments of one of his students. Muḥammad ibn Yusuf al-Birzālī (d. 1239), who was a scholar of ḥadīth and the patriarch of a prominent family of scholars that included his grandson, the famous historian 'Alam al-Dīn al-Birzālī (d. 1339), explained that he left Mecca to go to the Levant aiming to study Ibn Mājah's *Sunan*:

> There [in Damascus], I met al-shaykh Abū Muḥammad 'Abd al-Laṭīf al-Baghdādī, may God preserve him, and I knew that [Ibn Mājah's *Sunan*] was of his reporting (riwāyatih). So I asked him to read it with him and he accepted.[6]

Al-Birzālī asked al-Baghdādī to comment in more detail on the ḥadīth that formed the chapters on medicine in Ibn Mājah. He then added two traditions, rounding the number up to forty, and asked al-Baghdādī if he could write down this commentary. Although this commentary on the medical traditions was not authored by al-Baghdādī sensu stricto, he would have had the chance to read it and correct it, as it was composed with his permission and during his lifetime by his own student.

The most comprehensive biography of Muwaffaq al-Dīn al-Baghdādī survived in the biographical dictionary authored by Muwaffaq al-Dīn ibn Abī ʾUṣaybiʿah. Ibn Abī ʾUṣaybiʿah knew al-Baghdādī, who was a friend of Ibn Abī ʾUṣaybiʿah's grandfather and offered to teach the grandson. Ibn Abī ʾUṣaybiʿah himself did not have a particularly remarkable career, and his writings, outside of his dictionary, are mostly unknown. However, he was part of the medical milieu in Egypt and the Levant during the first half of the thirteenth century – a period that witnessed important political shifts and changes that also influenced the fortunes of medical dynasties at the time.[7] Ibn Abī Uṣaybiʿah's grandfather was a physician and was the first to carry the name for which his grandson would be known. The grandfather, who grew up and started his career in Damascus, moved to Cairo after Ṣalāḥ al-Dīn al-Ayyūbī (r. 1174–1193) consolidated his power and proclaimed the end of the Fatimid caliphate.[8] When the grandfather moved to Cairo, he reconnected with the celebrated physician Jamāl al-Dīn ibn Abī al-Ḥawāfir, who was one of the founders of a long-lasting and influential medical dynasty in Egypt that served Ayyubid and Mumluk courts for decades to come. Ibn Abī ʾUṣaybiʿah, the grandfather, was also friends with Mūsā ibn Maymūn al-Qurṭubī (Maimonides. d. 1204), who was a leading physician and scholar in Egypt at the time. His connections provided his sons, who would be Ibn Abī ʾUṣaybiʿah's father and uncle, with opportunities to study medicine with some of the best and most influential physicians of their time.

The connections between the Ibn Abī ʾUṣaybiʿah's small dynasty and the other major medical dynasties in Ayyubid-Mamluk Egypt, and the Levant seemed to flow from these early encounters and connections. Members of Ibn Abī ʾUṣaybiʿah's clan served in the most important hospitals (Bīmāristāns) in the region, including Bīmāristān al-Saqṭiyyīn built by the Fatimids in Cairo, and survived under the Ayyubids, and al-Bīmāristān al-Nāṣirī constructed by Ṣalāḥ al-Dīn al-Ayyūbī.[9] Descendants of the family may have worked in al-Bīmāristān al-Manṣūrī, which was built in 1285 by al-Manṣūr Qalawūn, but there is little information to confirm this.[10] In the Levant, they worked in al-Bimāristān al-Nūrī in Damascus and the Nūrī of Aleppo as well. Save for the uncle, Rashīd al-Dīn ʿAlī ibn Khalīfah, who had a long and detailed biography in his nephew's dictionary, the Ibnā Abī ʾUṣaybiʿah's service in the courts seemed infrequent and spotty. Regardless, the men of the family continued to be in direct contact with various members of the medical elite in Egypt and the Levant from at least the middle of the twelfth to the end of the thirteenth century. Muwaffaq al-Dīn's biographical dictionary was, in a way, a product of his and his family's position in this particular milieu – a position that enabled him to produce such respected work as well as shaped the work itself. Steeped in the medical milieu of the Levant and Egypt, Ibn Abī ʾUṣaybiʿah's biographical dictionary emerged as a testimony of his and his colleagues' views on the history and mythical foundations and figures of their profession as well as on the proper practice and behaviors that physicians needed to emulate.

Ibn Abī ʾUṣaybiʿah's dictionary was a rather comprehensive text that borrowed the structure of ṭabaqāt or generations that became common as early as the ninth century with the famous *Al-Ṭabaqāt al-Kubrā* by Ibn Saʿd (d. 845).[11] By the thirteenth century, many more ṭabaqāt volumes were in circulation as the genre came to be the central venue for documenting the histories of certain professions or certain groups of people, such as judges of certain schools of law (*madhhab*), ḥadīth reporters, Sufis, and Quran reciters, among many others.[12] Contemporary to Ibn Abī ʾUṣaybiʿah, the physician and bureaucrat Jamāl al-Dīn Abū al-Ḥasan al-Qifṭī (d. 1248) also wrote a biographical dictionary about physicians that Ibn Abī ʾUṣaybiʿah had access to and copied from.[13] Al-Qifṭī wrote another dictionary dedicated to grammarians (*al-nuḥāh*), perhaps in a nod to his other profession as a scribe. Both al-Qifṭī and Ibn Abī ʾUṣaybiʿah followed in the tradition of other authors of physicians' biographical dictionaries that extended as early as Ḥunyan ibn Isḥāq (d. 873), if not before. Naturally, both al-Qifṭī's and Ibn Abī ʾUṣaybiʿah's books were more voluminous than the earlier volumes, if only by virtue of including more physicians. Whereas al-Qifṭī seemed to rely heavily on Ibn al-Nadīm's (d. 990) Fihrist in many of the biographies about physicians of the tenth century and earlier, Ibn Abī ʾUṣaybiʿah seemed to employ a variety of other sources that came from different libraries of physicians and from conversations with his colleagues and friends.[14] Ibn Abī ʾUṣaybiʿah was also careful to document many of his sources, though definitely not all, and to make clear references to the people whom he spoke to or who helped edit his book. As such, the connections that Ibn Abī ʾUṣaybiʿah enjoyed among the elite physicians of his time were crucial in the making of his book. His sources were precisely the members of the major medical dynasties in the region and their friends and connections, along with the books that they owned or inherited. Moreover, Ibn Abī ʾUṣaybiʿah seemed to have written his voluminous dictionary in stages and to have sought the advice of many of his masters and colleagues, who helped in constructing his narratives and shared in the making of his book.

As such, Ibn Abī ʾUṣaybiʿah's book stands primarily as a representation of the elite medical environment in the thirteenth century. The sources from which this elite derived its history were the sources that Ibn Abī ʾUṣaybiʿah used – the direct swipes or subtle asides reminiscent of the animosities and alliances that shaped their environment as well as Ibn Abī ʾUṣaybiʿah's world and career. The values that this elite understood to be central in medical practice and to the life of a physician were emphasized and exemplified in the biographies. Furthermore, and perhaps most importantly, members of this elite were the editors and readers of the dictionary. Ibn Abī ʾUṣaybiʿah's narrative intended not only to provide a history of the medical profession through the various generations of its major practitioners. It also aimed to provide a professional and moralistic narrative that explained the most important values of the profession and provided through the stories of its more important and renowned practitioners, examples for how students should behave. In this context, the dictionary is a document that expressed Ibn Abī ʾUṣaybiʿah's own views about proper and moralistic practice and, for the purposes of this discussion, about the meaning of piety in medical practice and the behaviors and comportments worthy of pious physicians. The fact that this dictionary was read and edited by many of his colleagues and masters and that it remained a central text for centuries to come adds more weight to the relevance of Ibn Abī ʾUṣaybiʿah's views and how they corresponded to the general views of medical elites in his period. In this context as well, the volume dedicated to the physicians of Egypt and Levant, and particularly the physicians that Ibn Abī ʾUṣaybiʿah directly knew and encountered, carries even more relevance. For these biographies, Ibn Abī ʾUṣaybiʿah had access to a larger body of sources that he was able to employ, and he was in a position to express his preference and his editorial choices more concretely.

Al-Baghdādī's and Ibn Abī ʾUṣaybiʿah's near contemporary ʿAlāʾ al-Dīn ʿAlī ibn ʿAbd al-Karīm ibn Ṭarkhān al-Kaḥḥāl al-Ḥamawī (d. 1320) did not enjoy such an illustrious genealogy or similarly distinguished reputation. As seen from his name and from the very few and short biographies that survived about him, he was an oculist and may have practiced medicine as well. He likely descended from Hamat but eventually resided in Ṣafad. There, he was appointed the administrator of the state treasury (nāẓir Bayt al-Māl), a distinguished and respected position in the bureaucratic structures of the thirteenth and fourteenth centuries.[15] Unlike al-Baghdādī's extensive and impressive oeuvre, Ibn Ṭarkhān is known for only four books: two on ocular medicine, one that seems to be a biographical dictionary, and one on medical ḥadīths, which is his most famous and the only one that seems to have survived today. Ibn Ṭarkhān placed his book within the traditions of collections of forty ḥadīths, based on a prophetic tradition where the prophet promised heaven to any person who learns and teaches [as few as] forty of his traditions.[16] Many scholars, including Ibn Ṭarkhān, used this number as the basis of their composition, collecting forty traditions on one or more topics as a simple guide or a brief collection that could be easy to memorize. Ibn Ṭarkhān's book had two collections of forty traditions, the latter of which he claimed was more useful than the first.[17] He then added a few chapters that addressed a number of other important topics, such as the importance of medicine and the legality of seeking cure, all of which were based on traditions either mentioned in his two 40-item collections or drawn from others. Finally, he concluded the book with a rather detailed section on pharmacopeia, where he listed the names of various drug components alphabetically, including their uses and the traditions that they occurred in. Ibn Ṭarkhān explained in his introduction that he removed the isnāds from his traditions and only mentioned the major books that they occurred in, such as al-Bukhārī or Muslim, among others.[18]

In considering al-Baghdādī's and Ibn Ṭarkhān's books, it becomes clear that the presence of these books at the intersection of their authors' knowledge and careers in ḥadīth and medicine allowed them to present an argument for the place of medicine within a pietistic cosmology. As shown before, writing about ḥadīth was not merely an intellectual exercise where scholars worked with particular materials. Instead, it ostensibly entailed a specific pietistic orientation and maintained an acceptance and a propagation of the prophetic charisma as transmitted through the prophet's ḥadīths and his deeds.[19] In this framework, writing at the intersection of medicine and prophetic traditions, for a physician, entailed the positioning of medicine within an epistemic cosmology that reflected this pietistic orientation. Both authors intended to cast medicine as a worthy and pietistic endeavor in itself, or at least, one that belongs to the higher echelons of learning by highlighting its origins within the prophetic narrative and its place within the overall structures of pietistic and worthy knowledge.

As mentioned before, in her discussion of al-Baghdādī and Ibn Ṭarkhān, Irmeli Perho argued that they paved the road for later writings of prophetic medicine that were more focused and conversant in the Galenic tradition. Both books constituted a basis for the later and more celebrated writings of Ibn Qayyim al-Jawziyah and al-Dhahabī, among others, all of whom cited al-Baghdādī and Ibn Ṭarkhān on some of the more significant medical questions that they dealt with.[20] In addition to the impact of al-Baghdādī's and Ibn Ṭarkhān's medical knowledge and expertise on later prophetic medicine writings, their books engaged concretely with questions of piety and medical practice while also embodying, through their education and careers, the making of a pious and religiously educated medical practitioner. Similarly, Ibn Abī ʾUṣaybiʿah's book developed comparable narratives about the making of pious physicians. Although Ibn Abī Uṣaybiʾah's book has been used extensively by scholars as a source for the lives of many of his contemporaries or near-contemporaries,[21] the book's explicit message, as mentioned by the author, was to provide examples of good character and piety for physicians.[22] As such, Ibn Abī Uṣaybiʾah's biographies of revered figures served to provide models for behavior and to highlight what he and others in his milieu perceived to be the pious practice expected of physicians.

"Emulate the pious and knowledgeable": piety and biographies

In Muwaffaq al-Dīn ʿAbd al-Laṭīf al-Baghdādī's account of his own life, a few moments stand out as central to the narrative. The first is his childhood education. As a young boy, his father – a scholar of ḥadīth – sent him to study with the more prominent scholars of ḥadīth and language in Baghdad.[23] Throughout his life, al-Baghdādī and many of his contemporaries continued to appreciate his early ḥadīth training and the chains of transmission that he acquired.[24] Another influential moment came later in his life as al-Baghdādī encountered some of the figures that he thought changed his views and his life. He seemed to have been impressed the most by two people. The first was Ṣalāḥ al-Dīn al-Ayyūbī's vizier and adviser, al-Qāḍī al-Fāḍil (d. 1199), and the second was the Egyptian scholar Abū al-Qāsim al-Shāriʾī. Al-Baghdādī met al-Qāḍī al-Fāḍil in Ṣalāḥ al-Dīn's encampment near Acre during Ṣalāḥ al-Dīn's wars against the crusaders in the Levant.[25] Al-Baghdādī explained that, as al-Qāḍī al-Fāḍil was dictating two letters at the same time, the scholar asked al-Baghdādī about a few grammatical questions before offering him the opportunity to join the Ayyubid court in Damascus. When al-Baghdādī politely insisted on going to Egypt, al-Qāḍī al-Fāḍil gave him a note that guaranteed that the scholarly elites of Cairo welcomed him with open arms and showered him with gifts. It also allowed him to start a teaching career in Cairo, where he taught grammar and ḥadīth.[26]

Although al-Baghdādī seemed truly impressed by al-Qāḍī al-Fāḍil, his account also served to show his own stature and to draw attention to his own knowledge and expertise. This is not unusual for al-Baghdādī, who was known to be boastful and has been described by many of his biographers as, "A man whose claims [to knowledge] were more than his knowledge."[27] Others, like al-Jamāl al-Qifṭī, explained that al-Baghdādī made such huge claims to knowledge when he first arrived to Cairo that many students flocked to him; however, "[t]hen, he fell short and they [the students] abandoned him."[28] The second person who seemed to have impressed al-Baghdādī was Abū al-Qāsim al-Shāriʾī, who first introduced him to the philosophy of al-Farābī and to the works of Aristotle and other Greek philosophers. Al-Baghdādī, who had been a devotee of Ibn Sīnā before that, came to be gradually disillusioned by Ibn Sīnā's work. At the same time, he lost faith in alchemy and understood that it was a deluded endeavor. In his view, he survived from two major delusions (Ibn Sīnā and alchemy) that drove many people to their [intellectual and spiritual] demise.[29]

His self-serving aggrandizing tendencies aside, al-Baghdādī's narrative clarified what he considered to be central to his own carefully drawn persona: his knowledge of language, ḥadīth, and Quran and his career in critiquing Ibn Sīnā. Ḥadīth remained central to al-Baghdādī's career. It appears that he made his living mostly through teaching ḥadīth along with grammar. He also boasted a well-respected lineage in these sciences. Moreover, and to the same effect, his most important students were those who studied ḥadīth, grammar, and adab with him. In fact, most of the surviving autobiographical narrative that came to structure the conversation around al-Baghdādī's life – as later scholars continued to deal with his claims by affirming or refusing them – survived in the work of Ibn Abī Uṣaybiʾah, whose grandfather knew al-Baghdādī well and whose father and uncles studied grammar and ḥadīth with al-Baghdādī.[30] In other words, it was an offshoot of his ḥadīth and grammar intellectual descendants that preserved his autobiography. His critique of Ibn Sīnā and others whom he considered to be summarizers and commentators shaped most of his production in medicine and philosophy. He ridiculed Ibn Sīnā and rejected his works, criticizing philosophers and physicians for reading what he believed was inferior work. As Peter Pormann and N. Peter Joosse have shown, al-Baghdādī advocated for a return to Greek sources as opposed to relying on summaries and later commentaries. Pormann and Joosse have questioned the sincerity of this call because al-Baghdādī had also composed summaries of these texts.[31] As such, it appears that he may not have rejected the concept or the practice of writing and reading summaries as much as he detested specific authors and their works.

Primary sources do not show sufficient evidence to support al-Baghdadī's claims of a celebrated medical career. Ibn Abī Uṣaybiʾah explained that medicine came rather later in al-Baghdādī's career, beginning when he left for Damascus, likely in 1208. There, he started to be known for his work on medicine.[32] Interestingly, al-Baghdādī claimed that he taught some medicine in Cairo at al-Azhar, although he mentioned very little details. Al-Dhahabī and Ibn Shākir al-Kutubī, among others, seemed to affirm this particular order of al-Baghdādī's intellectual life as they consistently described him as first a grammarian and scholar of ḥadīth and then as a physician. Al-Baghdādī's animosity to Ibn Sīnā and his philosophy may have served him well with some of his contemporary ḥadīth scholars who objected to Ibn Sīnā along with other philosophers and theologians (*mutakalimūn*). However, among physicians, philosophers, and a growing number of legal scholars, such animosity may not have had similarly positive effects. Moreover, al-Baghdādī claimed that he learned medicine with the son of the famous physician Ibn al-Tilmīdh, of whom he spoke quite highly. However, Ibn al-Tilmīdh's son seemed to have had a rather mediocre reputation among the physicians of Egypt and the Levant, "Muwaffaq al-Dīn al-Baghdādī said that one of his masters, from whom he benefitted, was the son of Amīn al-Dawlah ibn al-Tilmīdh, and he expanded in describing him. This is because of his enthusiasm for Iraqis. Otherwise, Amīn al-Dawlah's son was not like that or even close to that."[33] It is not possible to know whether Ibn al-Tilmīdh's son was indeed a prominent physician. Most of our sources descend from the lineage of Ibn al-Tilmīdh himself, who had a rather strained relationship with his son. As such, most of the sources that reached us portray the son in a rather unforgiving light. In Egypt and the Levant, in the circles where Ibn Abī ʾUṣaybiʿah was active and around the various Bīmāristāns of the region, the reputation of Ibn al-Tilmīdh was stellar and his legacy was transmitted through his student Ibn al-Naqqāsh. However, Ibn al-Tilmīdh's son was rather scorned and considered to be a mediocre physician at best.[34] As such, being associated with Ibn al-Tilmīdh's son may not have been advantageous for al-Baghdādī.

In al-Baghdādī's narrative about his life, which was reported by Ibn Abī ʾUṣaybiʿah and cited by others, we encounter the making of a pious, educated physician. Although al-Baghdādī affirmed his deep interest and his keen attention to medical knowledge and practice, he gave equal attention to his knowledge and learning of ḥadīth, which constituted a good number of his writings. It is not possible to know with accuracy whether al-Qāḍī al-Fāḍil was indeed impressed with al-Baghdādī; however, the fact that al-Baghdādī relied on this encounter as evidence for his prominence, not as a physician but rather as a scholar of language, Quran, and ḥadīth, reveals the importance of these disciplines in the training and education of Muslim physicians at the time. Paulina B. Lewicka has argued that the thirteenth-century Levant witnessed the consolidation of pietistic attitudes among Muslim physicians. She explained how the rise of medical madrasas, which were built in Damascus, prevented physicians from engaging in philosophy and further consolidated the authority and prominence of religious scholars and religious Muslim physicians over the profession.[35] I have argued elsewhere that Lewicka's conclusions seem to overstate the importance of medical madrasas in this context as well as the increasing power of religious scholars and physicians.[36] Indeed, evidence suggests that interest in philosophy increased and that the physicians who founded and supervised these madrasas were themselves interested in and committed to philosophy. Moreover, there is no evidence that Muslim physicians dominated medical practice in any palpable fashion during this period. However, Lewicka's observation about the rising interest in religious sciences is accurate. The rise of ḥadīth sciences and its growing importance in the education of various members of the educated elites also affected the education and training of physicians such as al-Baghdādī, among many others. In the same context, the pietistic sensibilities engendered by such education and rooted in both earlier pietistic texts and Galenic ethics influenced the production of pious physicians, both as individuals and as symbols.

In the same context, Ibn Abī ʾUṣaybiʿah's biography of his uncle, Rashīd al-Dīn ibn Khalīfah, stands as another example of the production of the pious physician within biographical narratives.[37] Ibn Abī ʾUṣaybiʿah was evidently proud of his uncle, who seemed to have been the more famous physician of the family. He used the biography to explain much about his grandfather's life and his connections to major physicians in Egypt and Levant before delving into the details of his uncle's and his father's education and career. According to Ibn Abī ʾUṣaybiʿah, Rashīd al-Dīn was trained by the chief physician of the Egyptian realm, Jamāl al-Dīn ibn Abī al-Ḥawāfir. Rashīd al-Dīn accompanied the famous physician in the Bīmāristān and studied most of Galen's sixteen books with him. Rashīd al-Dīn also accompanied the renowned oculist Nafīs al-Dīn ibn al-Zubayr, who was the chief oculist in al-Bīmāristān al-Nāṣirī of Cairo at the time. As mentioned before, Rashīd al-Dīn's father, or Ibn Abī ʾUṣaybiʿah the grandfather, was friends with ʿAbd al-Laṭīf al-Baghdādī.[38] As such, Rashīd al-Dīn studied philosophy, particularly the works of Aristotle, as well as Arabic with al-Baghdādī. Rashīd al-Dīn moved then to Damascus and accompanied known physicians, such as Raḍiyy al-Dīn al-Raḥbī and Muhadhdhab al-Dīn ʿAbd al-Raḥīm al-Dakhwār in al-Bīmāristān al-Nūrī. Rashīd al-Dīn also continued his studies with ʿAbd al-Laṭīf al-Baghdādī as the latter moved to Damascus as well. According to Ibn Abī ʾUṣaybiʿah's account, the young Rashīd al-Dīn was only interested in "studying, learning, and complementing himself with virtues."[39] Rashīd al-Dīn learned the Quran by heart as a child; he also studied mathematics, astronomy, philosophy, and music and became a rather remarkable lute player.[40] In Damascus, Rashīd al-Dīn studied language and poetry with a number of leading Damascene litterateurs. According to his nephew, Rashīd al-Dīn also spoke and composed poetry in Persian.[41]

In Damascus, Rashīd al-Dīn met with the famous Sufi shaykh Ṣadr al-Dīn ibn Ḥamawayh. Ibn Abī ʾUṣaybiʿah was careful to record the exact date, which was the twentieth of Ramadan of the Hijri year 615 (1219 CE) when his uncle was given the Sufi mantle (*khurqah*) by his master and pronounced, as such, part of the shaykh's remarkable lineage that extended to the prophet through the imams ʿAlī al-Riḍā and his father and grandfather Musā al-Kādhim and Jaʿfar al-Ṣādiq.[42] Eleven months later, in Shaʿbān 616 (1220 CE), Rashīd al-Dīn died at the young age of thirty-eight and was buried with his father and brother in a Damascene cemetery.[43] Rashīd al-Dīn composed four books and three treatises, none of which have survived to my knowledge. The books included a book on medicine, where he "explained most generalities in medicine"[44] and one entitled *Ṭibb al-Sūq* or

"The Market Medicine," wherein Ibn Abī ʾUṣaybiʿah explained, "He composed for some of his students and includes mentions of common diseases, their causes and ways to treat them using simple and easily available materials."[45] He also composed a book on arithmetic and on surfaces. His treatises included ones on the pulse, comparing it to musical notations, on "the reason for which mountains were created," and one on medical cases and experimented drugs.

Just before detailing this short bibliography, Ibn Abī ʾUṣaybiʿah expounded upon what he described as some of his uncle's sayings and recommendations in wisdom (or philosophy) (*fī al-ḥikmah*). It is in these sayings, which Ibn Abī ʾUṣaybiʿah claimed to have heard directly from his uncle, that one can encounter Ibn Abī ʾUṣaybiʿah's views on the virtuous practice of medicine. The "sayings" were structured in short sentences that resembled aphorisms (*fuṣūl*), proverbs, or traditions of companions and pious men. Ibn Abī ʾUṣaybiʿah included similar aphorisms or words of wisdom in the biographies of a few other physicians, including ʿAbd al-Laṭif al-Baghdādī, among others. However, he claimed to be the only heir of his uncle's aphorisms and advice, which he heard from him and which were never written. With little mentions of medical practice and sparse advice in relation to medications, the majority of the sayings were focused on obeying God and living a good life worthy of physicians and scholars. As the sole heir to his uncle's wisdom, Ibn Abī ʾUṣaybiʿah was transmitting what he likely perceived as the epitome of the wisdom that his family embodied and the life that they aspired to. At the same time, and as will be seen later, Rashīd al-Dīn's sayings and aphorisms were similar in essence to those of Abd al-Laṭīf al-Baghdādī among other physicians that Ibn Abī ʾUṣaybiʿah worked with. Although these parallels may relate to the similar environ they inhabited and worked in, they also demonstrate a shared approach and outlook to the life seen as worthy of the learned.

One of the central pieces of advice that Rashīd al-Dīn repeated on several occasions was the need to follow the example of prophets, scholars, and wise men. For instance, in what Ibn Abī ʾUṣaybiʿah termed the recommendations for the daytime (*waṣiyat al-nahār*), Rashīd al-Dīn admonished, "Accept the advice of prophets and emulate the deeds of wise men (*ḥukamāʾ*)."[46] Later, he explained, "If you contemplate the movement and stillness of the virtuous (*al-fuḍalāʾ*), you will find much wisdom in them."[47] Similarly, one should "always accompany the masters [of knowledge and religion] (*al-mashāyikh*). You would either benefit from their knowledge or from their behavior," through emulating it. ʿAbd al-Laṭīf al-Baghdādī had similar advice to his readers, but he focused on emulating the prophet and the first generations of the prophet's companions:

> One should read histories and inspect biographies. As such, his short life would encompass the times of bygone nations and peoples [as if] he had encountered them and knew their good and bad. [. . .] You ought to emulate in your manner the manner of the first generation [of Muslims] (*al-ṣadr al-ʾawwal*). Thus, read the sira of the prophet and follow his deeds and his conditions, follow his traditions and emulate him as much as you can. If you come to know his manners in eating, drinking, dressing, sleeping, waking,

sickness, health and how he behaved towards God and with his spouses, companions and enemies, and did only little of that, you will be the happiest for it.[48]

Al-Baghdādī, a scholar of ḥadīth and sunna himself, was more emphatic in explaining the importance of emulating the prophet and the early companions as the central examples for pious life. Although his advice to learn about bygone nations and to read histories and biographies matched his interest in older texts, it also reflected the traditionalist paradigm that governed his thought and that conditioned pietistic behavior at the time.

For Rashīd al-Dīn, who was a Sufi and a follower of Ibn Ḥamawayh, scholars and religious leaders (*al-mashāyikh*) were God's favorites and were the conveyers of happiness and wellbeing for those who followed them. He explained:

- Be wary of hurting scholars for they are God's people.
- Any scholar, of real knowledge, who was ever done injustice, was made [a] victor by God and that who caused [the scholar] injustice would always be defeated.
- God has favorites that He guards with his eye that never sleeps. These are the scholars.
- Scholars are the real happy people.[49]

Although the identity of these scholars was not immediately made apparent, Rashīd al-Dīn's narrative showed that he was referring to scholars of religion and wisdom and those who followed the dictates of religion. In another aphorism, he explained that one should trust those who are knowledgeable in Islam and to avoid those who are knowledgeable and have certainty in other religions.[50] When elaborating on the nature of wisdom (*ḥikmah*), Rashīd al-Dīn explained that it was "following the orders of God."[51] To seek knowledge, one should attend to the revealed books of God, "because they have all the wisdom."[52]

Hinting briefly at discussions about Sufis and their commitment to the dictates of religion, particularly physical rituals and forms of worship, Rashīd al-Dīn was explicit in demanding that one should never "leave any of the physical worship for it is the best means to reach spiritual goals."[53] The focus on physical worship was a rather recurrent theme in the recommendations of a number of physicians mentioned by Ibn Abī 'Uṣaybiʿah and was connected to more profound views about limiting one's consumption of foods and drinks and access to various earthly pleasures. For instance, the biography of Ṣadaqah al-Sāmirī, who was a Samarian physician contemporary of Rashīd al-Dīn and who died ca. 1228, contained detailed discussion of fasting, which Ṣadaqah seemed to believe was a central practice for the pious and educated:

> Fasting is to prevent the body from food, the senses from errors, the limbs from vices and all of the body from whatever distracts from contemplating God. [. . .] Know that all good deeds can be seen [by people] except for

> fasting, which is only seen by God, because [fasting] is an act of the interior based on pure patience. Fasting is of three degrees: that of the commoners, which is preventing the belly and the pudendum from their passions; the fasting of the select, which is preventing hearing, vision, the tongue and all limbs from vices. Then, the fasting of the select among the select is for the heart to fast from all lowly concerns and earthly thoughts and stop anything except [contemplating] God.[54]

Rashīd al-Dīn was also emphatic in explaining that the human body needs very little to survive and that one should not follow passion or indulge. As such, one should strengthen his soul over his body and eat only the little that is sufficient to keep the body's power without increase. The increase should only be in the food of the soul.[55]

Rashīd al-Dīn had some advice for when one became knowledgeable enough to teach or to be known as a scholar, "If you arrive at the degree of teachers, do not withhold [knowledge] from those who deserve it. These are the smart, good-natured and wise. Withhold knowledge from all else."[56] The emerging scholar needed to behave in a particular way, according to al-Baghdādī. Excessive laughter, for instance, was a sign of triviality and was to be rejected. Similarly, excessive talk about matters of no concern to one's own scholarly pursuits were not proper for students. Silences when one's expertise or knowledge were being called for or referenced was not advised either. In short, moderation in speaking and laughter was required and expected. In the same way, a student was not to overly trust himself. Instead, one should consistently doubt himself and question his knowledge and his behavior. He should always try to know more and to behave better. Here, too, al-Baghdādī's recommendations were not based only on a heritage of medical ethics or of manners of physicians and elite scholars, but was also part of a long-standing literature on piety and pietistic performances. As Christopher Melchert explains, scholars of ḥadīth disliked laughter and joking and considered them signs of triviality and immaturity, if not impiety.[57] Smiling was encouraged, but laughter was not. Instead, a pensive and contemplative comportment that showed the gravity of knowledge and the enormity of the task of keeping God on one's mind all the time were more appropriate for the pious and for the scholar. Doubting oneself and constantly questioning one's behavior and commitment to divine demands were also important and recommended pious behaviors. Pious Muslims were encouraged not to feel satisfied with their work and worship and to always seek to do more.

This view on one's own behavior extended to other acts of explicit introspection that al-Baghdādī followed many other authors in explaining and recommending:

> You should reckon with yourself every night when you resign to your bed, look at what you have achieved of good and thank God for it, and look at what you have accrued of sins and ask God for forgiveness and repent. And then, you arrange for yourself the good that you plan to do in the following day and ask God to help you with it.[58]

In the same way, al-Baghdādī advised that one needed to consider his own feelings and his thoughts and remember that God sees all that is apparent or hidden. As such, one needs to strive to make what was hidden of his life as honorable and God-fearing as what was apparent. Ultimately, it was God who concealed what was concealed and He could reveal it to all people. Here, al-Baghdādī reiterated this introspective nature of Sunni piety that we discussed before. One was to be held accountable for thoughts and ideas and not only for deeds. One also needed to spend time thinking and reflecting on his own acts and to try to do his best to improve his behavior.

Rashīd al-Dīn and al-Baghdādī were also concerned with time and how young scholars could fall into the trap of wasting their time, which was a travesty in itself but also a sign of bad nurturing. Rashīd al-Dīn's advice started with one long paragraph described as the advice of the beginning of the day (*waṣiyyat awal al-nahār*) and another described as the advice of the beginning of the night (*waṣiyyat awal al-layl*). The two pieces of advice intended to provide a framework for action throughout the day and even during sleep. In the beginning of the day, one should consider their plans for the day and what they intended to do to follow God's orders. They should keep in mind that they will recount and consider their deeds at the end of the day and aim to act so that their good deeds exceed their bad deeds:

> Know that the virtuous is not one who remains in the natural state [of virtue] while away from harm. The virtuous is the one who remains in this state in the presence of harm. And abstaining from people is the best way to prevent harm.[59]

At night, one should consider their deeds from the day and reflect on what they did right or wrong. One should not be seduced to think and recount what they suffered from people throughout the day. This only leads to "wasting your time." Instead, one should think of good deeds and hope to do more good the following day. These thoughts provide for good dreams and visions that contribute to educating and training oneself even while asleep. As such, staying away from people and focusing one's time and effort on learning and on following God's orders were the key to the good life that Rashīd al-Dīn was advising. Ultimately, "If you fear for your money and never spend it except on what is important, then you should be more fearful for your time."[60] Here, Rashīd al-Dīn recalled Hippocrates's first aphorism, without mentioning him by name, explaining that knowledge is vast and one should dedicate all the time that they have to learning what they can.

In short, for both Rashīd al-Dīn and al-Baghdādī, among others, the best form of activity for a young physician or scholar was to emulate the prophet and the scholars of yore. Both al-Baghdādī and Rashīd al-Dīn insisted that learning from the writings of the ancients was superior to learning from their commentators and their summarizers, with al-Baghdādī the more forceful and insistent in this regard. They also explained that following the method of the companions and those of the early generations of Muslims was the best way to act and the best conduit to good living. In all cases, one should always abstain from seeking money or earthly rewards and should dedicate their lives to learning and acquiring virtue. For instance, al-Baghdādī insisted that seeking the favor of people of power or wealth was not consistent with either seeking God's favor or seeking knowledge. The attempt to acquire worldly possessions and to accumulate wealth and fame required attention and devotion of time and resources that a true seeker of knowledge could not afford, "I do not say that the world will turn away from the seeker of knowledge but that the seeker of knowledge turns away from the world."[61] If one dedicated himself to seeking knowledge and studied and wrote, the world would come to his door, as important people will hear of him and seek his nearness. To be sure, this is not only a question of time and dedication to scholarly endeavor. The rejection and renunciation of worldly possessions for higher pursuits were consistent themes in works on piety. People were encouraged to dismiss the value of worldly possessions and to focus instead on what truly mattered: good knowledge of God and worshipping Him.

Both scholars and others idolized the image of the hermit scholar who did not engage with people except when necessary and who sought one's own perfection and virtue. Of course, this might seem to contradict the fact that they both were physicians whose work naturally involved dealing with people. However, both physicians insisted that a physician should always focus on respecting himself and on following the honorable example of earlier physicians and of other pious people. Even in dealing with people, the learned ethical agent was introspective, concerned with their own perfection, and aware that they would be judged by God as individuals and based only on their deeds. The best way in life, Rashīd al-Dīn explained, was to avoid people.

Thus, piety, for al-Baghdādī, Rashīd al-Dīn, and many others, resided in emulating the prophet, learning about his life, and imitating his behavior. Although the piety of a scholar like al-Baghdādī eventually resembled and drew on the same resources that other people's piety drew on, a scholar had more responsibilities that were created by his knowledge, activities, and work. A scholar needed to devote himself to learning, whereas other people might engage in permissible activities with the aim of enrichment. Although these latter acts were legal, al-Baghdādī and others understood them to be of lower value than seeking useful knowledge in a pietistic manner. Scholars and students were more qualified to learn about the prophet and read carefully and diligently about his life and his sunna with the aim of both applying it to their lives and preserving it for others. In a way, the scholarly career of al-Baghdādī revolved around this particular form of epistemic piety. He learned prophetic traditions and spent the majority of his learning career invested in religious sciences and in learning about the prophet, his sunna, and about the Quran. Moreover, the majority of his writings were also about these topics. In this regard, al-Baghdādī's commentary on medical traditions and Ibn Ṭarkhān's collections of traditions, as discussed later, acquire a different meaning in view of these obligations of epistemic piety. There, these scholars intended to put all of their knowledge of ḥadīth as well as other earthly useful and religiously sanctioned knowledge to proper use by teaching people and invoking their pietistic feelings through instructing them about the prophet and his legacy.

Medicine in a pietistic cosmology

Muwaffaq al-Dīn al-Baghdādī's and Ibn Ṭarkhān's books were not intended to be books of medicine; rather, they were located firmly within the ḥadīth genre, despite the fact that their content was largely medical and was influenced by the authors' medical knowledge and practice. For al-Baghdādī, the actual author of the book, al-Birzālī, was not a physician but rather a scholar of ḥadīth. The selections and the choice of order was not of al-Baghdādī's or al-Birzālī's making, but was rather dependent on the choices made by Ibn Mājah in his *Sunan*. Ibn Ṭarkhān exhibited more control over the content of his book as he selected the traditions and added a few chapters to discuss issues that he believed to be important. However, as he explicitly remarked, the book was part of the forty-traditions genre, which was an important genre for ḥadīth that provided a venue for creating brief summaries intended to benefit large audiences. However, and as Pehro has explained, the medical experience and identity of the authors (or originators) are unmistakable.[62] They infused the texts with their medical knowledge and provided detailed commentaries that linked medical (Galenic) knowledge to the ḥadīths that they selected.

At another level, the two books positioned the two authors at the intersections of ḥadīth and medicine. For al-Baghdādī, the brief dictated commentary was perhaps the first commentary written on a section of Ibn Mājah's *Sunan*.[63] In fact, al-Birzālī explained that al-Baghdādī provided an oral commentary of the entire *Sunan*. However, only the medical part was recorded by al-Birzālī and there was no evidence that al-Baghdādī wrote the full commentary, as it did not appear on any of his bio-bibliographies. In embarking on this endeavor of reporting and commenting on Ibn Mājah, al-Baghdādī deployed his position as one of the reporters of Ibn Mājah's *Sunan*. However, the fact that only the commentary on the medical part was recorded and that al-Baghdādī's name did not make it to the list of Ibn Mājah's commentators reveals the relatively limited reputation that al-Baghdādī held within the circles of ḥadīth scholars. Moreover, the fact that al-Birzālī thought that the commentary on the medical chapter was the one most worthy of recording was due to al-Baghdādī's other professional interest and activity, namely medicine. As such, although al-Baghdādī's early education in ḥadīth enabled him to acquire a short isnād and authorized him to transmit and comment on Ibn Mājah, it was his medical reputation and career that conditioned the contours of his commentary and allowed it to survive. Similarly, Ibn Tarkhān's book was deployed at the intersection of his medical and religious professional identities, making claims to both disciplines and both readerships.

As seen in the previous chapters, medicine always occupied a privileged position among scholars of ḥadīth and law. Compilers and authors of ḥadīth collections dedicated chapters to medicine; other prominent scholars, such as Ibn al-Jawzī, composed books in medicine; and the tradition attributed to al-Shāfiʿī (and sometimes to the prophet), "knowledge is of two kinds: the knowledge of religion and knowledge of bodies," was ubiquitous and always taken to refer to medicine.[64] Although questions about the use of alcohol and other prohibited materials in treatment lingered for a long time, there is little evidence that these questions reflected on the worth of the profession as a whole or even on the Greco-Islamic version of the practice.[65] In fact, and perhaps as evidence for the prominence of medicine, religious scholars bemoaned what they perceived as non-Muslims dominating the medical profession and encouraged Muslims to pursue medical education and to work in medicine.[66] Al-Baghdādī and Ibn Tarkhān were not attempting to legitimize medical practice or to make a case for its legality. Instead, their books, particularly Ibn Ṭarkhān's, as will be seen later, attempted to locate medicine within the pietistic landscape, whereby learning and practicing medicine would be dignified by the prophetic example and by placing it within the inheritance of the prophet and his companions.

As a learned profession, there was probably more reason to attempt and provide a prophetic or pietistic lineage for medicine than would be the case for artisanal practices. Studying and teaching the sciences of revelation, prophetic traditions, and Islamic law were evidently at the top of this pietistic hierarchy because they implied (and required) a particular pietistic disposition from their practitioners. Other learned traditions occupied a lower rank but acquired their pietistic identity from being connected to the prophetic tradition.[67] Having significantly more editorial latitude in his book, Ibn Ṭarkhān was more forthright in his endeavor to place medicine within the pietistic landscape. He discussed this question through three main avenues: the origins of medical practice, the merits or outstanding qualities (*faḍl*) of medicine, and medicine's compatibility with intellect and religious law (*sharʿ*). He then addressed three other issues that also had implications on medicine's place and role in the pietistic landscape: the value and blessing of good health, the legality and pietistic implications of seeking cure, and the relationship of medicine to death, insofar that the latter is part of divine destiny. Ibn Ṭarkhān's book itself symbolized this connection between medicine, on one hand, and prophetic and revelatory sciences, on the other. As a book that relied on both, it was presented as occupying a higher pietistic and intellectual position than other writings that focused solely on medicine. In composing this book, Ibn Ṭarkhān exercised the pietistic impulse that he and others, like al-Baghdādī and Ibn Abī ʾUṣaybiʿah, thought was central to the making of pious physicians and medical practitioners.

The origin of medicine

The question of origins and originators of particular practices held special importance in the medieval intellectual landscape. Roy Mottahedeh has shown that such mythical genealogies for different practices played an important role in the organization of the epistemic landscape and allowed practitioners to claim exalted mythical origins that often went back to prophets or pious sages.[68] Medicine was definitely not an exception to this endeavor. In fact, physicians engaged in consistent affirmation of the role and importance of the fathers of the profession, the most prominent among whom were Hippocrates and Galen.[69] Ibn Ṭarkhān did not deviate much from this master narrative. In his view, Hippocrates stood as the central founder of medicine and he was, as such, given the first word in describing the origin of medicine. Here, however, Hippocrates's life and his work were not presented as the foundation for medicine, but rather, he was summoned to provide a testimony to the origin of medicine that went beyond him. Hippocrates's place in the medical genealogy was at once taken for granted and also deemed insufficient. There was no need to explain why he would be the very first person cited in the chapter on "The Origin of Medicine and That Who Initiated It (*fī bayān aṣl al-ṭibb wa dhikr al-wāḍi ʿ lahu*)," but Hippocrates was all but denied this position of originator and, instead, brought to testify that, "[medicine] is inspiration from God."[70] Hippocrates's framing statement is followed by a few suggestions:

> [Some] said, it was Seth, the son of Adam, who first brought medicine forth, and that he inherited it from Adam. It was also said that some saw medicines in a vision and then they used them and were cured. It was said that [medicine] was achieved by experimentation, and it was said by analogy, and it was said by coincidence.[71]

In these accounts, some of which Ibn Ṭarkhān seemed to return to later in his text, the narrative of medicine being an inspiration from God was emphasized through its descending from prophets or given to people through visions and coincidences. The question of coincidence was brought up again in words cited from Ḥunayn ibn Isḥāq, who explained that a woman from Egypt, who suffered from melancholy, happened to eat some medicinal plants by chance and was cured. Other origins referenced by Ibn Ṭarkhān included the people of India or "the magicians." Apart from these, Ibn Ṭarkhān returned to the theme of divine origin, "It was said that it was Hermes, who is the prophet Idrīs, who initiated all the crafts, philosophy and medicine and that he was the first who started medicine and wrote in it."[72] The divine origin was also cited through a prophetic tradition, which was cited by Abū Nuʾaym al-Isfahānī in his book on prophetic medicine. In this tradition the prophet narrated that whenever Solomon, the king and prophet, would pray, he would find a small plant growing in front of him. He would ask the plant what it was for. If it had a medicinal value, it would be written down. Ibn Ṭarkhān summarized this discussion, "Mostly, [medicine] was taught by God and through his revelation and inspiration. Then people added to it through experimentation and analogy."[73]

In addition to divine inspiration, Ibn Ṭarkhān followed another line of reasoning showing medicine as the product of innate behavior that was endowed by God. For instance, he explained, animals and humans seek food when they are hungry – hunger being a form of illness treated by food – and stop eating when they feel full, "These are all [forms of] medicine since it is the use of that which is good and the rejection of that which is bad. There is no meaning to medicine but this."[74] Other animals, Ibn Ṭarkhān explained, consumed materials that were not normally part of their diet in order to treat some problems. These included snakes, certain types of fish, and cats and other felines, among others. In consuming these materials, these animals were effectively using medicines inspired by God. Ibn Ṭarkhān's major point was that medicine was a common and natural behavior that God inspires all creatures to follow. He concluded this section with the verse, "Our Lord is He who gave everything its creation, then guided it."[75]

At the heart of Ibn Ṭarkhān's narrative, some operative definitions of medicine emerge. In his view, medicine was a pragmatic and effect-oriented practice that aimed to correct problems or ailments and to maintain health and comfort. Although knowledge of the human body and of various medications was undoubtedly part of medicine, they were foremost tools to achieve the central goal of treating patients and correcting ailments of the body. In this context, hunger, thirst, and other sorts of discomforts that affect the body did not differ much from other more complex diseases.[76] Ibn Ṭarkhān presented a view of medicine that seemed open to experimentation and that was linked to innate and unlearned practices of animals and humans. Al-Baghdādī, who presented a more theoretical commentary in his book, was in agreement. In his analysis of the first tradition, in which the prophet explained that God created a cure for every ailment, he distilled the rules of medicine to "treatment by opposites." He explained, however, that oftentimes such opposites are not readily available:

> We cannot always use [one thing] to treat its opposite for a number of [reasons]. We may be ignorant of [such opposite] since we do not know all medications or all the properties of a given medication. Also, what we know may not occur to us when we are working. It may be difficult to obtain [some of these medications], either because they are naturally rare or rare at this particular time. We may be able to obtain the medication but another thing related to the patient or to the time would prevent its [use].[77]

By highlighting the possible reasons for the lack of effective treatment, despite God's promise that every sickness has a treatment, al-Baghdādī provided a logical explanation for the shortcomings of learned medicine. Moreover, he implicitly argued for the importance of the study of medicine and for facilitating the exchange of medical materials in pursuant to God's promise of finding a cure for every ill.

In a similar vein, Ibn Ṭarkhān's discussion of medicine as part of innate behaviors that humans and animals alike engage in was part of a larger argument about the legality of, if not the obligation to, seek cure. Both Ibn Ṭarkhān and al-Baghdādī engaged with the view that tolerating pain and rejecting medicine is the more pious way to behave. For both of them, this view contradicts the fact that the prophet used medication and ordered people to make use of medicine. Moreover, both Ibn Ṭarkhān and al-Baghdādī argued that the rejection of medicine or of cure amounts to rejecting food:

> [A person holding this view] does not know that God, who created a disease, has also created a medicine to cure it; and He who created hunger has created

food as a medicine for it. Would this claimant abandon food as he abandons medicine? For hunger is also a disease.[78]

In Ibn Ṭarkhān's view, the innate nature of animals seeking a cure solidified the view that seeking a cure was not prohibited or disliked from a religious perspective.

The merits of medicine

Ibn Ṭarkhān was also interested in discussing the merits of medicine in comparison with other arts and practices. He first argued that any branch of knowledge acquired its merit based on the merit of its subject matter. Because medicine's subject matter was the human body, it was therefore one of the more distinguished branches of knowledge.[79] Here, the distinction awarded to the human body was part of how God honored humans and created them in the best possible form. Medicine, in Ibn Ṭarkhān's view, was a sunna because it was recommended and practiced by the prophet. He cited al-Shāfiʿī's ubiquitous tradition, "Knowledge is of two types: the knowledge of religion, and the knowledge of the body," which was often referenced in many works on medicine and piety. Similar to other compilers and authors, Ibn Ṭarkhān took "knowledge of the body" to mean medicine.[80] However, Ibn Ṭarkhān's view on medicine being a sunna was rather unique. At one level, he explained that, because the prophet has ordered people to seek treatment, a point that he would elaborate on later, then medicine is a sunna, "because he used it [medicine] and ordered it. There is no meaning for a sunna but this." He also cited another tradition where the prophet was reported to have said, "Five things are part of the sunna of prophets: shame, patience, cupping, *siwāk*,[81] and perfuming."[82] By referencing both cupping and *siwāk*, both of which are related to medical practice, the ḥadīth indicated to Ibn Ṭarkhān that medicine was indeed a prophetic sunna. Finally, he returned to the innate nature explaining that humans are created with a natural desire to protect themselves and maintain their health. Here, Ibn Ṭarkhān deployed the term sunna both in a legal and more generic sense. Legally, by linking medicine to the prophetic practice, he provided a space for it within the pietistic framework giving medical practice (or rather the use of medicine) an important spot in the religio-legal space. At another level, the literal meaning of the word *sunna* meant way or custom and referred to the divinely ordained custom of nature and of running the affairs of God's creature.[83] Thus, in Ibn Ṭarkhān's view, seeking cure and preserving health were ingrained in all creatures making them, and in turn medicine, the knowledge system that allowed for health part of God's custom or sunna.

Both al-Baghdādī and Ibn Ṭarkhān saw the importance of medicine being linked directly to the importance of health; therefore, the merits of medicine became linked to those of health. Health (*al-ṣiḥḥāh*) and wellbeing (*al-ʿāfiyah*) constituted important blessings that were endowed by God to his servants. Ibn Ṭarkhān marshalled a number of traditions, including a famous tradition reported by al-Bukhārī and many others where the prophet was reported to have said, "Two blessings that many people underestimate: health and free time."[84] Many scholars have commented on this tradition over the years, including Ibn al-Jawzī, who explained that the underestimation described in the tradition is related to people misusing their health and time and failing to use them for worship and for obeying the orders of God. Similar to wealth, which is coupled with health in a number of traditions, health was a blessing because of how it allowed the believers to worship more and to give more of their selves to God. Because health was seen as a blessing, medicine, in Ibn Ṭarkhān's view, was necessary as the main tool for preserving health, which is an obligation on Muslims in his view. Ibn Ṭarkhān argued that preserving one's health was a way of thanking God for this health and seeking his reward.

Medicine was also placed within a cosmology of death and hope. Ibn Ṭarkhān was keen on explaining that medicine did not aim to delay death or defy it – nor could it. In one tradition selected by Ibn Ṭarkhān, the prophet drew three lines. The first represented a human, the last his hopes and dreams, and the middle one his death or demise. The prophet explained that, as one worked for their hopes and dreams, their death would catch up with them.[85] In another tradition, the angels inquired of God how He planned to keep the numbers of humans in check, because they would procreate and fill the earth. God replied saying he had created death for them. When the angels responded that death would make their lives meaningless and futile, God explained that he had also created hope.[86] In these two traditions, Ibn Ṭarkhān seemed to bring together two pietistic dynamics: one of health and illness and one of death and hope. Although both illness and death represented manifest destinies that could not be evaded and (as will be explained later) a potential for reward, these manifest destinies were combined with blessings that God has given to people, namely health and hope. Both such blessings were fleeting but their presence was necessary for civilizing the earth (*iʿmār al-arḍ*) and establishing God's worship (*iqāmat shaʿāʾir allāh*). As such, medicine was the main tool to preserve health and it was part of the hope that allowed humans to thrive on earth and to worship God as He was owed. Discussing the merits of medicine, for Ibn Ṭarkhān, meant locating medicine within pietistic ontologies and epistemologies. At the ontological level, medicine was the hope that maintained humans on earth as they awaited their demise and the tool for them to protect their health and use to seek divine reward. Ontologically, medicine was a necessity for proper and pious living. Epistemologically, medicine was the study of the body and, in Ibn Ṭarkhān's view, came only second to the study of religion and religious law. In all cases, Ibn Ṭarkhān was insistent on explaining that medicine did not attempt or aim to violate divine will or to challenge predestined death. It was not trivial knowledge either. This merit, "as we have demonstrated, is indicated by the law and accepted by the intellect."[87]

Seeking cure and abstention

The question of health and its merit was also an intervention in a debate around the legality and the pietistic implications of seeking cure. In her work on prophetic medicine, Perho argued that there were some trends among mystics or Sufis but also among other scholars and religious figures that rejected seeking cure and considered it to be either impious or a violation of reliance on God.[88] As explained before, the question of withstanding illness and accepting the suffering without complaint was seen as a pietistic act that guaranteed further reward from God.[89] Although such reward was not in doubt, the implications were debated.

In this discussion about piety and seeking medical care, there were three distinct yet connected questions. First, was seeking cure in violation of reliance on God (*tawakkul*) or did it represent a violation or affront to divine will and fate? The answer to this question would define whether seeking cure or medical care was prohibited legally. A corollary of this question was related to the efficacy of medicine: Was earthly medicine at all effective, or was it simply a delusion because it was God who decided diseases and healing, independent and regardless of medicine? The second question, which assumed that medical care was not prohibited, probed the presence of precedence for medical care. In other words, although there might not be clear evidence for outlawing medical practice, it was still important to know if the prophet and his companions engaged in this practice or directly condoned it. Establishing that they did would establish the legality of the practice. If such legal precedence did not exist, legal scholars would have to find ways to determine legality. The third question assumed legality as discussed in the second question. However, it engaged with the question of piety. Although seeking cure may be legal and there may be direct evidence or precedence for it in the sunna of the prophet, it may not be the most pious choice for Muslims to make. The stakes for each of these questions, as well as the manner by which one could engage with them, were different, as was understood by al-Baghdādī and Ibn Tarkhan in their engagement with these questions.

Both al-Baghdādī and Ibn Ṭarkhān discussed the first question, whether seeking cure was a violation of *tawakkul* (reliance on God), in a number of places. Al-Baghdādī addressed this in his commentary on the first and second traditions. There, he explained that rejecting medicine was akin to rejecting food.[90] Ibn Ṭarkhān dealt with this question on two different levels. At one level, Ibn Ṭarkhān addressed what he referred to as the objections of Sufis and mystics. In the second tradition of his first forty traditions, where the prophet was reported to have said, "Every illness has a cure," Ibn Ṭarkhān explained that this tradition encouraged believers to seek medicine and cure:

> [The tradition] indicates preference for seeking cure. This is the view of al-Shāfiʿī and the majority of revered predecessors and the consensus of the followers. It also includes a response to those extremist Sufis who rejected cure saying, "everything is part of fate and predestination, and there is no need for [seeking] cure." This tradition and similar ones are arguments against them. We believe that God is the maker, and that cure is part of God's predestination. And that this is similar to the command to pray to God, or to take precautions against enemies, despite the fact that destiny does not change.[91]

In al-Baghdādī's and Ibn Ṭarkhān's view, the rejection of cure was related to a particular misconception of *tawakkul* or reliance on God. Should one simply accept the will of God and rely fully on him for treatment, or should one seek other forms of treatment that may seem to defy God's will or show reluctance in relying on him? In al-Baghdādī's commentary, the second tradition addressed this point with clarity, "The prophet was asked, '[We have] medications that we use to treat [ailments], and incantations that we incant [to treat ailments]. Do they prevent God's destiny? The prophet said, 'They are part of God's destiny.'"[92] In another tradition cited by Ibn Ṭarkhān, some companions told the prophet that they used to make use of medicine and other treatments before they became Muslims. Now, they preferred to rely on God and accept his will. The prophet responded that these medications are also part of God's will.[93] Emphasizing that medications were but part of God's destiny, Ibn Ṭarkhān explained that whether medications work or not remained in the hands of God. The physician was but a tool or a vessel that delivered God's will and destiny.

The second question, on whether one should rely on earthly medicines, did not, in fact, reject the possibility of treatment and did not argue that one needed to withstand illness. At the practical level, if diseases were willed by God as explained before, no medicine would be effective or would be able to help without God's will. At the same time, should God will healing, no medicine would be needed or required. If this indeed was the case, there was little value in enduring treatments or in even paying physicians because their intervention amounted to nothing. At the pietistic level, trusting in God and in His will seemed the more appropriate action to take. This intertwining of the practical and pietistic was part and parcel of discussions around *tawakkul* or reliance on God. Although the pietistic impulse was the main motivating factor, the practical claim was evidently present. For instance, in one tradition, a companion, sometimes reported to have been the first caliph Abū Bakr, was advised to consult with a physician while sick. The companion explained that he had seen a physician and that he advised him to pray and worship.[94] He referred to God as the physician. The doubts on the practical efficacy of medicine were also evident in a number of traditions where the companions asked the prophet whether there was any use in medicine. The prophet's answers to these questions presented medicine as a tool for God's will, as explained before.

Accusing extremist Sufis of propagating the notion that medicine violated God's will or that it was inconsequential, al-Baghdādī and Ibn Ṭarkhān argued that these Sufis failed to understand the proper meaning of *tawakkul*.[95] They explained that medicine was the means to deliver divine will and therefore was necessary:

> Reliance on God (*tawakkul*) does not contradict employing proper causes (*tasabbub*). That is because *tawakkul* is the heart's reliance on God, which does not contradict [employing] causes, which is mostly dependent on reliance. A healer, who is knowledgeable in medicine, would do what should be done and then rely on God and pray to him for his work to succeed. He is thus similar to a farmer who plows the earth, sows the seeds, wait and pray for God to reach his goals. A healer does the same: he delivers medicine and manages the patient with all his power and then employs reliance on God and prays to him for health to be achieved.[96]

Medicine was therefore a tool of God's destiny, and seeking cures was part of how God intended humans to live their lives. Reliance on God, then, meant or included the use of medicine and other tools for treatment. Al-Baghdādī retorted that abstaining from medicine was akin to abstaining from food, highlighting the absurdity in refusing to rely on or utilize the tools through which God delivers his will.

Although al-Baghdādī and Ibn Ṭarkhān provided ample evidence for the legality of seeking cure and marshalled legal precedence from the prophet's and companions' behavior to indicate that seeking medical care was legally permissible, there is no evidence that the legality of medicine was indeed in doubt. Legal precedence helped buttress claims about the importance and worthiness of medicine in the epistemic hierarchy and may have responded to some marginal views on the topic. Medicine was clearly a practice that was thought to be not only legal but also worthy of support through religious endowments or waqf, where religious scholars would admonish young Muslims to pursue careers in medicine. Nonetheless, the debates around the pietistic standing of seeking cure as opposed to withstanding illness were not uncommon or marginal. In addition to the anecdotes about Abū Bakr and ʿAlī ibn Abī Ṭālib, among others, opting for withstanding at the end of their lives, Aḥmad ibn Ḥanbal discussed this question directly and opined that "seeking cure is permitted but withstanding is a higher degree [of piety]."[97] Although this statement affirmed the legality of learning and practicing medicine, the notion that seeking cure was of a lesser pietistic rank than withstanding illness meant that medicine occupied a rather lower position in the overall epistemology of knowledge and practice. Here, the question was not related to fate or reliance on God (*tawakkul*) but rather focused on rejoicing in the potential for reward that came with illness and its place in this pietistic cosmology.

Ibn Ṭarkhān, who had more latitude in arguing this point and others as he selected his own traditions, did not doubt the importance and value of illness. In fact, he dedicated a chapter to the merits of ailments, where he cited many traditions about how illness provided penance and forgiveness and how it should be received with joy and acceptance.[98] Similar to many other scholars, Ibn Ṭarkhān concluded that the proper manner for believers in dealing with sickness was patience and acceptance.[99] Ibn Ṭarkhān's acceptance of the basic premise that governed the understanding of illness as a divine blessing did not prevent him from attempting to contextualize the accounts of Abū Bakr and Alī, among others. He argued that there might be four reasons for their rejecting cure, "either they were treated then they decided to stop."[100] In this case, their refusal was not indicative of a religious or pietistic preference for refusing treatment as a whole, but rather, it was a part of the general process of accepting treatment for a certain period and rejecting it at another time for various reasons, including the effectiveness of treatment for particular conditions. Ibn Ṭarkhān explained, "[their conditions] may have been chronic, and the effectiveness of the medications prescribed for it is only presumed *mawhūm* (i.e. not certain). It is reported, in explaining [their rejection of treatment] that they abstained from treating mysterious diseases, [which treatment was only] presumed."[101]

In the absence of an effective medication as attested by experience and medical knowledge, their decision to engage in untested or ineffective treatment or to completely refrain would have no implications on the question of seeking cure as a rule. Here, the efficacy of medical practice (or lack thereof) was brought in as a reason for accepting or rejecting treatment. In the same vein, Ibn Ṭarkhān hypothesized that God may have revealed to the two great companions that their demise was near and inevitable (*kūshifa bi qurb ajalihi*). This argument was reminiscent of the explanation given by Ibn Baṭṭāl in his commentary on Ṣaḥīḥ al-Bukhārī of the fact that the prophet rejected treatment on his deathbed. As explained before, Ibn Baṭṭāl argued that the prophet knew he was dying.[102]

In Ibn Ṭarkhān's view, the failure of treatment after some trying, the absence of an effective treatment, and the knowledge of one's approaching demise were important reasons for abandoning treatment and assuming the endurance stance. Accepting illness and enduring suffering would be more valuable if an effective treatment was known, or as Ibn Ḥanbal put it, "Treatment is a license and endurance is a higher degree of piety." Although treatment was part of God's fate and predestination much like diseases, one could always abstain from (rather than reject) treatment and assume a higher degree of submission to God's will. This submission to God's will was not based on framing medicine as a violation of destiny or a challenge to God. Instead, it is framed as part of renouncing the world and its goods (*zuhd*), a value that was respected by believers. There is no evidence of ambivalence in relation to the legality of medicine. Much evidence supported its legality, and scholars advocated for more Muslims to pursue medical careers. However, at the pietistic level, medicine occupied an ambivalent space that derived its ambivalence from its major subject: illness. At the same time, linking this abstention from treatment to questions of renunciation or zuhd meant that it was not available to all. Only a few were capable of achieving the degree of zuhd that would authorize a decision of abstaining from treatment.

Al-Baghdādī seemed to adopt a similar view in his discussion of leprosy. In the tradition that he commented on, the prophet advised people not to look intently at the leper. Al-Baghdādī brought in other traditions where the prophet refused to have audience with a leper. Both traditions seemed to indicate that leprosy was contagious and that one should not associate with a leper. Al-Baghdādī then followed with two other traditions that seemed to contradict the first two. In one tradition, the prophet took the hand of a leper, put it on a plate from which he was eating to indicate that he would share food with the leper, and said to his companions, "Eat with faith and reliance in God (*kulū thiqatan billāh wa tawakkulan ʾalā Allāh*)." The second tradition was one in which the prophet rejected contagion and attributed it to fate and destiny. Al-Baghdādī commented that these traditions, taken together, can seem confusing and contradictory, "once [the prophet] prohibits looking for a long time at a leper and refuses audience with him. At another time, he says '[There is] no contagion' and 'it is fate.' [Yet,] each of these traditions is trustworthy and, in their totality, they are also trustworthy."[103]

Al-Baghdādī explained that the prophet has spoken to each person according to their abilities:

> Some people are strong of faith and firm in belief, so [the prophet] talks to them in the vein of reliance on God (*tawakkul*). Some are not strong enough for this, so he talks to them by way of caution. And the prophet has done both; once by way of what he had of humanity and once by way of what he had of divine power, so that he would be taken as a guide in both, and each class of people would have a proof [that validates] their condition and fits their abilities.[104]

In the same way, seeking cure or abstaining from it could be understood as a matter of strength of faith and ability and as a matter of piety without legal implications. In this view, al-Baghdādī seemed to agree with Ibn Ḥanbal in allowing both decisions as legal but distinguishing rejecting contagion or abstaining from treatment as the more pious position.

In al-Baghdādī's and Ibn Ṭarkhān's framing, seeking cure was still an inferior degree of pietistic behavior than withstanding illness. However, by emphasizing examples of the prophet and companions in seeking cure as precedent, they aimed to present the act of abstaining from cure as an action that was not available to all and that required higher degrees of faith and belief. The view that both physicians presented was consistent with the pietistic ambivalence that characterized the production of illness in the pietistic landscape. This ambivalence allowed for the existence of diverse views around the best behavior pietistically and permitted the pious agent to choose and to change their views over time.

Piety and treatment

As seen before, for both Ibn Ṭarkhān and al-Baghdādī, the question of the place of medicine in relation to piety and whether or not seeking cure was a pietistic act took precedence over questions concerning the legality of medical practice and permissibility of learning and teaching medicine. Their engagement with the question of legality seemed to contribute to placing medicine within the prophetic precedence but did not necessarily carry immediate stakes. The piety question, however, carried important effects on the place of medicine in social and religious hierarchies. Ibn Ṭarkhān's interest in characterizing medicine as a craft intended for curing ailments allowed him to locate it within narratives of immediate utility and to engage in conversations concerning the value of health as a divine gift to humans that required protection and that conditioned specific acts of piety. Absent from this discussion is the value of theoretical knowledge as a conduit for such useful practice. Although this conversation is not particularly unheard of and was undertaken by many scholars, it was not one that Ibn Ṭarkhān or al-Baghdādī invested in. Furthermore, this view of medicine allowed Ibn Ṭarkhān to place learned/Galenic medicine within a cosmology that included a variety of other forms of treatment and that engaged with various forms of illness. For instance, in his discussion of a ḥadīth where the prophet offered to pray for the cure of a woman suffering from epilepsy, Ibn Ṭarkhān explained that prayers acted in a way similar to medications:

> [This tradition] is proof that prayer (*al-duʿā'*) acts like a healing medication in treating some diseases. [When this prayer] is by prophets or pious people, its blessing is greater, its act on the soul stronger, and [its effect] on the psychic faculties and their interactions remarkable.[105]

In another tradition, where the prophet was reported to have said, "Cure is in three things: a drink of honey, a cut by a copper, and a cautery by fire," Ibn Ṭarkhān proposed the possibility that the mention of cautery may have been indeed one of Quranic healing. He explained that some reporters narrated the tradition as ending with "a writing of a verse," referencing amulets made of Quranic verses.[106] He was also keen on deploying the prophet's practice of *ruqya* or incantations as a proof of the legitimacy and piety of seeking cure.[107] Ibn Ṭarkhān seemed to understand that there was a difference between the Quranic healing or incantations, on the one hand, and prescriptions by physicians, on the other. However, he was also insistent on counting medicine, seen as a craft for curing illnesses, as part of the same practice of incantations, prayers, and Quranic readings.

Similarly, he was interested in merging what he explained was spiritual medicine (*al- ṭibb al-rūḥānī*) and physical medicine (*al-ṭibb al-jismānī*). In discussing a tradition about "treating" sadness, worry, and sorrow, he affirmed:

> This tradition includes important indications, which include the permissibility of calling all spiritual symptoms (al-aʿrāḍ al-nafsāniyyah) diseases. This is because most physicians call them spiritual ailments. [The prophet] specified worry, sadness and grief because they relate to the future, present and past. Because, as we mentioned, worry is sadness for an evil that is anticipated to happen or for a good that is anticipated to be missed. And grief is for a matter that already happened, and sadness is what is between them.[108]

Similarly, he was keen on including the evil eye in his book and on providing physical description of its effect in a manner that reflected the logics of physical medicine:

> Some wisemen (*ḥukamā'*) claimed that an evil power emanates from the eye of the evil-eyer (*al- ʿā'in*) and reaches the evil-eyed (al-maʿīn) [causing] harm and destruction. They said this should not be discounted and that it is similar to the poisonous power that emanates from snakes, especially a certain type of snakes, which can hurt humans by looking at them. The evil eye is similar to this.[109]

In all these cases, medicine was not simply extended to include these various practices. Instead, it sought origins in these practices and used their solid place in the prophetic corpus to claim a similarly solid and recognizable space for Galenic practice as a branch or a type of these curing arts.

Within this cosmology of curing traditions, Ibn Ṭarkhān was aware of the potential differences and varying hierarchies between these cures. Narratives of possible or varying efficacy of different cures was not foreign to medical writings, where physicians and pharmacists discussed different treatments and categorized their varying efficacies.[110] Similarly, the notion of curable and incurable diseases (as well as diseases that can be cured with significant effort) was also articulated in medical writings as early as the ninth and tenth centuries. For instance, al-Rāzī explained in his *Letter to a Student* that a physician needed to understand the difference between these conditions and to set the expectations of his patients accordingly so as to escape blame when an incurable condition resulted in death.[111] Similar views were articulated by al-Ruhāwī in his book *On the Manners of Physicians* (*Adab al- Ṭabīb*).[112] For Ibn Ṭarkhān, as explained before, incurable conditions or conditions where cure had failed were occasions in which the choice to abstain from treatment and endure suffering was understandable, if not particularly encouraged. Similar to his suggested explanation of Abū Bakr's behavior in his sickness, he explained the prophet's advice to an epileptic woman, where the prophet advised her to withstand and gain heaven, as part of this view of incurable diseases.[113] Epilepsy, in Ibn Ṭarkhān's view, was a difficult disease to cure and, as such, the woman was advised to abstain from cures (including prayers) and to endure. At another level, Ibn Ṭarkhān compared certain prophetic recommendations to the advices and prescriptions of physicians, "[The prophet's] medicine is not like the medicine of physicians. That is because the prophet's medicine is certain and its benefits are assured with no doubt, while the physician's medicine is speculative (*maẓnūn*), so they are different."[114] Here, Ibn Ṭarkhān deployed the notion of certainty as a central difference between the prophet's and the physicians' medicine. Whereas the first is based on divine knowledge, and therefore is certain, physicians deployed their intellectual capacity and their knowledge to speculate with variable degrees of effectiveness, making it necessarily of a different, if not lesser, value.

Ibn Ṭarkhān came back to this question in various places. For instance, in his discussion of honey as a cure recommended by the prophet, he explained that the benefits of honey were mentioned in the Quran and were therefore certain:

> [the prophet said:] "use the two cures: honey and the Quran." In this saying, he combined human and divine medicine, the medicine of the bodies and the medicine of the souls, and the earthly and heavenly medications.[115]

Cupping offered another opportunity to assert this difference. Ibn Ṭarkhān explained that cupping is a cure of assured efficacy as compared to other medications and prescriptions. In addition to its being recommended by the prophet, it was more efficacious by virtue of its reaching the cause of illness directly and without mediation as it allowed the removal of excess or corrupt humors.[116] Other medications, he explained, took the route of the stomach and were digested and absorbed to the liver. Others crossed the skin before going to the intended organs through blood or other means. In both cases, the effect of medications was modulated by their route and by the various bodily materials that they encountered rendering their efficacy uncertain, or at least less certain than cupping. Therefore, cupping carried the certainty endowed by prophetic knowledge as well as that produced through the mechanics of physical medicine.

Efficacy was undoubtedly linked to causality. On one hand, causes explained how a particular treatment was or was not effective. On the other hand, a proper understanding of causality improved the efficacy of certain treatments as will be explained later. Causality played another important role at the pietistic level. As explained before, scholars writing on illnesses and on how pious Muslims should deal with their diseases insisted that proper behavior included a belief that God was the sole cause of diseases and also the sole origin of treatment. This attribution of full causality to God was necessary for obtaining reward and for gaining God's favor. Ibn Ṭarkhān reiterated the same point arguing that a belief in the spontaneous or innate efficacy of certain treatments or of the innate harm of certain diseases would be impious if not outright religiously prohibited.[117] One of the areas where causality seemed to be important was in the discussion of leprosy and other contagious diseases. Similar to what al-Baghdādī had done, Ibn Ṭarkhān mentioned a series of traditions that seemingly contradicted one another. In some, the prophet advised people not to stare at lepers and abstained from meeting them.[118] In others, he ate with them and he proclaimed, "There is no contagion."[119] Ibn Ṭarkhān suggested the explanation proposed by al-Baghdādī, which stated that the prophet provided examples for people of weaker or stronger faith and that he intended to demonstrate the range of acceptable behavior.[120] This, however, did not answer the question of contagion for Ibn Ṭarkhān, who explained that leprosy was a contagious and hereditary disease in the view of the people of medicine. Instead, he offered a different explanation for the prophetic proclamation:

> [The people] of *al-jāhiliyyah* (period before Islam) used to believe that contagious diseases were contagious in themselves without attributing any of these effects to God. Therefore, the prophet invalidated this belief by proclaiming "there is no contagion," while the other traditions offered guidance to avoiding what could often result in harm by the will of God and his destiny.[121]

In this view, the problem with a belief in contagion was not connected to whether diseases could be transmitted from one person to another or how these diseases could move; rather, it resided with the proper understanding of causality which placed God within the cosmology of diseases as the ultimate cause of events.

Ibn Ṭarkhān dealt in the same way with the contradicting traditions concerning incantations (*ruqya*). In some traditions, the prophet had prohibited al-ruqya, which were performed before Islam, and in others, he recommended and even practiced them himself.[122] In general, a ruqya was a series of words and phrases recited by a healer or someone familiar with the practice to treat a condition or a disease. The nature of these words, as well as the general practice, was something that scholars discussed at length, as explained before.[123] For Ibn Ṭarkhān, both the practice and the words were important. In his rather expansive view of medicine and the healing arts, Ibn Ṭarkhān considered arguments for the legality and effectiveness of al-ruqya to be connected to his overall point of the legality of seeking cure and of the preference for cure as opposed to withstanding ills. Al-ruqya functioned here as another form of treatment on par with the recipes prepared by Galenic practitioners. In considering the permissibility of ruqyas, Ibn Ṭarkhān used the same logic discussed before, contemplating how permitting ruqyas affected the understanding of causality:

> [This contradiction in traditions] may be because [the Arabs] used to believe that [ruqya] was beneficial owing to the nature of its words, as they used to believe in the *jahiliyyah*, [so the prophet prohibited it]. When [the Arabs] had truly believed and accepted God's law, he permitted them to use [ruqyas] while knowing that God is the origin of benefit and harm.[124]

Although Ibn Ṭarkhān insisted that God must be recognized as the source of all good and harm, he also accepted that there are some words and some medications that have particular qualities resulting in benefit and harm, "Know that there are words that have certain qualities and certain benefits, with the permission of God, which scholars have described in their books."[125] This seeming ambivalence placed God as the cause behind all causes while permitting different words, objects, and materials to exhibit certain qualities and to exert effects on other bodies without violating the will of God.

Materia prophetica

Based on this view of causality and effectiveness, Ibn Ṭarkhān discussed some specific treatments that were described and recommended by the prophet. In each of these treatments, he followed a rather consistent formula. First, he started by commenting on the tradition linguistically, explaining any difficult words. He also included other similar traditions that discussed the same topic or treatment. He then proceeded to explain and provide further evidence from prophetic traditions concerning the described treatment, adding details to its religious and pietistic value. Finally, he proceeded to use a Galenic medical explanation of the treatment, explaining its importance and value from a medical perspective. If needed, Ibn Ṭarkhān proceeded to explain any apparent contradictions – whether between the tradition and other traditions, as discussed before, or between the tradition and medical knowledge of the time. For instance, in the previous discussion of ruqya, he explained that using Quranic verses or words that invoke God and his prophet would be useful because they invoke God's mercy and request his help in cure. Using non-Arabic words, whose meanings are not clearly known, was prohibited because they may include polytheistic or otherwise prohibited references or invocations. In this context, he cited a number of traditions where the prophet asked people who used to practice ruqya before Islam to show or recite their ruqyas to him to judge whether they are permissible or not. In addition to the value and influence of words themselves, where the word of God is the most influential, Ibn Ṭarkhān explained that these incantations help the psychic faculties and strengthen patients who believed in the effectiveness of such treatment, allowing them to overcome diseases.

In another example, Ibn Ṭarkhān cited a tradition where the prophet advised one of his companions to pray when he suffered from a stomachache.[126] The tradition was also reported in Ibn Mājah's *Sunan* and, therefore, commented on by al-Baghdādī, whose comments seemed to have inspired Ibn Ṭarkhān. Both explained that prayers were beneficial for a variety of conditions for three main reasons; a divine one (*amr ilāhiyy*); a psychic one (*amr nafsiyy*); and a physical (natural) one (*amr ṭabīʿiyy*). The first was because praying was a form of worship and would, therefore, help a person remember God and seek his reward. The second related to how prayers distracted oneself from pain, allowing the innate power of nature to fight the disease. Al-Baghdādī explained that a good physician would always try to find ways to strengthen this innate power by strengthening the spirit.[127] Both al-Baghdādī and Ibn Ṭarkhān illustrated this point with the same anecdote:

> This [effect of prayers] is confirmed by an anecdote told about one of the descendants of ʿAlī (the prophet's cousin). [This man] suffered from an abscess that needed to be opened and drained but he refused to open it. So, [his attendants] let him start praying and then allowed the physician to open it. [The man] did not care [or feel it] because he was absorbed in worship.[128]

The anecdote mirrored the previously discussed one told by Ibn Abī al-Dunyā and others about ʿUrwa ibn al-Zubayr. In that anecdote, ʿUrwa, who refused to take a medication that would cloud his mind while his leg was being amputated, resorted, in one version, to prayer. In both cases, the pietistic performance of prayer involved full involvement of all senses that a person would not feel an abscess being opened or a limb being amputated. In the same vein, both al-Baghdādī and Ibn Ṭarkhān referenced a tradition where the prophet ordered those who visited a sick person to give him good tidings, "this does not change [fate], but it improves his feelings (*yuṭayyib nafs al-marīḍ*)."[129]

At the physical or natural level, prayer allowed for moving all parts of the body, exercising most of the muscles and internal organs. Al-Baghdādī explained, "I have seen a group of people [. . .] who were in good health. I looked into this and found that they prayed a lot."[130] Al-Baghdādī proceeded to explain how each movement in the prayer – from standing to sitting to bowing – moved specific organs and provided particular exercise to the body. Al-Baghdādī's rather extended commentary on this tradition discussed another tradition, in which the prophet said, "I have been made to like three things from this earthly world: good perfumes, women, and my true comfort is in prayer." Al-Baghdādī explained how perfumes and sexual intercourse were also useful for health and that they were desired, in part, because they allow a person to focus in his prayers, which is the ultimate goal and the most preferred for the prophet.[131]

As mentioned before, cupping played an important role in al-Baghdādī's and Ibn Ṭarkhān's narratives. In commenting on the tradition, "Cure is in three: honey, cupping and cautery," Ibn Ṭarkhān explained that these three ways of treatment were chosen by the prophet as examples because of their wide-ranging efficacy, but not because they were the only possible treatments for all conditions. He was not the only one who held this opinion. He cited the famous Maliki scholar Imām ʿAbd Allāh ibn Muḥammad al-Māzirī as saying in relation to this tradition:

> That is because diseases caused by overfilling are of three types: sanguine, biliary or melancholic. If they are sanguine, their treatment is through evacuating blood [by cupping or bloodletting.] If they are of the other types, their treatment is through laxation depending on their causative humor. It is as if the prophet used honey to refer to all laxatives.[132]

Al-Baghdādī's commentary included four traditions recommending cupping. In a rather brief comment, which Ibn Ṭarkhān copied as well, al-Baghdādī explained that cupping was more preferable to bloodletting, especially in hot regions like Arabia, and that it helped clean the surface of the body, which was more suitable for prevention. He then proceeded in explaining the various useful position and times for cupping, which were also explained in more details by Ibn Ṭarkhān.[133] Ibn Ṭarkhān cited other prophetic traditions as well as quotes from Ibn Sīnā's Qānūn to refer to the most beneficial parts of the body for cupping to achieve particular goals. Similarly, Ibn Ṭarkhān explained, using prophetic traditions as well as quotations from Ibn Sīnā, that cupping on the back of the head is harmful and leads to forgetfulness.

Fevers as a condition and honey as a treatment offered a rather different challenge because the prophetic traditions known about each of them seemed to contradict related medical views.[134] For instance, the prophet recommended that fevers be treated using water. He explained in various traditions that fever originated from hellfire, or resembled hellfire, and should be put out by water. For both Ibn Ṭarkhān and al-Baghdādī, this contradicted medical views, which reserved the use of water to a single type of fever: one caused by exposure to the sun and lasting for a day. Other types of fever required other treatments, and some were thought to be made worse with water. Both authors used the tradition to explain at length the various types of fever from a medical point of view and the various ways by which they could be treated. They then explained that the prophet may have referred to fevers caused by sun and heat because these were more common in Arabia.[135] Ibn Ṭarkhān concluded by discussing the pietistic value of fevers and quoted a number of traditions that indicated the rewards reserved to those who withstand the heat of fever.[136] At another level, Ibn Ṭarkhān was also interested in a tradition, in which the prophet said that fevers cleanse the body like fire purifies iron.[137] Although scholars such as Ibn Abī al-Dunyā and others understood this tradition to refer to sins, Ibn Ṭarkhān added another medical meaning by explaining how fevers cleaned and purified the body from various corrupt substances. In this context, both al-Baghdādī and Ibn Ṭarkhān opted to limit the applicability of the prophetic tradition to Arabia and to integrate it within a larger framework of medical knowledge.

The two scholars showed somewhat varying approaches when it came to honey. As shown before, honey was one of the major treatments that the prophet indicated and recommended. Both scholars understood that honey was used as a laxative, or in making laxatives, and therefore was not possible to use for all conditions. Moreover, the iconic tradition where the prophet recommended a man's brother to use honey for treating stomachache posed even more questions. The man's brother seemed to have suffered from diarrhea. His condition also was not improved upon using honey, prompting the prophet to declare, "God has spoken the truth and your brother's belly lied."[138] For both scholars, the medical justification for using honey, a laxative, in a condition of diarrhea was to further cleanse the body from whatever was causing the diarrhea in the first place. They both then asserted that the proclamation that honey is a cure for all ailments needed to be understood as referring to most ailments or to all ailments that require the use of laxatives.[139] In order to prove their points, they brought in a number of examples that showed that these omissions were linguistically correct. Although both scholars attempted to mitigate the apparent differences between the prophetic corpus represented by this iconic tradition and practical medical traditions, Ibn Ṭarkhān went back to affirm the curative value of honey as certain and assured as opposed to the recommendations offered by physicians. As explained before, honey, cupping, and other materials recommended by the prophet emanated, in Ibn Ṭarkhān's view, from divine wisdom and were, therefore, based on certain and unquestionable knowledge.[140] This view cast the explanations offered by Ibn Ṭarkhān in a different light. Although he presented arguments that explained these contradictions, he was clear in his view that prophetic knowledge reigned supreme because of the certainty with which it was imbued.

For al-Baghdādī, dealing with potential differences and apparent contradictions was not new. In fact, his most important book in ḥadīth was in the genre of *mukhtalif al-ḥadīth*, which addressed potential contradictions and looked to explain how these contradictions existed in the prophetic corpus. Placing this discussion within the traditions and views of the genre of *mukhtalif al-ḥadīth* allows for a better understanding of how the authors understood their work and their explanations. Authors in these writings operated under the premise of the need to maintain the coherence of the corpus descending from the prophet, the expansion of which was valuable to scholars of law and ḥadīth alike.[141] At the same time, such corpus could not withstand contradictions and required deep reflections in order to better understand the reasons behind these seeming contradictions. Although in some cases the resolution to these contradictions was through pronouncing one tradition as inauthentic, this was rarely done.[142] Instead, in the majority of cases authors of this genre attempted to maintain the integrity of the corpus by explaining contradictions through invoking abrogation, special cases and circumstances, omissions, or various other interpretative and exegetical tools. Ibn Ṭarkhān did not have al-Baghdādī's track record in this genre or in the sciences of ḥadīth in general; however, his writing showed his familiarity and knowledge of ḥadīth, and his explanations and comments, some of which he derived from al-Baghdādī, were signs of his comfort in the genres of ḥadīth, including *mukhtalif al-ḥadīth*.

In the same way, al-Baghdādī and Ibn Ṭarkhān operated with the intention of maintaining the integrity of the medical and prophetic corpuses and with the premise that contradictions were not possible between two corpuses that were imbued with significant degrees of certainty. Yet similar to how discussions of contradicting ḥadīths entertained a diverse and malleable view of certainty about whether the prophet said or did a particular tradition and operated with a pragmatic and formalistic definition of truth, al-Baghdādī and Ibn Ṭarkhān wrote with an open mind to the construction of certainty, explaining that a number of prophetic traditions may have referred to specific circumstances or contained linguistically sanctioned omissions, symbols, and metaphors. At the same time, both scholars, especially Ibn Ṭarkhān, were keen on establishing a clear hierarchy that placed prophetic knowledge above medical knowledge. The first was ultimately the product of revelation, whereas the latter was a product of speculation.

Conclusion

Did physicians have to be pious? The answer to this question, which lies at the foundation of this chapter, relies primarily on the definition we use for the word pious. Although the Arabic adjectives *muttaqī* and *taqiyy* were used sometimes to describe physicians, they do not capture the entire landscape of piety in this period. Along with these two adjectives, phrases that denote fear of God and commitment to religious obligations, regardless of their nature, and others that emphasized renunciation (zuhd) as well as self-control and discipline were deployed to describe the forms of piety that physicians performed. If piety here is understood to denote certain social performances that condition the production of ethical and proper agents, then being part of the educated elites required a certain level of piety. Belonging to the learned required an avowed disinterest in the matters of this world, a rejection of the control of passion, and a commitment to higher causes that included a lifelong commitment to learning as well as commitment to the dictates of religion. As seen in Chapter 4, such commitments stemmed in part from Galenic Hellenistic ethics and acquired important Islamicate meanings at the hands of scholars like Ibn al-Jawzī, among others. In addition to the volumes of spiritual medicine, these social and epistemic virtues extended to many other ethical writings in various genres. Physicians, as members of the learned elites, espoused these views and ostensibly aimed to recreate this mode of living.

At another level, physicians, similar to other professionals, needed to grapple with the peculiarities of their own profession and the pietistic questions that this profession posed. In the first chapter, we encountered how scholars of ḥadīth, at an early stage of the professional development of the group later known as *ahl al-ḥadīth*, tackled the connection between adab and ḥadīth and provided pietistic explanations to the journey that many of them took from adab and other earthly endeavors to ḥadīth. In the process, they re-created the study of ḥadīth as an endeavor that embodied the prophetic message and argued for the unparalleled importance of ḥadīth in the Islamicate context. Physicians faced similar tasks of producing their profession in a pietistic language. This did not mean that all physicians were pious or that medicine mattered only in so far that it was a religious or pietistic endeavor. Rather, this meant that medical practitioners, along with almost all other learned professionals, worked to place their profession within a pietistic hierarchy that imbued their work with social and epistemic capital. Importantly, this also did not mean that only physicians were concerned with this effort. Many scholars and authors, whether or not writing religious texts, were invested in the categorization of knowledge in general, and some of them paid special attention to medicine – such as Ibn al-Jawzī. In this context, al-Baghdādī, Ibn Abī ʾUṣaybiʿah, and Ibn Ṭarkhān represent important examples of physicians uniquely equipped and positioned to intervene in this question of whether and how to be a pious physician. In this context, al-Baghdādī and Ibn Ṭarkhān's commitment to religious and linguistic training both professionally and through their writings on medicine and ḥadīth made them important examples of physicians uniquely equipped and placed to intervene in this question.

For these physicians, the life of the pious physician was one rooted in continuous learning and sincere following and emulation of the masters of the profession and of the symbols of religious authority. Like all others, they considered imitating the prophet and his companions to be the best approach to piety. At another level, emulating sources of intellectual and pietistic authority contributed to a larger intellectual and professional orientation, where the fathers of the profession were recast as both figures of professional excellence and pietistic authority. In all cases, physicians needed to learn the history of the prophet and his companions, as well as those of Hippocrates and Galen and others. They needed to embody their wise and pious learning by following their advice and emulating their behavior. This emulation was part of a continuous and consistent endeavor of self-fashioning, whereby physicians needed to manage their time, occupy themselves with study and thought, and focus on the improvement of themselves. This attitude of constant self-improvement and the strive for perfection was also part of the ethical formation of educated elites at the time, as seen in Chapter 4.

At another level, these authors aimed to situate medicine within the religious and pietistic hierarchy – a placement that influenced the prestige of their profession and their work. In this regard, they insisted on the role of medicine as a guard of good health and as an endowed nature with which God equipped different beings. Yet these physicians were also interested in maintaining the pietistic ambivalence around illness – suffering was to be welcomed, patience was praised and recommended, and treatment was still commended as a way of following the prophet's sunna. In this context, these scholars expanded the meaning of treatment to include not only Galenic preparations or even modes of diet modifications. They also included prayers, incantations, the Quran, and many other means of treatment. In this medico-pietistic narrative, the meaning of medicine expanded to included not only the learned medical practice but also any other form of healing. At stake was not which medicine was to be used, but whether healing arts were themselves pious. This discussion invoked a deeper conversation about the effectiveness of medicines and whether using prescriptions and preparations was efficacious. In other words, these authors engaged with the question of whether material objects, or even prayers and incantations, could be thought of as useful or helpful and whether believing in their efficacy was in any way impious.

Piety, in Ibn Ṭarkhān's view, did not rely on rejecting the role of objects or words but on the proper orientation and perception of the role of God in this cosmology and, as explained before, in holding and accepting pietistic ambivalence with devotion. In this view, pious Muslims were to understand that certain words had some particular qualities, and that this was particularly true for "[t]he word of God, from which originates all good and to which all good is attributed."[143] This was also true for a number of physical treatments, especially those described by the prophet like cupping, honey, black seed, and others. Yet pious Muslims also needed to believe that all effects were possible because of God's will and that words or other forms of treatment had no inherent effect without His desire: "In general, all incantations and readings are but a supplication to God to grant wellness because of such request, in the same way that He grants wellness because of the medication that he created and destined."[144] Ibn Ṭarkhān used the same logic, which rooted the religious question in the proper belief in the cause of illness and improvement, to explain a tradition in which the prophet was reported to have said, "Whoever used cautery or ruqya absolved himself from reliance on God (*tawakkul*)."[145] In Ibn Ṭarkhān's view, the key question was whether one believes in the value of these procedures on their own independent from God's will or whether one believed in them as tools to bring about God's ultimate will and destiny. For him, the latter was consistent with reliance on God and with pietistic practice.[146]

The same pietistic ambivalence extended to the question of contagion, where the prophet could be seen as permitting people to avoid lepers or escape from the plague and yet, at the same time, also prohibiting them from believing that diseases were innately contagious. Furthermore, the prophet also encouraged Muslims to rely on God's will and to continue to deal with lepers and others.[147] In all these cases, the orders, as explained by Ibn Ṭarkhān, were aimed at protecting pious Muslims from possible delusions that might endanger their faith. By prohibiting people from entering a town afflicted by plague and prohibiting them from leaving it, there would be little risk in people believing that their fate relied on their escape or failure to do so. In the same way, a person getting leprosy after eating with or staring at a leper might be deluded into thinking that this was caused by contagion, without considering God's role and his will, "If this person falls sick, he might think to himself that the sickness was caused by contagion. So he gets deluded (*yuftan*)."[148] Here, the deployment of *fitna* (lit. and in this context, seduction) to indicate the risk of delusion and bad belief highlighted the introspective nature of this pietistic discourse and underlined how such discourse was premised on a continuous process of purifying thoughts and beliefs – even if these thoughts did not manifest in acts.

As a member of the learned elite, a pious physician needed to represent the ethics of sovereignty over the self and to embody moderation and renunciation. He, as learned physicians were almost always men, needed to understand the place of his practice within a pietistic hierarchy. Such understanding meant, first, accepting the superiority of religious and revealed knowledge even when this knowledge was directly related to medical practice. In this context, finding, organizing, and commenting on prophetic traditions that focused on illness, medicine, and healing was in part a performance of epistemic piety whereby epistemic agents organized their knowledge around pietistic habits, texts, and literatures and also an investment in the connection between one's intellectual and professional interest and religious texts and discourses. To be sure, not all physicians engaged in this practice of epistemic and professional piety. In fact, and seeing that the majority of physicians were not Muslim, it is reasonable to say that at least a plurality of physicians did not adopt the views presented by al-Baghdādī and others. Nonetheless, the practice of epistemic piety and the attendant pietistic performances described earlier were deeply connected to Galenic and Hellenistic ethics and, consequently, were constitutive of the urban elite ethic of the time. Thus, these epistemic practices and pietistic performances likely influenced the behaviors of many more physicians than merely those who self-proclaimed as 'pious.'

Notes

1 Ibn Abī Uṣaybi'ah and Najjār, 4: 242.
2 Ibn Mājah (d. 887) was a scholar of ḥadīth who studied with some of the prominent figures in ḥadīth in the ninth century, including Ibn Abī Shaybah. His *Sunan* was the last to be recognized by a growing number of Sunni scholars as one of the most trustworthy books along with al-Bukhārī's, Muslim's, al-Nasāʾī's, Abū Dāwūd's, and al-Tirmidhī's. Brown explained that one of the more attractive qualities of Ibn Mājah's collection was that he included many traditions that did not exist in the previous books expanding what legal scholars can rely on in their work. Brown, "Canonization of Ibn Mâjah."
3 Brown, "Canonization of Ibn Mâjah," 175–6.
4 Kutubī et al., 2: 10. Abū Zarʿah al-Maqdisī (later known as al-Rāzī, see al-Dhahabī, 20: 503) is to be differentiated from the famous and celebrated scholar of ḥadīth, Abū Zarʿah al-Rāzī (d. 878), who was a much more celebrated and influential scholar. The latter was claimed to have praised Ibn Mājah's *Sunan*, a claim doubted by al-Dhahabī and others but one that helped Ibn Mājah's *Sunan* to gain acceptance. See Brown.
5 Scholars of law and ḥadīth valued short isnāds (chains of transmission) for a number of reasons. On one hand, shorter isnāds indicated fewer opportunities for falsification and more reliability. On the other hand, and perhaps more importantly, a shorter isnād was a closer connection to the prophet himself. See Mirza, "The Peoples' Hadith," 63. See also Sayeed, "Women and Ḥadīth Transmission." Sayeed explains how women, especially those who survived into old age, played an important role in shortening chains of transmissions, adding to their importance in ḥadīth circles.
6 Al-Birzālī, *Kitāb al-Arbaʿīn al-Ṭibbiyyah al-Mustakhrajah min Sunan Ibn Mājah wa Sharḥaha lil-ʿAllāmah ʿAbd al-Laṭīf al-Baghdādī*, 3.
7 Ragab, *The Medieval Islamic Hospital*.
8 Ibn Abī Uṣaybi'ah and Najjār, 4: 338.
9 Ragab, *The Medieval Islamic Hospital*.
10 Ibn Abī Uṣaybi'ah and Najjār, 4: 339–40.

11 See Cooperson, *Classical Arabic Biography*. Roded, *Women in Islamic Biographical Collections*.
12 Makdisi, "'Ṭabaqāt'-Biography."
13 Qifṭī, *Tārīkh*.
14 Ragab, *The Medieval Islamic Hospital*.
15 Al-Kaḥḥāl, *Al-Aḥkām al-Nabawīyah fī al-Ṣināʻah al- Ṭibbīyah*.
16 On the *arbaʿīn* (forty) literature in ḥadīth, see Alavi, "Concept of Arba'īn;" and, "Arba'in Literature."
17 Al-Kaḥḥāl, *Al-Aḥkām al-Nabawīyah*.
18 Ibid.
19 Melchert, "Piety of the Hadith Folk." See also Begg, "Hadith as a Means of Routinizing Charisma."
20 Perho, *The Prophet's Medicine*, 56–7.
21 See, for instance, Pormann's excellent analysis of Ibn Abī ʾUṣaybiʿah's biographies as sources for earlier medical practice: Pormann, "Islamic Hospitals." See also Behrens-Abouseif, "Physician in Arab Biographies;" Qaṭāyah, *Al- Ṭabīb al-ʻArabī ʻalī Ibn Riḍwān, raʾīs Aṭibbāʾ Miṣr*; Zuʻbī, *Aṭibbāʾ min al-Tārīkh*.
22 Ibn Abī Uṣaybiʻah and Najjār.
23 In his biography of ʿAbd al-Laṭīf al-Baghdādī, Ibn Abī ʾUṣaybiʿah copied much of al-Baghdādī's biography from one composed by al-Baghdādī himself. Ibn Abī ʾUṣaybiʿah had access to a copy in al-Baghdādī's own handwriting on account of al-Baghdādī's friendship with Ibn Abī ʾUṣaybiʿah's grandfather and father. See Ibn Abī ʾUṣaybiʿah, *ʻUyūn al-Anbāʼ fī Ṭabaqāt al-ʼAṭibbā*, 4: 213.
24 Berkey explains about thirteenth- to fourteenth-century Cairo, "It became routine for scholars to bring their children with them to sessions in which a collection of ḥadīth or some other book was being recited, and for the presiding shaykh to issue ijāzas to the children as well," (Berkey, *The Transmission of Knowledge in Medieval Cairo*, 32). On children's education, see Gil'adi, *Children of Islam*, 42–59.
25 Ibn Abī Uṣaybiʻah and ʻĀmir Najjār, *Kitāb ʻUyūn al-Anbāʾ fī Ṭabaqāt al-Aṭibbāʾ*, 4: 226–7.
26 On ʿAbd al-Laṭīf al-Baghdādī's life and a summary of his autobiography copied by Ibn Abī ʾUṣaybiʿah, see Stern, "A Collection of Treatises by 'Abd al-Laṭīf al-Baghdādī," 53–70. See also Toorawa, "Al-Baghdadi's Education and Instruction." On al-Baghdādī's travels, see Toorawa, "Travel in the Medieval Islamic World." On his work and scholarship, see Pormann and Joosse, "Decline and Decadence;" Shalem, "Experientia and Auctoritas."
27 Muḥammad ibn Shākir Kutubī et al., *Fawāt al-Wafayāt*, 2: 10.
28 Al-Dhahabī, *Siyar Aʻlām al-Nubalāʾ*, 22: 322.
29 Ibn Abī Uṣaybiʻah and Najjār, 4: 229. See also Joosse, "'Unmasking the Craft.'"
30 Ibn Abī Uṣaybiʻah and Najjār, 4: 213 and 4: 341. Ibn Abī ʾUṣaybiʿah's father and uncle studied Aristotle's works with al-Baghdādī as well. However, they studied philosophy and Aristotle's work with Sadīd al-Dīn al-Manṭiqī.
31 Pormann and Joosse.
32 Ibn Abī Uṣaybiʻah and Najjār, 4: 211.
33 Ibid., 4: 218.
34 Ragab, *The Medieval Islamic Hospital*.
35 See Lewicka, "Medicine for Muslims?"
36 Ibid., 163–70.
37 Ibn Abī Uṣaybiʻah and Najjār, 4: 338.
38 Ibid., 4: 339–40.
39 Ibid., 4: 341.
40 Ibid., 4: 348.
41 Ibid., 4: 342–3.
42 Ibid.

43 Ibid., 4: 373.
44 Ibid., 4: 374.
45 Ibid., 4: 374.
46 Ibid., 4: 356.
47 Ibid., 4: 366.
48 Ibid., 4: 237–8.
49 Ibid., 4: 361.
50 Ibid., 4: 362.
51 Ibid., 4: 364.
52 Ibid., 4: 366.
53 Ibid., 4: 367.
54 Ibid., 4: 296–7.
55 Ibid., 4: 364.
56 Ibid., 4: 359.
57 Melchert, "Piety of the Hadith Folk."
58 Ibn Abī Uṣaybiʿah and Najjār, 4: 236.
59 Ibid., 4: 356.
60 Ibid., 4: 364.
61 Ibid., 4: 239.
62 Perho, 57.
63 The first known commentary (*sharḥ*) of Ibn Mājah's *Sunan* was authored by ʿAlāʾ al-Dīn Mughlaṭāy (d. 1361). See Brown, "Canonization of Ibn Mājah," 173.
64 See Chapters 1, 2, and 3 for more details.
65 A cursory examination of medical textbooks from the ninth century on shows that the attitudes of physicians changed towards the use of religiously prohibited materials. Alcohol remained a central question well into the fifteenth century and beyond. However, pork seemed to have disappeared from medical writings. For instance, Ibn Rabbān al-Ṭabarī's (d. 870) *Fridaws al-Ḥikmah*, which was one of the earliest medical textbooks that survived, included advice to use pork as a suitable light food for weaning infants, (Al-Ṭabarī and Jindī, *Firdaws al-Ḥikmah fī al-Ṭibb*) this advice was hardly found later. In fact, religious writings about medicine did not even engage with the use of swine, which seems to have disappeared from common usage.
66 See Lewicka, *Medicine for Muslims?* and, Ragab, *The Medieval Islamic Hospital*, 163–70.
67 See Heck, "Hierarchy of Knowledge."
68 Mottahedeh, "Some Islamic Views."
69 Different biographical dictionaries of physicians started with a discussion of the origin of medicine and the identity of those who first devised the practice. In addition to Ibn Abī ʾUṣaybiʿah, see for instance Qifṭī, *Tārīkh al-Ḥukamāʾ*; and, Ibn Juljul and Sayyid, *Ṭabaqāt al-Aṭibbāʾ wa-al-Ḥukamāʾ*.
70 Al-Kaḥḥāl, 211.
71 Ibid., 211.
72 Ibid., 212.
73 Ibid., 212.
74 Ibid., 213.
75 [Q20: 50].
76 Compare this, for instance, to Ibn Sīnā's definition of medicine in the introduction of his Canon, "Medicine is a science by which the conditions of the human body, in terms of what is healthy [for it] and what causes it to lose health, are known." Ibn Sīnā was aware that this definition put more emphasis on the theoretical. He continued, "One might say that medicine is divided into [theoretical] consideration and practice, and that you have made it all theoretical when you call it a science *ʿilm*. We say that it is said that some crafts are theoretical and others are practical [. . .]. And medicine includes both." (Avicenna, *Kitāb al-Qānūn fī al-Ṭibb*, 1).

77 Al-Birzālī, 5.
78 Ibid., 5–6.
79 Using the subject matter as a measure for developing a hierarchy of knowledge was rather common, and was the one used by Ibn al-Nadīm, for instance, in his *Fihrist* (Ibn al-Nadim, *Al-Fihrist*). See Heck, "The Hierarchy of Knowledge in Islamic Civilization."
80 Al-Kaḥḥāl, 215.
81 This referred to cleaning teeth with a twig mostly from *Arak* trees (*Salvadora persica*). The prophet was reported to recommend cleaning teeth after meals and before prayers.
82 Ibid., 215.
83 This idea of *sunnat allāh* (or the custom of God) was repeated in the Quran and ḥadīth in several occasions. See, for instance, "This is a custom of God (sunna) with those who passed away before. And thou wilt never find in a custom of God any substitution." [Q33: 62] among many others.
84 Ibid.
85 Al-Kaḥḥāl.
86 Ibid.
87 Ibid.
88 Perho, 65–7. The question of *tawakkul*, sometimes translated as 'reliance on God' or 'fatalism,' was discussed by a number of authors in various contexts. See, for instance, Hamdy, "Islam, Fatalism, and Medical Intervention;" Lewisohn, "Way of Tawakkul;" Burrell, "Trust in Divine Providence;" and Kayani, King, and Fleiter, "Fatalism and Road Safety."
89 See Chapter 3 for more details.
90 Al-Birzālī.
91 Al-Kaḥḥāl, 59.
92 Al-Birzālī, 6.
93 Al-Kaḥḥāl.
94 As seen before, this tradition was always recalled in discussions about seeking cure. For instance, and as discussed in Chapter 3, Ibn Baṭṭāl recalled this tradition in his commentary on al-Bukhārī, Ibn Baṭṭāl, Sharḥ Ṣaḥīḥ al-Bukhārī.
95 This was also in line with similar attacks against Sufis at the time, see Anjum, "Sufism Without Mysticism?" and, Ramli, "Rise of Early Sufism."
96 Al-Kaḥḥāl, 328–29.
97 Ibid.
98 Al-Kaḥḥāl, 233–44.
99 Ibid., 242.
100 Ibid., 330.
101 Ibid., 330.
102 See Chapter 3.
103 Al-Birzālī, 36.
104 Ibid., 37.
105 Al-Kaḥḥāl, 99.
106 Ibid., 104.
107 Ibid., 119.
108 Ibid., 316.
109 Ibid., 283.
110 See, for instance, Alvarez-Millán, "Medieval Islamic Medical Literature". Alvarez-Millan explained how al-Rāzī's *mujarrabāt* or experimented preparations made a clear claim to tried efficacy.
111 Al-Rāzī, *Akhlāq al-Ṭabīb*.
112 Ruhāwī, *Adab al-Ṭabīb*.
113 Al-Kaḥḥāl, 98–9.

114 Ibid., 77.
115 Ibid., 77.
116 Ibid., 271.
117 Ibid., 59.
118 Ibid., 147–8.
119 Ibid., 148, 150.
120 Ibid., 153.
121 Ibid., 150–1.
122 Ibid., 123–8.
123 See Chapter 1 for more details.
124 Al-Kaḥḥāl, 125.
125 Ibid., 125.
126 Ibid., 267. The same tradition was also reported by Abū Nuʿaym al-Asfahānī in his *Prophetic Medicine* (al-Aṣbahānī, 32).
127 Al-Birzālī, 38.
128 Al-Kaḥḥāl, 267.
129 Ibn Mājah included this tradition in his treatise on funerals, where he also compiled traditions related to visiting patients. It was recalled by al-Baghdādī in his commentary but was not part of the treatise on medicine, which he was commenting on, Al-Birzālī, 38; and, Al-Kaḥḥāl, 267–8.
130 Al-Birzālī, 39.
131 Ibid., 40–1.
132 Kaḥḥāl, 102–3.
133 Al-Birzālī, 34–5.
134 See the discussion about fevers in Chapter 3.
135 Al-Kaḥḥāl, 64.
136 Ibid., 65–8.
137 Ibid., 68.
138 Ibid., 75.
139 Ibid., 102–3.
140 Ibid., 77.
141 See Brown, "Critical Rigor vs. Juridical Pragmatism."
142 Relying on meaning or content to reject a particular tradition was often referred to as *matn* criticism – a practice in ḥadīth sciences that became common starting perhaps in the thirteenth and fourteenth centuries. Brown has argued convincingly that this form of criticism was practiced in the early period of ḥadīth science history, albeit without naming it as such. See Brown, "Matn Criticism."
143 Ibid., 125.
144 Ibid., 117.
145 Ibid., 275.
146 Ibid., 275.
147 Ibid., 151.
148 Ibid., 153.

Coda

This book is invested in three main pursuits: piety, patienthood, and medieval Islam. Each of these concepts provides important points of departure for elaborate investigations in a variety of directions. Here, I have explored each locus only to the point where it intersects with the other two. Limiting this investigation to these intersections presented certain challenges and opportunities. Foremost is the undeniable fact that these intersections cannot provide a full understanding of such categories. A full understanding of these categories requires a deeper investigation into the networks of meanings and symbols that construct these categories, which spread over various genres and relied on different languages, traditions, and epistemic practices. At the same time, this admittedly more modest pursuit of looking into the intersection of these three categories offers the opportunity to dive deeper into a particularly rich area for investigation that can furnish important insights on the various meanings of these three categories beyond their intersection. I argue that the practices, traditions, and spaces of patienthood taking place in the medieval and classical Islamic context provided an important accentuation of the modes in which piety engaged with embodied practices and performances. Furthermore, this space and temporal (historical) period was key in the making of authoritative discourses on piety and patienthood in the medieval period and beyond.

As a coda to this volume, I will reflect and meditate on these three categories, ruminating on these intersections and exploring possibilities that this book's investigation may have opened or could have overlooked.

Piety

Piety is a term that has a long and elaborate history in the study of religion. I took piety in this book as a translation of the term *taqwā*, which indicates fear from and reverence to God.[1] If seen from the contours of this term, piety is not only ubiquitous in Islamic writings from the medieval period and until today; it is also a central concept that governs how Muslims were instructed to understand their obligations to God and to their community. Piety here is not an equivalent of religious law or another expression of the religious obligations that Muslims needed to fulfill. Instead, it hovers over this sphere of legality, creating the environment in which the worth of deeds is adjudicated depending on the intentions of those who undertake these deeds.[2] Moreover, piety represents what lies beyond the law as a practice that engages more concretely with the making of the religious self.[3]

As a font of embodied as well as intellectual practice, piety acts as a locus for investigating the process through which religion, as a set of texts, practices, and institutions constantly in a hermeneutical dynamic of reproduction, manifests in the lives of the religious. In this book, piety is a practice of self-making that informs traditions of understanding oneself in relation to God, the prophet, and society. Here, piety stands as a site for exploring a temporality of anticipation – the affect that is awaited and constantly in a process of remaking and realization but almost never fully accomplished.[4] For the pious, we are never pious enough. This anticipatory, suspicious, if not paranoid, temporality that governs the production of piety is rooted in the enunciatory function of pietistic performances, as evidence of seeking, attempting, and reaching but never of accomplishing. Pietistic performances are indeed communicative acts that condition certain forms of reception, rely on identifiable lexicon, and engender a space of self-making.[5] Piety cannot be reduced to what was done or achieved or to what is required, legal, permitted, or prohibited. Instead, it functions precisely in this anticipatory space that works to condition the affects from whence acts and thoughts emerge.[6] As a social lexicon, piety is an inspirational script. It works to condition the future of action and thought by implicating the past and engaging the present. The pious, as a category of social recognition, is therefore in a constant state of self-realization, and they are judged not on following the letters of law or tradition, but for their reverence to them.

As such, piety is not only a religious phenomenon but rather a sociocultural category of discipline. The rules of self-making apply in relation to various social and cultural activities and positions from medicine to politics to religion and ethics. Yet in its function as a lexicon of sociocultural worth, piety is constructed in shared materials and resources and rooted in communal understandings and practices.[7] As such, and in this book, the investigation of piety hinges on these two interconnecting valences: anticipation and archival construction. In its anticipatory valence, piety transcends the questions of the legal and prohibited and those of right and duty. It functions to construct the infrastructure in which acts of following the law or conforming to the rules become acts of ritualized reverence and appreciation.[8] At the same time, in its nature as a process of archival construction, piety involves semantic negotiations where networks of meanings are distributed on certain symbols and where shared narratives, stories, recommendations, and acts form an archive that is at once dynamic and malleable and also legible and interpretable. The pious is made and remade at these intersections and through a self-making endeavor that is rooted in unachievable futurity that acquires meaning through comprehensible iterations.

In this view, piety is deeply connected to self-care. In his work on self-care, Foucault explained how concepts of care were rooted in Hellenistic or Greco-Roman understandings of the body as a constant work in progress and of selfhood as an endeavor toward modes of perfection.[9] This ethic of self-care conditioned processes of self-reflection and investigation, whereby individuals needed to understand themselves and contend with their desires and passions.[10] It also created iterative modes of self-education and training where free men performed their perfection through the constant endeavor toward perfection itself. In other words, in Foucault's view, self-care constituted ritualized social and individual performances that produced particular meanings and identities rooted in embodied discourses of observance and care.[11] In this book, piety acquires similar dimensions at a number of levels. At one level, piety was an iterative process whereby the pursuit of pietistic behaviors was in itself pietistic. At another level, piety required strict modes of self-awareness where the pious agent needed to observe themselves and understand the motives behind their deeds. Ultimately, these motives and intentions were the central component of pietistic performance, on which hinged divine reward.

This mode of observance demanded and facilitated the development of introspective subjectivities where the pious agent performed themselves as self-obsessed and disinterested in the praise of the blame of others. Although pietistic acts were, by definition, outwardly in that they were directed to God who existed outside the self, they served to draw the pietistic agent closer to God, who now came to occupy a position that was physically between the pious agent and the world. As seen before, pietistic writings about illness explained how visiting a patient would indeed be a visit to God who resided with the patient (Chapter 3). In this context, the visit, although remaining an outward act of piety that involved another person, was transformed into an interior reflection about God and his presence. One was visiting God, and the visited patient became the occasion for this encounter with God. Another tradition that circulated widely explained how money given in charity fell in the hand of God before falling in the hands of beggars. The tradition narrated how pious companions would dip the money they give in charity in perfume, explaining that these coins were indeed being dropped in God's hands.

At another level, this pietistic performance of self-care was a value in itself. Although God came to occupy the position of a party to these pietistic exchanges, pietistic narratives insisted on the fact that God did not need any of these practices.[12] God's acceptance of these acts and His intervention in their performance was a conduit for one to develop the pietistic habits that are necessary for good and proper living.[13] More importantly, there was never enough piety. As such, the process of seeking to learn and understand and to teach oneself how to behave and think in a pietistic manner was in itself an act of piety that required its own self-reflection and its own patterns of observance.[14] As shown before, the notion of collecting ḥadīth and of learning about the behavior of the prophet for the purposes of emulating him exemplified this form of piety.[15] As such, considering piety as self-care allows for a deeper understanding of the processual nature of pietistic practice and for the futuristic and anticipatory temporality in which piety operates.

At the same time, and as explained before, piety did not only operate in the future but also in the past, building on examples and developing from narratives of precedence. Here, Annemarie Schimmel, following Armand Abel, proposed the concept of *imitatio Muhammadi* as a mode of thinking about this overarching character of Islamic piety, which relied heavily on imitating and emulating the prophet:

> But it was through this imitation of Muhammad's actions as transmitted through the ḥadīth that Islamic life assumed a unique uniformity in social behavior, a fact that has always impressed visitors to all parts of the Muslim world. It is also visible, for instance, in the hagiography of Muslim saints. For, as Frithjof Schuon says: "This 'Muhammadan' character of the virtues . . . explains the relatively impersonal style of the saints; there are no other virtues than those of Muhammad, so they can only be repeated in those who follow his example; it is through them that the Prophet lives in his community."[16]

In this view, the past of the pietistic performance is rooted in ḥadīth as a testimony to the practice of the prophet and a key to understanding how the prophet performed his life.

Abel and Schimmel's mobilization of *imitatio Christi* in their coining of the term *imitatio Muhammadi* to understand this practice of emulating the prophet is a useful starting point for a deeper investigation into the making of the Islamic practice of emulation. In particular, it is useful for this present investigation, which is invested in the period where the *emulatable* image of Muḥammad emerged with the production of ḥadīth collections and books on zuhd (renunciation) and *raqāʾiq* (exhortations). Here, I argued that the image of Muḥammad emerged in an historical process that could be traced through the writings of Ibn Saʿd and many others who followed him.[17] At the same time, I also argued that this interest in the details of Muḥammad's life emerged, in part, at the intersection of the encyclopedic culture of adab, with its varying interests, and the legal debates that aimed to establish prophetic authority and to create a temporal break with the immediate past for the benefit of constructing a more distant ideal.[18] This process of the historical making of Muḥammad as an object of veneration and a character with detailed contours was key to making Muḥammad *emulatable.*

At another level, *imitatio Muhammadi* differs from *imitatio Christi* in its intentionally fragmented nature. Ḥadīth, by virtue of its narrative structure and its historical connection to adab, was never composed of long and connected narratives.[19] Instead, it was made of *petits recits* (or little narratives), which were collected and culled from various sources and deployed for a variety of reasons and to serve various purposes. To borrow Jean-Francois Lyotard's analytic, the structures of ḥadīth exhibited aversion to a controlling grand narrative.[20] Although a meta-narrative that underscored the infallibility or the religious and intellectual authority of the prophet developed over time, it only served as a background to the web of little narratives – localized, limited, event focused, and occasion sensitive – that constituted the body of ḥadīth. In this view, Muḥammad, as an *emulatable* character, was the product of an archive of these little narratives – a picture that is intentionally fragmented and that provides meaning only at two levels: at the meta-level as a discourse about prophethood that is devoid of details and at the micro-level as localized, event-focused narratives. At the same time, the legacy of Muḥammad, as protected and reported in ḥadīth, was never unified, purified, or simply reduced to the canonical or trustworthy.[21] In fact, and as discussed before, although legal scholars attempted to create tools to adjudicate the comparative legal and normative authority of particular traditions, pietistic writings, sometimes authored by the same scholars, continued to accept a much wider spectrum of ḥadīths and showed significant tolerance of the requirements of authenticity.[22]

As such, the role of the ḥadīth scholar was one of collecting, curating, and deploying these little narratives in a variety of situations and for different purposes. The piety that resulted from this particular archive was one that is equally fragmented and intentionally piecemealed. In fact, it is the fragmented nature of this piety that provided it with significant strength and endowed this archive with staying power over the centuries. In the absence of a grand narrative, and in accepting this fragmented nature of the archive as a manifestation of the pietistic performance of salvaging the prophet's legacy, contradictory positions could coexist and thrive. In fact, I argue in this book that the idea of ambivalence and the need to hold contradictory, paradoxical, or ambivalent positions in tension was at the heart of the performance of Islamic piety, especially in relation to illness.[23] Escaping this ambivalence and attempting to construct a singular position was sometimes, but not always, necessary in law but was hardly attempted in pietistic narratives, which thrived on the multiplicity of views that one could choose from and invested in a pietistic economy where not all could perform all acts and where more was almost always possible and recommended. Here, I argue that the narrative nature of this pietistic corpus was key to the development of this peculiar form of pietistic habitus: an ambivalent one.

Patienthood

Similar to piety, patienthood is equally futuristic and anticipatory. I have thought of patienthood in this book not simply as an epistemic category that endows individual moments of illness with meaning and supplies individual patients with resources for communication. It is also a category of future certainties that acquire meaning through previous iterations, whether affecting the self or the other, and through epistemic systems of normalcy and health constructed around scientific, religious, and other sociocultural discourses. Patienthood is therefore a process that invites active subscription and investment. To subscribe to a particular mode of patienthood is to engage in a constant process of self-investigation that anticipates the next illness or disease and that affirms, even through doubting, the connected narratives of normalcy and health. As opposed to sickness, patienthood is an open-ended ritual practice whereby those branded or subscribed to the state of illness – past, present, and future – invest in the reincarnation of this state and in its inscription on their bodies – both as a general category of embodied existence, or as a particular iteration of social selfhood. Patienthood is therefore the ever-changing answer to the question of how, not why, we get sick. In this view, patienthood is also premised on an iterative process of self-care where accepting or rejecting illness and preparing for it or protecting oneself against it are rooted in a constant process of observing oneself in relation to normalcy and in considering how the body acted and behaved.[24]

At another level, and in the context of this study, I have argued that patienthood was an occasion for the production of a ritualistic space that was endowed with the presence of God, often portrayed in a physical sense.[25] As mentioned before, God was seen as present in the company of the sick awaiting visitors. This was also a reason why it was recommended to ask the sick to pray for their visitors as they were party to this continuous process of divine presence. In the Islamic context, God revealed the rituals by which he preferred to be worshipped. For instance, in the story of Adam and Eve, God revealed to Adam the words which he used to pray for forgiveness. In the same way, God revealed the various rituals that the prophet used and instructed his nation to follow in their worship. In this context, the call-and-response structure that animated the pietistic practice of patienthood was reminiscent of these revealed worship-words and further emphasized the space of illness as a ritualistic one.[26]

In addition, patienthood conditioned a particular form of piety, as explained before. Here, patienthood invoked an epistemic investigation into causes and results and motivated decisions about seeking or rejecting cure. This investigation of causality, which ended with God as the ultimate cause of illness, developed into a process of recognition that mirrored the admission of God's unity and supremacy over creation. It also emphasized the ambivalent nature of the pietistic endeavor by focusing on the need to recognize and accept God as the cause of illness while refraining from blaming him. In the same vein, the question of seeking cure was also portrayed pietistically, but not legally, as one that carried layers of ambivalence that depended on one's ability to withstand, the nature of one's diseases, and the type of sins that one believed they had committed.[27] Finally, as the recognition of correct causality mirrored the process of recognizing God's unity and power, the space of patienthood was one that encouraged significant modes of self-reflection as one was to question their thoughts to ensure that they were not visited by doubt and that the pietistic ambivalence that they cultivated was not undermined by their affliction.[28]

Diseases, however, were not only physical. Spiritual patienthood, a different form of patienthood, was also investigated and accrued a significant amount of pietistic writings. Here, it is instructive to recall Foucault's understanding of the nature of medicalization in self-care as a discursive mode that engaged forms of knowledge and experience in discourses of normalcy and imbued it with the power and authority of medical narratives.[29] Spiritual diseases stood as part of ethical discourses that aimed for the continuous perfection of the self through control, moderation, and rational thought, which was understood as subjecting the spirit to the control of the intellect. Here, the causality structure was different from physical ills. Although physical ills needed to be directly attributed to God, pietistic writings instructed that spiritual ills were part of human nature. In fact, some argued that these spiritual ills emerged from divinely endowed qualities that aimed to protect and save the body. Hunger, and the resulting gluttony, were meant to ensure that the body consumed its needs. Sex and the attendant promiscuity or excessive passion were necessary for the maintenance of humans on earth. Even anger was necessary to allow one to fight for their existence. As such, the spiritual ills were rather deviations from the divinely endowed good nature, which needed to be protected by the intellect and by the dictates of religious law.[30]

These two modes of patienthood, physical and spiritual, provoke important questions about the individual's sovereignty over their body and spirit. On one hand, physical patienthood demonstrated that sovereignty over the physical body was always limited and incomplete. One was responsible for the way they used their bodies, but the body ultimately belonged to God and was even called upon to testify against its owners in the Day of Judgement.[31] The piety that physical patienthood engendered was one rooted in accepting this lack of control and deficient sovereignty over the body and in realizing that God controlled the fate of the body in this world and in the next. The manifestation of this acceptance of incomplete sovereignty was through patience and surrender to God's will. This is why the discussion of seeking cure ultimately revolved around whether cure demonstrated a form of rejection of God's will. Although God would ultimately determine whether a cure would work, the question concerned whether seeking cure was, in a way, an attempt to escape God's control or subvert the divine sovereign order.[32]

On the other hand, spiritual patienthood was rooted in the individual's failure to exercise their divinely endowed sovereignty. Spiritual diseases were not to be tolerated or accepted but to be prevented and cured as soon as possible. Here, the individual, perceived as an ethical agent that stood outside the body, the spirit, and, at times, even the intellect, exerted their sovereignty as arbiters and were to exercise their power by following the dictates of religious law and God's commandments. The pietistic energy here was directed not to accepting an incomplete sovereignty as part of the servitude to God, but rather in asserting sovereignty over the spirit as part of what distinguished humans from animals and as part of one's responsibility in this world. Self-reflection here acquired a more powerful meaning as one reflected and monitored the spirit for which one was responsible. It was therefore natural for authors of spiritual medicine to move from this discussion to discussing one's responsibility to their wives, children, and slaves. Here, too, the order of the world as endowed by God placed specific actors in particular positions and endowed them with certain responsibilities that they needed to fulfill.

The line that separated the practices of pietistic sovereignty also separated the different gendered forms of sovereignty. Physical patienthood was presented as a space of pietistic practice for people of all genders and ages. Women were used as examples of good and commendable behavior. They, too, were to be visited and God was present in their company. Because physical patienthood demanded admission of missing or incomplete sovereignty as a pietistic practice, it was fully available to those whose sovereignty over their bodies was already restricted by gendered, racial, sexual, social, religious, political, and financial structures, among others. Spiritual patienthood, on the other hand, was only available to those who enjoyed a socially sanctioned practice of sovereignty: essentially, freemen.[33]

Ultimately, patienthood, as a mode of self-reflection and self-care, intersected with piety, which addressed the same questions and engendered similar practices. In fact, as piety was indeed a social virtue that crossed sectarian and religious lines, patienthood was possible to articulate only at the intersection of pietistic and medical discourses. Although the experience of illness and the space of patienthood was not based only on these pietistic concerns, such concerns, and the archive that constructed them, were key to the making of patienthood during this period.

Medieval Islam

In meditating on the category of medieval Islam, I do not wish to provide a justification for the study of this period by invoking its utility and relevance to contemporary or presentist concerns. The relevance, utility, and legitimacy of this study have been demonstrated by many scholars of Islamic studies throughout the history of the discipline. Instead, I aim to interrogate the deployment of this category in the contemporary as a mode of describing, analyzing, and disciplining Islam as a religion and as a religio-ethnic identity. "Medieval" and "medievalism" are categories endowed with moral significance. Throughout the colonial and postcolonial period, and particularly in the post-9/11 world, the descriptive "medieval" has been deployed to present Islam, and those who carry it as a belief or as an identity, as belonging to the past, lacking in the requirements of modern living, and as savage, backward, and barbaric. Here, "medieval" is not descriptive of chronology but rather a requirement of a moral historiography that attributes worth in relation to the modern Euro-American.[34] In this context, "medieval Islam" becomes the diagnostic that justifies marginalization, securitization, and exclusion as it has served to justify colonization before. As a specter that haunts the contemporary, "medieval Islam" is defined as an identity and as a state of being that demands apology and justification on the part of Muslims. This moral deployment of the term "medieval" renders it superfluous as it integrates within the meaning of Islam itself. Islam, in this discourse, is medieval, and "medieval Islam" is a redundancy at best and a complacency at worst.

In this context, the study of medieval Islam can be a subversive act in its endeavor to recapture the word medieval as a descriptive of chronology that is devoid of moralization. Although the term lies within the European chronology, the study of medieval Islam should aim to animate the dating of "medieval" as a mode of subverting and resisting its moral significance and its deployment in securitized discourses. As such, I argue that the study of medieval Islam carries an emancipatory potential in locating Muslims as beings with history rather than fossils frozen in history. By adding to the details and knowledge of how medieval Islam is a version and not an essence, a history and not a Platonic form, the study of medieval Islam provides a texture that serves to liberate contemporary Muslims from the authoritative and normative identity that renders them an other and justifies their policing and their colonization.

In this context, the narrativistic nature of the texts I engaged in this book and their composition of little narratives that resist purification, unification, or consolidation, animates them, and in turn, animates the medieval Islam that they construct, as objects of continuous hermeneutics. I argue that the nature of this pietistic archive is one that is rooted in curating, editing, arranging, and configuring. It is also a narrative form that demands these operations and a pietistic text that places worth in these epistemic practices of curating and interpreting. At the same time, I argue that the ambivalent nature of this pietistic discourse renders hermeneutics not only possible but often necessary, and not only at the authoritative and learned level, but also at the level of the daily and individual. Although this particular archive acquired the staying power that its revelatory claims underwrite and was endowed with the attendant intellectual and epistemic authority, this power and this authority could only manifest through consistent processes of curating and editing that continuously changed the nature and the meaning of this archive.

Indeed, I argue that this archive produced in the Islamic classical period – a period that chronologically maps on the medieval – does indeed have influence on the contemporary and has claims on the pietistic practices of contemporary Muslims. However, this influence can only be achieved through a hermeneutic that is necessarily contemporary. At the same time, the archive's revelatory claims work to obfuscate these processes of hermeneutics in order to channel the staying power of the text over time. In investigating this archive, its modes of construction, and the connected manners of argumentation and hermeneutics, I aimed to uncover how it functioned and continues to function, precisely, as an archive: one that acquires its legitimacy by its connection to the past but lacks the ability to construct meanings except by the modes of arrangement of the present. To be sure, this work does not claim to investigate all the various modes of hermeneutics that were deployed to arrange this archive, choosing to focus on a rather early period where this archive was compiled and where the traditions of hermeneutics were developed. In doing so, it looks at only a sliver of what this archive contains and peaks at but a single card in its branching catalog. Far more modest in its hopes, this work aspires to the production of a new scholarly font that highlights the historically specific and contemporarily relevant archive of medieval or classical Islam. It also aims to place itself as a statement of subversion for the contemporary mode of deployment of medieval or classical Islam as an overarching, overpowering identity that failed or escaped the process of interpretation.

In this context, piety, as it intersects with the bodily practice of patienthood, presented an opportunity to locate the medieval Islamic archive at the intersection of the embodied, localized, and "little" in response to its deployment as disembodied, universal, and grand.

Notes

1 Jafri, "Particularity and Universality;" Ohlander, "Fear of God (Taqwā);" Christopher Melchert, "Exaggerated Fear."

2 Powers, "Interiors, Intentions, and the "Spirituality.'"
3 Sheikh, "Sources of Selfhood and Technologies." See also Schofer, "Ethical Formation and Subjection."
4 Here, I am drawing on works on queer temporality and the notions of anticipation and nonrealization. See, for instance, Dinshaw et al., "Theorizing Queer Temporalities"; Halberstam, "Queer Temporality and Postmodern Geographies" and *In a Queer Time and Place*; and Sedgwick, *Touching Feeling*.
5 See Sedgwick, *Touching Feeling*. See also Weheliye, *Habeas Viscus*.
6 See, for instance, Ibn al-Jawzī's discussion of training oneself as shown in Chapter 4. In one of Ibn al-Jawzī's anecdotes, a pious man explained that he drove his spirit to piety while it screamed long enough until he was able to drive it to piety while it celebrated. Here and in other places, narratives of self-formation were key to the discussion of pietistic performance.
7 See discussions of pietistic institutions, for instance, in Talmon-Heller, *Islamic Piety in Medieval Syria*.
8 See, for instance, Ibn Baṭṭāl's discussion of the difference between the legal and pious in relation to seeking cure (Chapter 3). Similarly, Ibn Tarkhān engaged with Ibn Ḥanbal's differentiation between pious and legal behavior in relation to seeking medical care (Chapter 5).
9 Foucault, *The History of Sexuality, vol. 3*.
10 See Chapter 4.
11 Foucault, *The History of Sexuality, vol. 3*.
12 Al-Kūfī, *Kitāb al-Zuhd*.
13 Ibn Al-Jawzī, *Al-Ṭibb al-Rūḥānī*.
14 See, for instance, the discussion on the piety of ḥadīth students in Chapter 1. See also Al-Rāmhurmuzī, *Al-Muḥaddith al-Fāṣil Bayna al-Rāwī wa al-Wā'ī*; Melchert, "Piety of the Hadith Folk."
15 See Chapter 1.
16 Schimmel, *And Muhammad Is His Messenger*.
17 Chapter 1.
18 Chapter 1.
19 Sperl, "Man's 'Hollow Core;'" Khalidi, *Images of Muhammad*.
20 Lyotard, *The Postmodern Condition*.
21 See, for instance, the resistance to the efforts of al-Bukhārī and Muslim ibn al-Ḥajjāj in constructing a corpus of authentic ḥadīth, Brown, *The Canonization of al-Bukhārī and Muslim*.
22 Chapter 1. See also Brown, "Did the Prophet Say It or Not?"
23 Chapter 3.
24 See Kleinman, *Patients and Healers in the Context of Culture* and *The Illness Narratives*.
25 Chapter 3.
26 Chapter 3.
27 Chapter 3.
28 Chapter 3.
29 Foucault, *The History of Sexuality, vol. 3*.
30 Chapter 4.
31 Chapter 3. See also Hamdy, *Our Bodies Belong to God*.
32 Chapter 3.
33 Chapter 4.
34 Ragab, "Monsters and Patients."

Bibliography

Abbott, Nabia. "Hadith Literature – II: Collection and Transmission of Hadith." *Arabic Literature to the End of the Umayyad Period* (1983): 289–98.

Abd Allāh, Maḥmūd Sayyid, and Muḥammad ʻAbd al-Sattār Uthmān. *Madāfin Ḥukkām Miṣr Al-Islāmīyah Bi-Madīnat Al-Qāhirah.* Alexandria: Dār al-Wafā' li-Dunyā al-Ṭibāʻah wa-al-Nashr, 2004.

Abū Dāwūd, al-Ḥāfiẓ Sulayman ibn al-Ashʾath al-Azdī. *Sunan Abī Dāwūd.* Beirut: al-Maktabah al-ʾAṣriyyah, 2009.

Adamson, Peter. "Platonic Pleasures in Epicurus and Al-Rāzī." In *In the Age of al-Farābī: Arabic Philosophy in the Fourth-Tenth Century*, edited by Peter Adamson, 71–97. London: Warburg Institute, 2008.

———. "Avicenna and His Commentators on Human and Divine Self-Intellection." *The Arabic, Hebrew and Latin Reception of Avicenna's Metaphysics* (2011): 97–122.

———. "Abū Bakr Al-Rāzī on Animals." *Archiv für Geschichte der Philosophie* 94, no. 3 (2012): 249–73.

———. "Abū Bakr Al-Rāzī (D. 925), the Spiritual Medicine." In *The Oxford Handbook of Islamic Philosophy*, edited by Khaled El-Rouayheb and Sabine Schmidtke, 63–82. Oxford: Oxford University Press, 2016.

———. "Health in Arabic Ethical Works." In *Health*, edited by Peter Adamson. Oxford: Oxford Univeristy Press, Forthcoming.

Afsaruddin, Asma. *Excellence and Precedence: Medieval Islamic Discourse on Legitimate Leadership.* Leiden: Brill, 2002.

Aguadé, Jorge. "Some Remarks About Sectarian Movements in Al-Andalus." *Studia Islamica*, no. 64 (1986): 53–77.

Aigle, Denise. "Les Autorités Religieuses dans l'Islam Médiéval. Essai." In *Les Autorités Religieuses Entre Charismes Et Hiérarchie. Edited by Denise Aigle*, 17–40. Turnhout: Brepols, 2011.

ʻAlā' al-Dīn al-Kaḥḥāl, ʻAlī ibn ʻAbd al-Karīm. *Al-Aḥkām Al-Nabawīyah Fī Al-Ṣināʻah Al-Ṭibbīyah.* Edited by Aḥmad ʻAbd al-Ghanī al-Najūlī Jamal. al-Ṭabʻah 1. ed. Beirut and Kuwait: Maktabat Ibn Kathīr; Dār Ibn Ḥazm lil-Ṭibāʻah wa-al-Nashr wa-al-Tawzīʻ, 2003.

Alajmi, Abdulhadi, and Khaled Keshk. "Umayyad Ideology and the Recurrence of the Past/Ideología omeya y el recurso al pasado." *Anaquel de Estudios Árabes* 24 (2013): 7.

Alavi, Khalid. "The Concept of Arba'īn and Its Basis in the Islamic Tradition." *Islamic Studies* 22, no. 3 (1983): 71–93.

———."A Brief Survey of Arba' in Literature (up to the Time of al-Nawawi)." *Islamic Studies* 23, no. 2 (1984): 67–82.

Alghani, Jalal. "Mediaeval Arabic Love Theory Between Dissonance and Consonance: Abū Bakr Muḥammad Ibn Zakariyyā, Al-Rāzī and His Argument Against, Ishq." *Acta Orientalia* 67, no. 3 (2014): 273–87.

Amir-Moezzi, Mohammad Ali. "Seul L'homme de Dieu Est Humain: Theologie et Anthropologie Mystique à Travers L'exégèse Imamite Ancienne (Aspects de l'Imamologie Duodécimaine IV)." *Arabica* 45, no. 2 (1998): 193–214.

———. *The Divine Guide in Early Shi'ism: The Sources of Esotericism in Islam*. New York: SUNY Press, 2016.

Anjum, Ovamir. "Sufism Without Mysticism? Ibn Qayyim al-Ǧawziyyah's Objectives in 'Madāriǧ al-Sālikīn.'" *Oriente Moderno* 90, no. 1 (2010): 161–88.

Anjum, Tanvir. "Sufism in History and Its Relationship with Power." *Islamic Studies* 45, no. 2 (2006): 221–68.

Al-Anṣārī, Abū Yūsuf Ya'qūb ibn Ibrāhīm. *Kitāb al-Āthār*. Haydar Abad: Lajnat Iḥyā' al-Ma'ārif al-Nu'mānīyah, 1937.

Arjomand, Said Amir. "The Constitution of Medina: A Sociolegal Interpretation of Muhammad's Acts of Foundation of the Umma." *International Journal of Middle East Studies* 41, no. 4 (2009): 555–75.

Arkoun, Mohammed. *Contribution á L'étude de L'humanisme Arabe Au Ive/Xe Siècle: Miskawayh (320/325–421)*. Vol. 12. Paris: Vrin, 1970.

———. *Humanisme Arabe Au Iv/Xe Siecle*. Paris: Vrin, 1982.

Al-Aṣbahānī, Abū Nu'aym Aḥmad ibn 'Abd Allāh. *Al-Ṭibb Al-Nabawiyy*. Beirut: Dār Ibn Ḥazm, 2006.

Ashtiany, Julia. *Abbasid Belles Lettres*. Vol. 2. Cambridge: Cambridge University Press, 1990.

Assef, Qais. "Le Soufisme et Les Soufis Selon Ibn Taymiyya." *Bulletin d'études orientales* 60, no. 1 (2012): 91–121.

Avicenna. *Kitāb al-Qānūn fī al-Ṭibb*. Romae: In Typographia medicae, 1593.

Al-Azmeh, Aziz. "Rhetoric for the Senses: A Consideration of Muslim Paradise Narratives." *Journal of Arabic Literature* 26, no. 3 (1995): 215–31.

Bacharach, Jere L. "Marwanid Umayyad Building Activities: Speculations on Patronage." *Muqarnas* 13 (1996).

Al-Balkhī, Aḥmad ibn Sahl. *Maṣāliḥ Al-Abdān Wa-Al-Anfus*. Edited by Mahmoud Maṣrī and Ahmed al-Khayyat. Cairo: Ma'had al-Makhtutat al-'Arabiyyah, 2005.

Bar-Asher, Meir M. "Quelques Aspects de L'éthique D'abū-Bakr Al-Rāzī Et Ses Origines dans L'œuvre de Galien (Première Partie)." *Studia Islamica* (1989): 5–38.

Bauer, Karen. "Emotion in the Qur'an: An Overview." *Journal of Qur'anic Studies* 19, no. 2 (2017): 1–30.

Bauhng, Victor Jongjin. "Early Sīra Material and the Battle of Badr." *SOAS (School of Oriental and African Studies)* (2012).

Begg, Rashid. "Hadith as a Means of Routinizing Charisma." *Religion and Theology* 19, nos. 1–2 (2012): 110–21.

Behrens-Abouseif, Doris. "The Image of the Physician in Arab Biographies of the Post-Classical Age." *Der Islam; Zeitschrift für Geschichte und Kultur des Islamischen Orients* 66 (1989): 331.

Bellamy, James A. "The Makārim al-Akhlāq by Ibn Ab?'L-Dunyā (A Preliminary Study)." *The Muslim World* 53, no. 2 (1963): 106–19.

Berkey, Jonathan Porter. *The Transmission of Knowledge in Medieval Cairo: A Social History of Islamic Education*. Princeton: Princeton University Press, 2014.

Bernabé-Pons, Luis F. "Taqiyya, Niyya y el Islam de los Moriscos." *Al-Qanṭara* 34, no. 2 (2013): 491–527.

Biesterfeldt, Hans Hinrich. "Medieval Arabic Encyclopedias of Science and Philosophy." In *The Medieval Hebrew Encyclopedias of Science and Philosophy*, edited by Steven Harvey, 77–98. Dordercht, Boston: Kluwer Academic Publishers, 2000.

Bin Ramli, Harith. "The Rise of Early Sufism: A Survey of Recent Scholarship on Its Social Dimensions." *History Compass* 8, no. 11 (2010): 1299–315.

Al-Birzālī, Muḥammad ibn Yusuf. *Kitāb al-Arbaʾīn al-Ṭibbiyyah al-Mustakhrajah min Sunan Ibn Mājah wa Sharḥaha lil-ʾAllāmah ʾAbd al-Laṭīf al-Baghdādī*. Titwan, Morocco: Lisān al- Dīn, 1951.

Bonebakker, Seeger A. "Adab and the Concept of Belles-Lettres." In *Abbasid Belles-Lettres*, edited by Julia Ashtiany, 16–30. Cambridge: Cambridge University Press, 1990.

Bonner, Michael. "The Kitāb al-Kasb Attributed to al-Shaybānī: Poverty, Surplus, and the Circulation of Wealth." *Journal of the American Oriental Society* 121, no. 3 (2001/07).

Bosworth, Clifford Edmund. "A Pioneer Arabic Encyclopedia of the Sciences: Al-Khwarizmi's Key of the Sciences." *Isis* 54, no. 1 (1963): 97–111.

Brockopp, Jonathan. "Contradictory Evidence and the Exemplary Scholar: The Lives of Sahnun B. Saʿ Id (D. 854)." *International Journal of Middle East Studies* 43, no. 1 (2011): 115–32.

Brown, Jonathan. *The Canonization of al-Bukhārī and Muslim: The Formation and Function of the Sunnī Ḥadīth Canon: Islamic History and Civilization*. Vol. V. 69. Leiden and Boston: Brill, 2007.

———. "Critical Rigor vs. Juridical Pragmatism: How Legal Theorists and Ḥadīth Scholars Approached the Backgrowth of 'Isnāds' in the Genre of 'Ilal al-Ḥadīth." *Islamic Law and Society* (2007): 1–41.

———. "How We Know Early Hadīth Critics Did Matn Criticism and Why It's So Hard to Find." *Islamic Law and Society* 15, no. 2 (2008): 143–84.

———. "Did the Prophet Say It or Not? The Literal, Historical, and Effective truth of Ḥadīths in Early Sunnism." *Journal of the American Oriental Society* 129, no. 2 (2009): 259–85.

———. "The Canonization of Ibn Mâjah: Authenticity Vs. Utility in the Formation of the Sunni Ḥadîth Canon." *Revue des mondes musulmans et de la Méditerranée*, no. 129 (2011): 169–81.

———. "Even If It's Not True It's True: Using Unreliable Hadīths in Sunni Islam." *Islamic Law and Society* 18, no. 1 (2011): 1–52.

———. "Faithful Dissenters: Sunni Skepticism About the Miracles of Saints." *Journal of Sufi Studies* 1, no. 2 (2012): 123–68.

Brunelle, Carolyn Anne. "From Text to Law: Islamic Legal Theory and the Practical Hermeneutics of Abū Jaʿfar Aḥmad al-Ṭaḥāwī (d. 321/933)." (2016).

Al-Bukhārī, Muḥammad ibn Ismāʻīl. *Ṣaḥīḥ al-Bukhārī*. Cairo: al-Maṭbaʻah al-Amīrīyah, 1896.

Burge, Stephen. "Angels, Ritual and Sacred Space in Islam." *Comparative Islamic Studies* 5, no. 2 (2009).

———. "Reading Between the Lines: The Compilation of Ḥadīt and the Authorial Voice." *Arabica* 58, no. 3 (2011): 168–97.

———. *Angels in Islam: Jalal Al-Din Al-Suyuti's Al-Haba'ik Fi Akhbar Al-Mala'ik*. Vol. 31. London: Routledge, 2015.

———. "Myth, Meaning and the Order of Words: Reading Hadith Collections with Northrop Frye and the Development of Compilation Criticism." *Islam and Christian – Muslim Relations* 27, no. 2 (2016): 213–28.

Burrell, David B. *Towards a Jewish-Christian-Muslim Theology*. Chichester; Malden, MA: Wiley-Blackwell, 2011.

Chabbi, Jacqueline. "Remarques Sur Le Développement Historique Des Mouvements Ascétiques Et Mystiques Au Khurasan: Iiie/Ixe Siècle-Ive/Xe Siècle." *Studia Islamica* (1977): 5–72.

Chittick, William C. "Mysticism Versus Philosophy in Earlier Islamic History: The Al – Tūsi, Al – Qūnawi Correspondence." *Religious Studies* 17, no. 1 (1981): 87–104.

Conrad, Lawrence I. "Tāʿūn and Wabāʾ Conceptions of Plague and Pestilence in Early Islam." *Journal of the Economic and Social History of the Orient* 25, no. 3 (1982): 268–307.

Cooperson, Michael. "Ibn Ḥanbal and Bishr Al-Ḥāfī: A Case Study in Biographical Traditions." *Studia Islamica* (1997): 71–101.

———. *Classical Arabic Biography: The Heirs of the Prophets in the Age of al-Ma'mun.* Cambridge: Cambridge University Press, 2000.

Corbin, Henry. "The Theory of Visionary Knowledge in Islamic Philosophy." *Temenos* 8 (1987): 224–37.

Daaïf, Lahcen. "Dévots et Renonçants: L'autre Catégorie de Forgeurs de Hadiths." *Arabica* 57, no. 2 (2010): 201–50.

Denaro, Roberta. "The Most Beautiful Body: The Physical Dimension in Martyrdom Narratives." *Annali Sezione Orientale* 77, nos. 1–2 (2017): 97–115.

Al-Dhahabī, Muḥammad ibn Aḥmad ibn ʿUthmān. *Siyar Aʿlām al-Nubalāʾ*. Beirut: Muʾassasat al-Risālah, 2001.

Dickinson, Eerik. *The Development of Early Sunnite Ḥadīth Criticism: The Taqdima of Ibn Abī Ḥātim al-Rāzī (240/854–327/938)*. Vol. 38. Brill, 2001.

Dols, Michael W. *Essay Review: Islam and Medicine: Health and Medicine in the Islamic Tradition: Change and Identity*. London, England, UK: Sage Publications, 1988.

———. *Majnūn: The Madman in Medieval Islamic Society*. Edited by Diana E. Immisch. Oxford: Oxford University Press, 1992.

Drory, Rina. "The Abbasid Construction of the Jahiliyya: Cultural Authority in the Making." *Studia islamica*, no. 83 (1996): 33–49.

Druart, Thérèse-Anne. "The Ethics of Al-Razi (865–925?)." *Medieval Philosophy & Theology* 6, no. 1 (1997): 47–71.

Duderija, Adis. "Toward a Methodology of Understanding the Nature and Scope of the Concept of Sunnah." *Arab Law Quarterly* 21, no. 3 (2007): 269–80.

———. "Evolution in the Canonical Sunni Hadith Body of Literature and the Concept of an Authentic Hadith During the Formative Period of Islamic Ought as Based on Recent Western Scholarship." *Arab Law Quarterly* 23, no. 4 (2009/09/01): 389–415.

———. *The Sunna and Its Status in Islamic Law: The Search for a Sound Hadith.* New York, NY: Palgrave Macmillan, 2015.

Dutton, Yasin. "ʿAmal V. Ḥadīth in Islamic Law: The Case of Sadl Al-Yadayn (Holding One's Hands by One's Sides) When Doing the Prayer." *Islamic Law and Society* 3, no. 1 (1996): 13–40.

———. *The Origins of Islamic Law: The Qur'an, the Muwaṭṭa' and Madinan 'amal.* London: Routledge Curzon, 2002.

Eichner, Heidrun. "Essence and Existence: Thirteenth-Century Perspectives in Arabic-Islamic Philosophy and Theology." *The Arabic, Hebrew and Latin Reception of Avicenna's Metaphysics* (2012): 123–52.

Eisenlohr, Patrick. "Technologies of the Spirit: Devotional Islam, Sound Reproduction and the Dialectics of Mediation and Immediacy in Mauritius." *Anthropological Theory* 9, no. 3 (2009): 273–96.

El-Cheikh, Nadia M. "Describing the Other to Get at the Self: Byzantine Women in Arabic Sources." *Journal of the Economic and Social History of the Orient* 40, no. 2 (1997): 239–50.

El-Shamsy, Ahmed. *The Canonization of Islamic Law: A Social and Intellectual History*. Cambridge: Cambridge University Press, 2013.

Endress, Gerhard. *The Works of Yahyā Ibn'adī: An Analytical Inventory*. 1. Aufl. ed. Wiesbaden: Reichert, 1977.

Faizer, Rizwi S. "Muhammad and the Medinan Jews: A Comparison of the Texts of Ibn Ishaq's Kitab Sirat Rasul Sllah with al-Waqidi's Kitab al-Maghazi." *International Journal of Middle East Studies* 28, no. 4 (1996/11/01): 463–89.

Fancy, Nahyan. *Science and Religion in Mamluk Egypt: Ibn al-Nafis, Pulmonary Transit and Bodily Resurrection (Culture and Civilization in the Middle East)*. London: Routledge, 2013.

Fathi, Asghar. "The Islamic Pulpit as a Medium of Political Communication." *Journal for the Scientific Study of Religion* (1981): 163–72.

Fierro, Maribel. "Studies on the History of Maliki Hadith Scholarship and Jurisprudence in North Africa up to the 5th Century Ah. Bio-Bibliographical Notices from the Library of the Qairawan Mosque." Consejo Superior de Investigaciones Cientificas, Instituto de Filologia: Duque de Medinaceli, 6, 28014 Madrid, Spain, 1998.

———. "Islamic Law in Al-Andalus." *Islamic Law and Society* 7, no. 2 (2000): 119–21.

———. "Proto-Malikis, Malikis and Reformed Malikis in Al-Andalus." *The Islamic School of Law: Evolution, Devolution, and Progress* (2005): 57–76.

———. "Local and Global in Hadīth Literature: The Case of Al-Andalus." *The Transmission and Dynamics of the Textual Sources of Islam: Essays in Honour of Harald Motzki*, edited by C.H.M. Versteegh, Nicolet Boekhoff-van der Voort and Joas Wagemakers (2011): 63–90.

Forcada, Miquel. "Ibn Bājja on Medicine and Medical Experience." *Arabic Sciences and Philosophy* 21 (2011): 111–48.

Frank, Tamar. "'Taṣawwuf Is. . . ': On a Type of Mystical Aphorism." *Journal of the American Oriental Society* (1984): 73–80.

Al-Geyoushi, Muhmmad Ibraheem. "Al-Hakim Al-Tirmidhi: His Works and Thoughts." *Islamic Quarterly* 14, no. 4 (1970): 159.

———. "Al-Tirmidhi's Conception of the Struggle Between 'Qalb' and 'Nafs'." *Islamic Quarterly* 18, no. 3 (1974): 3.

Gil'adi, Avner. "'Ṣabr' (Steadfastness) of Bereaved Parents: A Motif in Medieval Muslim Consolation Treatises and Some Parallels in Jewish Writings." *The Jewish Quarterly Review* (1989): 35–48.

———. *Children of Islam: Concepts of Childhood in Medieval Muslim Society*. London: Palgrave Macmillan, 1992.

Gobillot, Geneviève. "Patience (Ṣabr) et Rétribution des Mérites: Gratitude (shukr) et Aptitude au Bonheur Selon al-Ḥakīm al-Tirmidhī (m. 318/930)." *Studia Islamica* (1994): 51–78.

Goodman, Lenn Evan. "The Epicurean Ethic of Muḥammad Ibn Zakariyâ'ar-Râzî." *Studia Islamica* (1971): 5–26.

———. "How Epicurean Was Rāzī?" *Studia Graeco-Arabica* 5 (2015): 247–80.

Görke, Andreas, Harald Motzki, and Gregor Schoeler. "First Century Sources for the Life of Muḥammad? A Debate." *Der Islam* 89, nos. 1–2 (2012): 2–59.

Graham, William A. "Traditionalism in Islam: An Essay in Interpretation." *The Journal of Interdisciplinary History* 23, no. 3 (1993): 495–522.

Griffin, Kit. "Notes on the Moroccan Sensorium." *Anthropologica* (1990): 107–11.

Griffith, Sidney H. "Yaḥyā B. 'Adī 'S (D. 974) Kitāb Tahdhīb Alakhlāq." In *The Oxford Handbook of Islamic Philosophy*, edited by Khaled El-Rouayheb and Sabine Schmidtke. Oxford: Oxford University Press, 2016.

Haeri, Niloofar. "The Sincere Subject: Mediation and Interiority Among a Group of Muslim Women in Iran." *HAU: Journal of Ethnographic Theory* 7, no. 1 (2017): 139–61.

———. "Unbundling Sincerity: Language, Mediation, and Interiority in Comparative Perspective." *HAU: Journal of Ethnographic Theory* 7, no. 1 (2017): 123–38.

Hagemann, Hannah-Lena. *History and Memory: Khārijism in Early Islamic Historiography*. Edinburgh: University of Edinburgh, 2014.

Al-Ḥakīm al-Tirmidhī, Abū ʿAbd Allāh Muḥammad ibn ʿAlī. *Adab al-Nafs*. Edited by Aḥmad ʿAbd al-Raḥīm al-Sāyiḥ. Cairo: al-Dar al-Misriyyah al-Libnaniyyah, 1993.

Hallaq, Wael B. "The Authenticity of Prophetic Ḥadîth: A Pseudo-Problem." *Studia Islamica*, no. 89 (1999): 75–90.

Hamdy, Sherine F. "Islam, Fatalism, and Medical Intervention: Lessons from Egypt on the Cultivation of Forbearance (Ṣabr) and Reliance on God (Tawakkul)." *Anthropological Quarterly* 82, no. 1 (2009): 173–96.

Heck, Paul L. "The Hierarchy of Knowledge in Islamic Civilization." *Arabica* 49, no. 1 (2002): 27–54.

Herzfeld, Ernst. "Damascus: Studies in Architecture: I." *Ars Islamica* 9 (1942/01/01): 1–53.

Hinds, Martin. "'Maghazi' and 'Sira' in Early Islamic Scholarship." Paper presented at the La vie du prophete Mahomet: colloque de Strasbourg, 1980.

Hirschkind, Charles. "Is There a Secular Body?" *Cultural Anthropology* 26, no. 4 (2011): 633–47.

Hoffman-Ladd, Valerie J. "Mysticism and Sexuality in Sufi Thought and Life." *Mystics Quarterly* 18, no. 3 (1992): 82–93.

Ibn ʿAbd Rabbih, Abū ʿUmar Shahāb al-Dīn Aḥmad ibn Muḥammad. *Al-ʿAqd al-Farīd*. Beirut: Dār al-Kutub al-ʿIlmiyyah, 1983.

Ibn Abī al-Dunyā, al-Ḥāfiẓ Abū Bakr ʿAbd Allāh ibn Muḥammad. *Kitāb al-ʿAql wa Faḍlihi*. Edited by Lutfī Muḥammad al-Ṣaghīr. Riyadh: Dar al-Rayah, 1989.

———. *Al-Maraḍ wa al-Kaffārāt*. Mumbai: al-Dār al-Salafiyyah, 1991.

———. *Mudārāt al-Nās*. Edited by Muḥammad khayr Yusuf. Beirut: Dar Ibn Ḥazm, 1998.

Ibn Abī Shaybah, Abū Bakr ʿAbd Allāh ibn Mūḥammad. *Al-Kitāb al-Muṣannaf fī al-Aḥādīth wa al-Āthār*. Edited by Kamāl Yūsif al-Ḥūt. Riyadh: Maktabat al-Rushd, 1988.

———. *Kitāb al-Adab*. Beirut: Dār al-Bashāʾir al-Islāmiyyah, 1999.

Ibn Abī Uṣaybi'ah, Aḥmad ibn al-Qāsim, and 'Āmir Najjār. *Kitāb 'Uyūn al-Anbāʾ fī Ṭabaqāt al-Aṭibbāʾ*. Cairo: al-Hayʾah al-Miṣrīyah al-'Āmmah lil-Kitāb, 2001.

Ibn ʿAsākir, ʿAlī ibn al-Ḥasan. *Tārīkh Madinat Damashq*. Edited by Muhib al-Dīn Al-Amrawy. Beirut: Dar al-Fikr, 1995.

Ibn al-Athīr, 'Izz al-Dīn. *Al-Kāmil fī al-Tārīkh*. Edited by Muḥammad Dabbūs. Cairo: al-Hay'ah al-Miṣrīyah al-'Āmmah lil-Kitāb, 2006.

Ibn Bābawayh al-Qummī, Muḥammad ibn 'Alī. *'Uyūn Akhbār al-Riḍā*. al-Najaf: Maṭba'ah al-Ḥaydarīyah, 1970.

Ibn Basṭām, ʿAbd Allāh ibn Sābūr, and Al-Ḥusayn ibn Sābūr Ibn Basṭām. *Ṭibb al-Aʾimmah*. Edited by Muḥammad Mahdī al-Sayyid Ḥasan. Najaf: al-Maktabah al-Ḥaydariyyah, 1965.

Ibn Baṭṭāl, Abū al-Ḥasan ʾAlī ibn Khalaf. Sharḥ Ṣaḥīḥ al-Bukhārī. Riyadh: Maktabat al-Rushd, 2003.

Ibn al-Farḍī, ʿAbd Allāh ibn Muḥammad ibn Naṣr al-Azdī. *Tārīkh ʿUlamāʾ al-Andalus*. Cairo: Maktabat al-Khānjī, 1988.

Ibn Ḥibbān, Abū Ḥātim Muḥammad. *Rawdat al-ʿUqalāʾ wa Nuzhat al-Fuḍalāʾ*. Edited by Muḥammad Abd al-Ḥamīd, Muḥammad Hamza and Muḥammad al-Fiqī. Beirut: Dar al-Kutub al-'Ilmiyyah, 1955.

———. *Al-Sīrah al-Nabawiyyah wa Akhbār al-Khulafā'*. Beirut:al-Maktabah al-Thaqafi yyah, 1996.

Ibn Ḥabīb al-Qurṭubī, 'Abd al-Malik ibn Ḥabīb ibn Sulaymān. *Al-Mukhtaṣar fī al-Ṭibb*. Beirut: Dār al-Kutub al-'Ilmiyyah, 1998.

Ibn Ḥanbal, Aḥmad ibn Muḥammad. *Kitāb al-Sunnah*. Mecca: al-Matba'ah al-Salafiyyah, 1930.

———. *Al-Musnad*. Edited by Aḥmad Muḥammad Shākir. al-Ṭab'ah 4. ed. Cairo: Dār al-Ma'ārif, 1951.

———. *Kitāb al-Zuhd*. Edited by Muḥammad Sharaf. Beirut: Dar al-Nahda al-'Arabiyya, 1981.

Ibn al-Jarrāḥ, Wakī'. *Ṣaḥīḥ Kitāb al-Zuhd*. Edited by Abd al-Raḥman Al-Faryawā'ī. Beirut: Mu'assat al-Kutub al-Thaqafiyyah, 1993.

Ibn al-Jawzī, Abū al-Faraj 'Abd al-Raḥmān ibn 'Alī. *Al-Shifā' fī Mawā'iẓ al-Mulūk wa al-Khulafā'*. Edited by Fouad Abdelmonem Ahmad. Alexandria: Dar al-Da'wah, 1978.

———. *Al-Tibb al-Rūḥānī*. Cairo: Maktabat al-Thaqafah al-Diniyyah, 1986.

———. *Dhamm al-Hawā*. Edited by Khaled Abdel Latif Al-'Alami. Beirut: Dar al-Kitab al-Arabi, 1998.

———. *Ṣifat al-Ṣafwah*. Edited by Ahmed Ali. Cairo: Dar al-Hadith, 2009.

———. *Luqat al-Manāfi' fī 'ilm al-Ṭibb*. Edited by Marzuq Ali Ibrahim. Cairo: Dar al-Kutub, 2010.

Ibn Al-Jazzar. *Ibn al-Jazzar on Fevers: A Critical Edition of Zad al-Musafir wa-Qut al-Hadir: Provisions for the Travelers and Nourishment for the Sedentary, Bk. 7, Chs. 1–6: The Original Arabic Text*. Edited by Gerrit BOS. London: Kegan Paul International, 2000.

Ibn Juljul, Sulaymān ibn Ḥassān, and Fu'ād Sayyid. *Ṭabaqāt al-Aṭibbā' wa-al-Ḥukamā'*. Textes Et Traductions D'auteurs Orientaux. Cairo: nstitut Français D'archéologie Orientale, 1955.

Ibn Mājah, Muḥammad ibn Yazīd. *Sunan Ibn Mājah*. Beirut: Dar al-Kutub al-Ilmiyyah, 1998.

Ibn Marthad, 'Alqamah, and Ibn Abī Ḥātim al-Rāzī. *Zuhd al-Thamāniyah min al-Tābi'īn*. Edited by Abd al-Raḥman Al-Faryawā'ī Medina. KSA: Maktabat al-Dar, 1984.

Ibn al-Nadīm, Mohammed ibn Ishaq. *Al-Fihrist* [L'Index]. Beyrouth: Khiat, 1964.

Ibn Qayyim al-Jawzīyah, Muḥammad ibn Abī Bakr. *Al-Ṭibb al-Nabawī*. Edited by Muḥammad Fatḥī Abū Bakr. Cairo: Al-Dar al-masriah al-lubnaniah, 1989.

Ibn Qutaybah, 'Abd Allāh ibn Muslim. *Kitāb al-Ma'ārif*. Edited by Muḥmmad Ismā'īl 'Abd Allāh Ṣāwī. Cairo: al-Maṭba'ah al-Islamīah, 1934.

———. *Ta'wīl Mukhtalaf al-Ḥadīth*. Beirut: al-Maktab al-Islāmī, 1999.

Ibn Rāshid Al-Azdī, Mu'ammir. *Al-Jāmi'*. Beirut: al-Maktab al-Islāmī, 1982.

Ibn Sa'd, Abū 'Abd Allāh Muḥammad. *Al-Ṭabaqāt al-Kubrā*. Beirut: Dār al-Kutub al-'Ilmiyyah, 1990.

———. *Al-Mutamim li-Tabaqāt Ibn Sa'd*. Ta'if, KSA: Al-Ṣiddīq, 1993.

Ibn al-Sunnī, Aḥmad ibn Muḥammad. "Al-Ṭibb Al-Nabawī." Suleymaniye, Fatih 03585. Manuscript, n.d.

Ibn 'Umayrah, Aḥmad ibn Yaḥyā. *Bughyat al-Multamis fī Tārīkh Ahl al-Andalus*. Cairo: Dār al-Kitāb al-'Arabī, 1967.

Idris, Hady Roger. "Réflexions Sûr Le Malikisme Sous Les Umayyades D'espagne." *Atti* 2 (1967): 397–414.

Israeli, Isaac, and Muḥammad Ṣabbāḥ. *Kitāb al-Aghdhiyah wa-al-Adwiyah*. al-Ṭab'at 1. ed. Bayrūt: Mu'assasat 'Izz al-Dīn, 1992.

Jones, John Marsden B. "The Chronology of the Maghāzī – A Textual Survey." *Bulletin of the School of Oriental and African Studies* 19, no. 2 (1957): 245–80.

———. "Ibn Isḥāq and al-Wāqidī: The Dream of 'Ātika and the Raid to Nakhla in Relation to the Charge of Plagiarism." *Bulletin of the School of Oriental and African Studies* 22, no. 1 (1959): 41–51.

———. "The Maghazi Literature." *Arabic Literature to the End of the Umayyad Period* (1983): 344–51.

Joosse, N. Peter. " 'Unmasking the Craft': Abd al-Laṭīf al-Baghdādī's Views on Alchemy and Alchemists." In *Islamic Thought in the Middle Ages*, 301–18. Leiden, Boston: Brill, 2008.

Jouili, Jeanette S., and Annelies Moors. "Introduction: Islamic Sounds and the Politics of Listening." *Anthropological Quarterly* 87, no. 4 (2014): 977–88.

Juynboll, Gualterus H.A. *Muslim Tradition: Studies in Chronology, Provenance and Authorship of Early Hadıth.* Cambridge: Cambridge University Press, 1983.

Al-Kashkarī, Ya'qūb. *Kunnāsh fī al-Ṭibb*. Edited by Fuat Sezgin and Kütüphanesi Süleymaniye Umumî. Frānkfurt am Main: Ma'had Tārīkh al-'Ulūm al-'Arabīyah wa-al-Islāmīyah, 1985.

Katz, Marion Holmes. *Prayer in Islamic Thought and Practice*. Cambridge: Cambridge University Press, 2013.

Kayani, Ahsan, Mark J. King, and Judy J. Fleiter. "Fatalism and Road Safety in Developing Countries, with a Focus on Pakistan." *Journal of the Australasian College of Road Safety* 22, no. 2 (2011): 41–7.

Khalek, Nancy. "Medieval Biographical Literature and the Companions of Muḥammad." *Der Islam* 91, no. 2 (2014): 272–94.

Khalidi, Tarif. *Arabic Historical Thought in the Classical Period.* Cambridge: Cambridge University Press, 1994.

———. *Images of Muhammad: Narratives of the Prophet in Islam Across the Centuries.* New York: Random House LLC, 2009.

———. "Premodern Arabic/Islamic Historical Writing." In *A Companion to Global Historical Thought*, edited by Prasenjit Duara, Viren Murthy and Andrew Sartori, 78–91. Chichster; West Sussex; Malden, MA: Wiley Blackwell, 2014.

Khalil, Atif. "Is God Obliged to Answer Prayers of Petition (Du'a)?: The Response of Classical Sufis and Qur'anic Exegetes." *The Journal of Medieval Religious Cultures* 37, no. 2 (2011): 93–109.

Khan, Hussain Ahmad. " 'The People of My Generation Are Best': Conceptualizing Testimony in Early Islam (9th and 10th Centuries)." *Journal of Social Sciences & Humanities (1994–7046)* 24, no. 1 (2015).

Khan, Ruqayya Yasmine. " 'The Chambir of My Thought': Self and Conduct in an Early Islamic Ethical Treatise." *History of Religions* 49, no. 1 (2009): 27–47.

Al-Khaṭīb al-Baghdādī, Abū Bakr Aḥmad ibn Thābit. *Tārīkh Madinat al-Salām*. Beirut: Dār al-Gharb al-Islāmī, 2001.

Khoury, Nuha N.N. "The Dome of the Rock, the Ka'ba, and Ghumdan: Arab Myths and Umayyad Monuments." *Muqarnas* (1993): 57–65.

Al-Khwānsārī al-Aṣbahānī, Muḥammad Bāqir al-Mūsawī. *Rawdāt al-Jannāt fī Aḥwāl al-'Ulamā' wa al-Sādāt*. Beirut: al-Dār al-Islāmiyyah, 1991.

Kilpatrick, Hilary. "A Genre in Classical Arabic Literature: The Adab Encyclopedia." Paper presented at the Union Européenne des Arabisants et Islamisants: 10th Congress, Edinburgh, 9–16 September, 1982.

Kinberg, Leah. "What Is Meant by Zuhd." *Studia Islamica*, no. 61 (1985): 27–44.

Al-Kirmānī, Ḥamīd al-Dīn. *Al-Aqwāl al-Dhahabiyyah*. Edited by Salāḥ al-Sāwī. Tehran: Imperial Iranian Academy, 1977.

Kister, M.J. "The Sirah Literature." In *Arabic Literature to the End of the Umayyad Period*, 352–67. Cambridge: Cambridge University Press, 1983.

———. " 'And He Was Born Circumcised': Some Notes on Circumcision in Hadith." *Oriens* 34 (1994): 10–30.

Kleinman, Arthur. *Patients and Healers in the Context of Culture: An Exploration of the Borderland Between Anthropology, Medicine, and Psychiatry*. Vol. 3. Berkeley: University of California Press, 1980.

———. *The Illness Narratives: Suffering, Healing, and the Human Condition*. Basic Books, 1988.

Koetschet, Pauline. "Galien, Al-Rāzī, Et L'éternité Du Monde. Les Fragments Du Traité Sur La Démonstration, Iv, Dans Les Doutes Sur Galien." *Arabic Sciences and Philosophy* 25, no. 2 (2015): 167–98.

Kohlberg, Etan. *The Attitude of the Imami-shi'is to the Companions of the Prophet*. Oxford: University of Oxford, 1971.

———. "Some Imāmī-shī'ī Views on Taqiyya." *Journal of the American Oriental Society* (1975): 395–402.

———. "Some Zaydi Views on the Companions of the Prophet." *Bulletin of the School of Oriental and African Studies* 39, no. 1 (1976): 91–8.

Kraus, Paul. "Raziana Ii: Extrait Du Kitāb A'lām Al-Nubuwwa D'abū Ḥātim Al-Rāzī." In *Muḥammad Ibn Zakarīyā 'Ar-Rāzī (D. 313/925): Texts and Studies*, edited by Fuat Sezgin, Māzin Amāwī, Carl Ehrig-Eggert and E. Neubauer. Frankfurt am Main: Institute for the History of Arabic-Islamic Science at the Johann Wolfgang Goethe University, 1999.

Al-Kūfī, Hannād ibn al-Sarī. *Kitāb al-Zuhd*. Edited by Abd al-Raḥman Al-Faryawā'ī. Kuwait: Dar al-Khulafa, 1985.

Al-Kutubī, Muḥammad ibn Shākir, 'Alī Muḥammad Mu'awwaḍ, 'Ādil Aḥmad 'Abd al-Mawjūd, and Khallikān Ibn. *Fawāt al-Wafayāt*. al-Ṭab'ah 1. ed. 2 vols. Bayrūt: Dār al-Kutub al-'Ilmīyah, 2000.

Lagrange, Frederic. "The Obscenity of the Vizir." In *Islamicate Sexualities*, edited by Kathryn Babayan and Afsaneh Najmabadi, 161–203. Cambridge, MA: Harvard University Press, 2008.

Lalani, Arzina R. *Degrees of Excellence: A Fatimid Treatise on Leadership in Islam*. London: I. B. Tauris, 2009.

Lev, Efraim. "An Early Fragment of Ibn Jazlah's Tabulated Manual 'Taqwīm Al-Abdān' from the Cairo Genizah (T-S Ar.R1.137)." *Journal of the Royal Asiatic Society* 24, no. 2 (2014): 189–223.

Lev, Efraim, and Zohar Amar. " 'Fossils' of Practical Medical Knowledge from Medieval Cairo." *Journal of Ethnopharmacology* 119, no. 1 (2008): 24–40.

Lev, Efraim, and Leigh Chipman. *Medical Prescriptions in the Cambridge Genizah Collections: Practical Medicine and Pharmacology in Medieval Egypt: Cambridge Genizah Studies*. Leiden; Boston: Brill, 2012.

Lewicka, Paulina. *Medicine for Muslims? Islamic Theologians, Non-muslim Physicians and the Medical Culture of the Mamluk Near East*. History and Society During the Mamluk Era (1250–1517). Bonn: Annemarie Schimmel Kolleg Working Papers, 2012.

Lewisohn, Leonard. "The Way of Tawakkul: The Ideal of Trust in God in Classical Persian Sufism." *Islamic Culture* 73, no. 2 (1999): 27–62.

Librande, Leonard. "Ibn Abī al-Dunyā: Certainty and Morality." *Studia Islamica*, nos. 100–101 (2005): 5–42.

Livingston, John W. "Science and the Occult in the Thinking of Ibn Qayyim al-Jawziyya." *Journal of the American Oriental Society* 112, no. 4 (1992): 598–610.

Lucas, Scott C. *Constructive Critics, Ḥadīth Literature, and the Articulation of Sunnī Islam: The Legacy of the Generation of Ibn Sa'd, Ibn Ma'īn, and Ibn Ḥanbal*. Vol. 51. Leiden; Boston: Brill, 2004.

———. "Where Are the Legal Hadīth? A Study of the Musannaf of Ibn Abī Shayba." *Islamic Law and Society* 15, no. 3 (2008): 283–314.

Mahmood, Saba. "Ethics and Piety." In *A Companion to Moral Anthropology*, edited by Didier Fassin, 221–41. Chichester; West Sussex: Wiley Blackwell, 2012.

Makdisi, George. "'Ṭabaqāt'-Biography: Law and Orthodoxy in Classical Islam." *Islamic Studies* 32, no. 4 (1993): 371–96.

Malamud, Margaret. "Gender and Spiritual Self-Fashioning: The Master-Disciple Relationship in Classical Sufism." *Journal of the American Academy of Religion* 64, no. 1 (1996): 89–117.

Marín, Manuela. "The Early Development of Zuhd in al-Andalus." *ShiÆa Islam, Sects, and Sufism: Historical Dimensions, Religious Practice and Methodological Considerations* (1992): 83–94.

Al-Marūzī, 'Abd Allāh ibn al-Mubārak. *Kitāb al-Zuhd*. Edited by Ḥabīb al-Raḥmān al-A'ẓamī. Beirut: Dar al-Kutub al-'Ilmiyyah, 2004.

Al-Māwardī, Abū al-Ḥasan 'Alī ibn Muḥammad. *Adab al-Dunyā wa al-Dīn*. Beirut: al-Hayat, 1986.

McAuliffe, Jane Dammen, and Bidgoli Mohammad Taqi Diyari. "Assessing the Isra'iliyyat: An Exegetical Conundrum." *Pazhuhesh-Dini*, no. 23 (2012): 23–63.

Melchert, Christopher. "The Transition from Asceticism to Mysticism at the Middle of the Ninth Century CE." *Studia Islamica*, no. 83 (1996): 51–70.

———. "Bukhārī and Early Hadith Criticism." *Journal of the American Oriental Society* (2001): 7–19.

———. "The Piety of the Hadith Folk." *International Journal of Middle East Studies* 34, no. 3 (2002): 425–39.

———. "Aḥmad Ibn Ḥanbal's Book of Renunciation." *Der Islam* 85, no. 2 (2011): 345–59.

———. "Exaggerated Fear in the Early Islamic Renunciant Tradition." *Journal of the Royal Asiatic Society* 21, no. 3 (2011): 283–300.

Merguerian, Gayane Karen, and Afsaneh Najmabadi. "Zulaykha and Yusuf: Whose 'Best Story'?" *International Journal of Middle East Studies*, no. 29 (1997): 485–508.

Millán, Cristina Álvarez. "Practice Versus Theory: Tenth-Century Case Histories from the Islamic Middle East." *Social History of Medicine* 13, no. 2 (2000): 293–306.

———. "Medical Anecdotes in Ibn Juljul's Biographical Dictionary." *Suhayl. International Journal for the History of the Exact and Natural Sciences in Islamic Civilisation* 4 (2004): 141–58.

———. "The Case History in Medieval Islamic Medical Literature: Tajārib and Mujarrabāt as Source." *Medical history* 54, no. 2 (2010): 195–214.

Mirza, Sarah Z. "The Peoples' Hadith: Evidence for Popular Tradition on Hadith as Physical Object in the First Centuries of Islam." *Arabica* 63, nos. 1–2 (2016): 30–63.

Miskawayh, Abū 'Alī Aḥmad ibn Muḥammad. *Tahdhīb Al-Akhlāq*. Edited by 'Imad al-Hilālī. Beirut: Manshurat al-Jamal, 2011.

Al-Miṣrī, 'Abd Allāh ibn Wahb. *Al-Kitāb al-Jāmi'*. Edited by Ḥasan Ḥussayn Abū al-Khayr. Riyadh: Dār Ibn al-Jawzī, 1995.

Mohaghegh, Mehdi. "Notes on the 'Spiritual Physic' of Al-Razi." *Studia Islamica*, no. 26 (1967): 5–22.

Moosa, Ebrahim. *Ghazali and the Poetics of Imagination*. Chapel Hill, NC: University of North Carolina Press, 2005.

Morrison, Robert. *Islam and Science: The Intellectual Career of Nizam al-Din al-Nisaburi*. London: Routledge, 2007.

Moscoso, Javier. *Pain: A Cultural History*. New York, NY: Palgrave Macmillan, 2012.

Mottahedeh, Roy. "Some Islamic Views of the Pre-islamic Past." *Harvard Middle Eastern and Islamic Review*, no. 1 (1994): 17–26.

———. *Loyalty and Leadership in an Early Islamic Society*. London: I. B. Tauris, 2001.

Motzki, Harald. "The Muṣannaf of ʿAbd al-Razzāq al-Sanʿānī as a Source of Authentic Aḥādīth of the First Century A.H." *Journal of Near Eastern Studies* 50, no. 1 (1991/01/01): 1–21.

Al-Mundhirī, al-Ḥāfiẓ Zakiyy al-Dīn ʾAbd al-ʾAẓīm. *Al-Targhīb wa wl-Tarhīb*. Edited by Ibrāhīm Shams al-Dīn. Beirut: Dār al-Kutub al-ʾIlmiyyah, 2003.

Musa, Aisha Y. "Al-Shāfi'ī, the Ḥadīth, and the Concept of the Duality of Revelation." *Islamic Studies* (2007): 163–97.

———. *Ḥadīth as Scripture: Discussions on the Authority of Prophetic Traditions in Islam*. 1st ed. New York, NY: Palgrave Macmillan, 2008.

Muslim ibn al-Ḥajjāj, al-Qushayrī. *Ṣaḥīḥ Muslim*. al-Ṭab'ah 1. ed. Istanbul: al-Maṭba'ah al-'Āmirah fī Dār al-Khilāfah al-'Alīyah, 1911.

Al-Najāshī, Aḥmad ibn 'Alī. *Rijāl al-Najāshī: Aḥad al-Uṣūl al-Rijālīyah*. Edited by Muḥammad Jawād Nāʾīnī. al-Ṭab'ah 1. ed. Beirut: Dār al-Adwāʾ, 1988.

Nasr, Seyyed Hossein. "Intellect and Intuition: Their Relationship from the Islamic Perspective." *Studies in Comparative Religion* 13, no. 1 (1982).

Nasr, Seyyed Hossein, and Oliver Leaman. *History of Islamic Philosophy*. Routledge History of World Philosophies. London and New York: Routledge, 1996.

Newby, Gordon D. "Imitating Muhammad in Two Genres: Mimesis and Problems of Genre in Sirah and Sunnah." *Medieval Encounters* 3, no. 3 (1997): 266–83.

Newman, Andrew J. *Islamic Medical Wisdom: The Tibb Al-A'imma*. London: Muhammdi Trust, 1991.

———. "Baqir Al-Majlisi and Islamicate Medicine: Safavid Medical Theory and Practice Re-Examined." *Society and Culture in the Early Modern Middle East: Studies on Iran in the Safavid Period* (2003): 371–96.

———. "The Recovery of the Past: Ibn Bābawayh, Bāqir Al-Majlisī and Safawid Medical Discourse." *Iran* 50, no. 1 (2012): 109–27.

Northrup, Linda. "Qalawun's Patronage of the Medical Sciences in Thirteenth-century Egypt." *Mamluk Studies Review* 5 (2001): 119–40.

O'Banion, Patrick J. " 'They Will Know Our Hearts': Practicing the Art of Dissimulation on the Islamic Periphery." *Journal of Early Modern History* 20, no. 2 (2016): 193–217.

O'Kane, John, and Bernd Radtke. *The Concept of Sainthood in Early Islamic Mysticism: Two Works by Al-Hakim Al-Tirmidhi-an Annotated Translation with Introduction*. London: Routledge, 2013.

Olsan, Lea T. "Charms and Prayers in Medieval Medical Theory and Practice." *Social History of Medicine* 16, no. 3 (2003): 343–66.

Orfali, Bilal. "A Sketch Map of Arabic Poetry Anthologies up to the Fall of Baghdad." *Journal of Arabic Literature* 43, no. 1 (2012): 29–59.

Osman, Amr. "ʿAdālat al-Ṣaḥāba: The Construction of a Religious Doctrine." *Arabica* 60, nos. 3–4 (2013): 272–305.

Pellat, Charles. *The Life and Works of Jāḥiẓ*. Berkeley: University of California Press, 1969.

Perho, Irmeli. *The Prophet's Medicine: A Creation of the Muslim Traditionalist Scholars*. Helsinki: The Finnish Oriental Society, 1995.

Picken, Gavin N. *The Concept of Sunna in the Early Shāfi 'ī Madhhab*. New York: Palgrave Macmillan, 2015.

Pormann, Peter E. "Islamic Hospitals in the Time of al-Muqtadir." In *Abbasid Studies II: Occasional Papers of the School of Abbasid Studies, leuven, 28 june-1 july 2004*, edited by John A. Nawas, 337–81. Leuven: Uitgeverij Peeters en Departement Oosterse Studies, 2010.

Pormann, Peter E., and N. Peter Joosse. "Decline and Decadence in Iraq and Syria after the Age of Avicenna?: 'Abd al-Latif al-Baghdadi (1162–1231) Between Myth and History." *Bulletin of the History of Medicine* 84, no. 1 (2010): 1–29.

Powers, David S. *Zayd*. Philadelphia: University of Pennsylvania Press, 2014.

Powers, Paul R. "Interiors, Intentions, and the 'Spirituality' of Islamic Ritual Practice." *Journal of the American Academy of Religion* 72, no. 2 (2004): 425–59.

Qaṭāyah, Salmān. *Al-Ṭabīb al-'Arabī 'Alī Ibn Riḍwān, Ra'īs Aṭibbā' Miṣr, 376 h/986 m-460 h/1067 m*. al-Ṭab'ah 1. ed. Bayrūt: al-Mu'assasah al-'Arabīyah lil-Dirāsāt wa-al-Nashr, 1983.

Al-Qifṭī, 'Alī ibn Yūsuf. *Tārīkh al-Ḥukamā'*. Leipzig: Dieterich'sche Verlagsbuchhandlung, 1912.

Al-Qurtubi, Muhammad ibn Ahmad, and Aisha Abdurrahman Bewley. *Tafsir Al-Qurtubi: Classical Commentary of the Holy Quran*. London: Dar al-Taqwa, 2003.

Radtke, Bernd. "Al-Hakim al-Tirmidhi on Miracles." *GAS* 1 (2000): 653–9.

Ragab, Ahmed. "Epistemic Authority of Women in the Medieval Middle East." *HAWWA: Journal of Women of the Middle East and the Islamic World* 8, no. 2 (2010): 181–216.

———. *The Medieval Islamic Hospital: Medicine, Religion and Charity*. Cambridge: Cambridge University Press, 2015.

———. "One, Two, or Many Sexes: Sex Differentiation in Medieval Islamicate Medical Thought." *Journal of the History of Sexuality* 24, no. 3 (2015): 428–54.

Rahman, Fazlur. *Health and Medicine in the Islamic Tradition: Change and Identity*. New York: Crossroad, 1987.

Raisuddin, Anm. "Baqī b: Makhlad al-Qurṭubī (201–276/816–889) and His Contribution to the Study of Ḥadīth Literature in Spain." *Islamic Studies* 27, no. 2 (1988): 161–8.

Al-Rāmhurmuzī, al-Ḥasan ibn 'Abd al-Raḥmān. *Al-Muḥaddith al-Fāṣil Bayna al-Rāwī wa al-Wā'ī*. Edited by Muḥammad 'Ajjāj Khaṭīb. Beirut: Dār al-Fikr, 1984.

Rashed, Marwan. "Abū Bakr Al-Rāzī Et La Prophétie." *Mélanges de la Institute Dominicain d'Etudes Orientales du Caire* 27 (2008): 169–82.

Al-Rāzī, Abū Bakr. *Akhlāq al-Ṭabīb*. Cairo: Maktabat Dār al-Turāth, 1977.

———. *Al-Ṭibb al-Rūḥānī*. Edited by 'Abd al-Laṭīf al-'Abd. Cairo: Maktabat al-Nahdah al-Misriyyah, 1978.

———. *Ṭabīb man lā Ṭabīb la-hu, aw, man lā Yaḥduruhu al-Ṭabīb*. Edited by Muḥammad Rakābī Rashīdī. Silsilat Ṭibb Al-I'shāb. al-Ṭab'ah 1. ed. al-Qāhirah: Dār Rakābī, 1998.

———. *Al-Ḥāwī fī al-Ṭibb*. Edited by Muḥammad Muḥammad Ismail. Beirut: Dār al-Kutub al-'Ilmiyyah, 2000.

Al-Rāzī, Abū Ḥātim Aḥmad ibn Ḥamdān. *A'lām al-Nubuwwa fī al-Radd 'alā al-Mulḥid Abū Bakr al-Rāzī*. Edited by George Ṭarābīshī. Beirut: Dār al-Sāqī, 2003.

Al-Rāzī, Ibn Abī Ḥātim. *Tafsīr Ibn Abī Ḥātim*. Riyadh: Maktabat Nizar Mustafa al-Bāz, 1999.

Richardson, Kristina L. *Difference and Disability in the Medieval Islamic World: Blighted Bodies*. Edinburgh: Edinburgh University Press, 2012.

Rippin, Andrew. "The Exegetical Genre 'Asbāb al-Nuzūl': A Bibliographical and Terminological Survey." *Bulletin of the School of Oriental and African Studies, University of London* 48, no. 1 (1985): 1–15.

———. *The Qur'an and Its Interpretative Tradition*. Burlington: Ashgate, 2001.

Robinson, Chase F. "History and Heilsgeschichte in Early Islam: Some Observations on Prophetic History and Biography." *History and Religion: Narrating a Religious Past* 68 (2015): 119.

Roded, Ruth. *Women in Islamic Biographical Collections: From Ibn Sa'd to Who's Who*. London: Lynne Rienner Publishers, 1994.

Rose, Paul Lawrence. "Muhammad, the Jews and the Constitution of Medina: Retrieving the Historical Kernel." *Der Islam* 86, no. 1 (2011): 1–29.

Al-Ruhāwī, Isḥāq ibn 'Alī. *Adab al-Ṭabīb*. Frankfurt: Institute of Arabic and Islamic Sciences, 1985.

Rustomji, Nerina. "Early Views of Paradise in Islam." *Religion Compass* 4, no. 3 (2010): 166–75.

Sadan, Joseph. "An Admirable and Ridiculous Hero: Some Notes on the Bedouin in Medieval Arabic Belles Lettres, on a Chapter of Adab by al-Râghib al-Iṣfahânî, and on a Literary Model in which Admiration and Mockery Coexist." *Poetics Today* (1989): 471–92.

Salem, Feryal. *The Emergence of Early Sufi Piety and Sunnī Scholasticism*. Leiden: Brill, 2016.

Al-Ṣan'ānī, 'Abd al-Razzāq ibn Hammām. *Al-Muṣannaf*. Beirut: al-Maktab al-Islāmī, 1983.

———. *Al-Amālī fī Āthār al-Ṣaḥābah*. Riyadh: Maktabat al-Sā'ī, 1989.

Sánchez, Ignacio. "Reading Adab as Fiqh: Al-Ǧaḥiẓ's Singing-Girls and the Limits of Legal Reasoning (Qiyās)." *Bulletin d'études orientales*, no. Tome LX (2012): 203–21.

Sayeed, Asma. "Women and Ḥadīth Transmission Two Case Studies from Mamluk Damascus." *Studia Islamica* (2002): 71–94.

Schacht, Joseph. *The Origins of Muhammadan Jurisprudence*. Oxford: Clarendon Press, 1959.

Schimmel, Annemarie. *Mystical Dimensions of Islam*. Chapel Hill, NC: University of North Carolina Press, 1975.

———. *My Soul Is a Woman: The Feminine in Islam*. New York: Bloomsbury, 2003.

———. *And Muhammad Is His Messenger: The Veneration of the Prophet in Islamic Piety*. Chapel Hill, NC: University of North Carolina Press, 2014.

Schofer, Jonathan Wyn. *The Making of a Sage: A Study in Rabbinic Ethics*. Madison: University of Wisconsin Press, 2005.

———. "Embodiment and Virtue in a Comparative Perspective." *Journal of Religious Ethics* 35, no. 4 (2007): 715–28.

———. *Confronting Vulnerability: The Body and the Divine in Rabbinic Ethics*. Chicago: University of Chicago Press, 2010.

———. "Ethical Formation and Subjection." *Numen* 59, no. 1 (2012): 1–31.

Al-Shāfi'ī, Muḥammad ibn Idrīs. *Al-Risālah*. Edited by Aḥmad Muḥammad Shākir. Cairo: Maṭba'at Muṣṭafā al-Ḥalabi, 1938.

Shalem, Avinoam. "Experientia and Auctoritas: 'Abd al-Latif al-Baghdadi's Kitāb al-Ifāda wa'l-I'tibār and the Birth of the Critical Gaze." *Muqarnas Online* 32, no. 1 (2015): 197–212.

Al-Shaybānī, Muḥammad ibn al-Ḥasan. *Kitāb al-Āthār*. Edited by Abū al-Wafā Al-Afghānī. Beirut: Dār al-Kutub al-'Ilmiyyah, 1993.

Shefer-Mossensohn, Miri, and K. Abou Hershkovitz. "Early Muslim Medicine and the Indian Context: A Reinterpretation." *Medieval Encounters* 19, no. 3 (2013): 274–99.

Shoemaker, Stephen J. *The Death of a Prophet: The End of Muhammad's Life and the Beginnings of Islam*. Philadelphia: University of Pennsylvania Press, 2011.

Sirry, Munim. "Pious Muslims in the Making: A Closer Look at Narratives of Ascetic Conversion." *Arabica* 57, no. 4 (2010): 437–54.

Sizgoric, Thomas. "Narrative and Community in Islamic Late Antiquity." *Past & Present*, no. 185 (2004): 9–42.

Spellberg, Denise A. *Politics, Gender and the Islamic Past: The Legacy of Aisha Bint Abi Bakr*. New York: Columbia University Press, 1994.

Sperl, Stefan. "Man's 'Hollow Core': Ethics and Aesthetics in Ḥadīth Literature and Classical Arabic Adab." *Bulletin of the School of Oriental and African Studies* 70, no. 3 (2007): 459–86.

Stearns, Justin K. *Infectious Ideas: Contagion in Premodern Islamic and Christian Thought in the Western Mediterranean*. Baltimore: Johns Hopkins University Press, 2011.

———. "All Beneficial Knowledge Is Revealed." *Islamic Law and Society* 21, nos. 1–2 (2014): 49–80.

Stern, Samuel Miklos. "A Collection of Treatises by 'Abd al-Laṭīf al-Baghdādī." *Islamic Studies* 1, no. 1 (1962): 53–70.

Stowasser, Barbara Freyer. *Women in the Qur'an, Traditions, and Interpretation*. New York: Oxford University Press, 1994.

Stroumsa, Sarah. *Freethinkers of Medieval Islam: Ibn Al-Rawāndī, Abū Bakr Al-Rāzī and Their Impact on Islamic Thought*. Vol. 35. Leiden; Boston: Brill, 1999.

Sviri, Sara. "Hakim Tirmidhi and the Malamati Movement in Early Sufism." *The Heritage of Sufism* 1 (1993): 583–613.

Al-Ṭabarī, Abū Ja'far Muḥammad ibn Jarīr. *Tārikh al-Rusul wa al-Mulūk*. Cairo: Dār al-Ma'ārif, 1969.

———. *Tafsīr al-Ṭabarī: Jāmi' al-Bayān 'an Ta'wīl Āy al-Qur'ān*. Edited by Abdallah Abdel Mohsen al-Turkī. Cairo: Hajr, 2001.

Al-Ṭabarī, 'Alī ibn Sahl Rabbān. *Firdaws al-Ḥikmah fī al-Ṭibb*. Edited by 'Abd al-Karīm Sāmī Jindī. Bayrūt, Lubnān: Dār al-Kutub al-'Ilmīyah, 2002.

Ṭāshkubrī'zādah, Aḥmad ibn Muṣṭafá. *Risālat al-Shifā' li-Adwā' al-Wabā'*. Cairo: al-Maṭba'ah al-Wahbīyah, 1875.

Temel, Ahmet. *The Missing Link in the History of Islamic Legal Theory: The Development of Usū al-Fiqh Between al-Shāfi 'ī and al-Jassās During the 3rd/9th and Early 4th/10th Centuries*. Santa Barbara: University of California, 2014.

Thurlkill, Mary F. *Chosen Among Women: Mary and Fatima in Medieval Christianity and Shiite Islam*. Notre Dame, IN: University of Notre Dame Press, 2008.

Al-Ṭihrānī, Aghā Bazrak. *Al-Dhari'ah ilā Taṣānīf al-Shi'ah*. Beirut: Dār al-Aḍwā', 1983.

Al-Tirmidhī, Muḥammad ibn 'Īsā ibn Sawrah. *Al-Shamā'il al-Muḥammadīyah wa al-Khaṣā'il al-Muṣṭafawwīyah*. Beirut: Dār al-Kutub al-'Ilmīyyah, 1996.

———. *Al-Jāmi' al-Kabīr*. Beirut: al-Gharb al-Islāmī, 1998.

Tokatly, Vardit. "The Alām Al-Hadīth of Al-Khattābī: A Commentary on Al-Bukhārī's Sahīh or a Polemical Treatise?" *Studia Islamica* 92 (2001): 53–91.

Toorawa, Shawkat M. "A Portrait of Abd al-Latīf al-Baghdadi's Education and Instruction." *Law and Education in Medieval Islam: Studies in Memory of Professor George Makdisi: Oxford: EJW Gibb Memorial Trust Series* (2004): 91–109.

———. "Travel in the Medieval Islamic World: The Importance of Patronage as Illustrated by 'Abd al-Latif al-Baghdadi (d. 629/1231)(and other littérateurs)." In *Eastward Bound: Travel and Travellers (1050–1550)*, edited by Rosamund Allen, 53–69. Manchester: Manchester University Press, 2004.

Tor, Deborah. "Historical Representations of Yaʿqūb b. al-Layth: A Reappraisal." *Journal of the Royal Asiatic Society* 12, no. 3 (2002): 247–75.

Tottoli, Roberto. "Origin and Use of the Term Isrāʾīliyyāt in Muslim Literature." *Arabica* (1999): 193–210.

Al-Ṭūsī, Shaykh al-Ṭāʾifah Muḥammad ibn al-Ḥasan. *Al-Tibyān fī Tafsīr al-Qurʾān*. al-Najaf: al-Maṭbaʿah al-ʿIlmīyah, 1959.

ʿUmrajī, Aḥmad Shawqī Ibrāhīm. *Al-Muʿtazilah fī Baghdād wa-Atharuhum fī al-Ḥayāh al-Fikrīyah wa-al-Siyāsīyah: Min Khilāfat al-Maʾmūn Ḥattá Wafāt al-Mutawakkil ʿalá Allāh min Sanat 198–247 H/813–861 M*. Cairo: Madbuli, 2000.

Urban, Elizabeth. "The Identity Crisis of Abū Bakra: Mawlā of the Prophet, or Polemical Tool?" In *The Lineaments of Islam*, 119–49. Leiden; Boston: Brill, 2012.

Vallat, Philippe. "Between Hellenism, Islam, and Christianity: Abū Bakr Al-Rāzī and His Controversies with Contemporary Muʿtazilite Theologians as Reported by the Ashʿarite Theologian and Philosopher Fakhr Al-Dīn Al-Rāzī." *Ideas in Motion in Baghdad and Beyond: Philosophical and Theological Exchanges Between Christians and Muslims in the Third/Ninth and Fourth/Tenth Centuries* (2015): 178.

Walker, Paul E. *Hamid Al-Din Al-Kirmani: Ismaili Thought in the Age of Al-Hakim*. Vol. 3. London: I. B. Tauris, 1999.

———. "The Relationship Between Chief Qāḍī and Chief Dāʿī Under the Fatimids." In *Speaking for Islam*, edited by Gudrun Kramer and Sabine Schmidtke, 70–94. Leiden: Brill, 2006.

———. *Master of the Age: An Islamic Treatise on the Necessity of the Imamate*. London: I. B. Tauris, 2007.

Webb, Peter A. *Creating Arab Origins: Muslim Constructions of al-Jāhiliyya and Arab History*. London: University of London, 2014.

Wisnovsky, Robert. "Essence and Existence in the Eleventh-and Twelfth-Century Islamic East (Masˇriq): A Sketch." *The Arabic, Hebrew and Latin Reception of Avicenna's Metaphysics* 7 (2012): 27.

———. "New Philosophical Texts of Yaḥyā Ibn ʿadī: A Supplement to Endress' Analytical Inventory." In *Islamic Philosophy, Science, Culture, and Religion: Studies in Honor of Dimitri Gutas*, 307–26. Leiden; Boston: Brill, 2012.

Yaldiz, Yunus. *The Afterlife in Mind: Piety and Renunciatory Practice in the 2nd/8th-and Early 3rd/9th-century Books of Renunciation (Kutub al-Zuhd)*. Dissertation, Utrecht University, 2016.

Zakharia, Katia. "Imru'al-Qays, 'Porte-étendard des Poètes vers le Feu', dans le Livre de la Poésie et des Poètes d'Ibn Qutayba." *Arabica* (2009): 192–234.

Zaman, Muhammad Qasim. "Maghāzī and the Muhaddithūn: Reconsidering the Treatment of 'Historical' Materials in Early Collections of Hadith." *International Journal of Middle East Studies* 28, no. 1 (1996): 1–18.

Zinger, Oded. "Tradition and Medicine on the Wings of a Fly." *Arabica* 63, nos. 1–2 (2016): 89–117.

Zuʿbī, Maḥmūd. *Aṭibbāʾ min al-Tārīkh: Al-Asrār wa-Taqwīm al-Adillah*. al-Ṭabʿah 1. ed. ʿAmmān: Wizārat al-Thaqāfah, 2004.

Zuhrī, Muḥammad ibn Muslim. *Al-Maghāzī al-Nabawīyah*. Dimashq: Dār al-Fikr, 1980.

Index